Dasgupta's
Recent Advances in
Obstetrics and Gynecology

Dasgupta's Recent Advances in Obstetrics and Gynecology

Volume 13

Editor

Nandita Palshetkar MD FCPS FICOG FRCOG (UK)
Professor Emeritus in Obstetrics and Gynecology
DY Patil School of Medicine
Navi Mumbai, Maharashtra, India
Infertility Specialist, Lilavati Hospital IVF Center, Mumbai
Scientific Director and Co-Founder, Bloom IVF
Scientific Director and Co-Founder, BAUFICI Genetics
President, Indian
Society of Assisted Reproduction (2022–2024)
President, Association of Maharashtra Obstetric
and Gynaecological Societies (2020–2022)
Past President, FOGSI, IAGE, MOGS and MSR

Co-Editors

Rohan Palshetkar MS (Obs & Gyne) FRM ADRME BDRME
Professor
DY Patil School of Medicine
Navi Mumbai, Maharashtra, India
Head of Unit, Bloom IVF, Nerul
Consultant, Sir HN Reliance Foundation Hospital, Surya Hospital
Breach Candy, Palshetkar Patil Nursing Home
Chairperson, FOGSI Young Talent Promotion
Committee (2024–2027)
Treasurer, AMOGS; Joint Treasurer, MAGE;
Managing Committee Member, MSR & MOGS

Pratik Tambe MD FICOG
ART Consultant and Gynec Endoscopic Surgeon
Department of Obstetrics and Gynecology
Ashirwad IVF
Mumbai, Maharashtra, India
Chair, AMOGS Endocrinology Committee
Governing Council Member, ICOG
Managing Committee Member, ISAR, MSR, MOGS

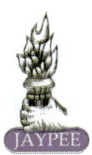

JAYPEE BROTHERS MEDICAL PUBLISHERS
The Health Sciences Publisher
New Delhi | London

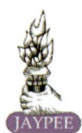 **Jaypee Brothers Medical Publishers (P) Ltd.**

Headquarters
Jaypee Brothers Medical Publishers (P) Ltd
EMCA House, 23/23-B
Ansari Road, Daryaganj
New Delhi 110 002, India
Landline: +91-11-23272143, +91-11-23272703
+91-11-23282021, +91-11-23245672
Email: jaypee@jaypeebrothers.com

Corporate Office
Jaypee Brothers Medical Publishers (P) Ltd
4838/24, Ansari Road, Daryaganj
New Delhi 110 002, India
Phone: +91-11-43574357
Fax: +91-11-43574314
Email: jaypee@jaypeebrothers.com

Overseas Office
JP Medical Ltd.
83, Victoria Street, London
SW1H 0HW (UK)
Phone: +44 20 3170 8910
Fax: +44 (0)20 3008 6180
Email: info@jpmedpub.com

Website: www.jaypeebrothers.com
Website: www.jaypeedigital.com

© 2024, Jaypee Brothers Medical Publishers

The views and opinions expressed in this book are solely those of the original contributor(s)/author(s) and do not necessarily represent those of editor(s) or publisher of the book.

All rights reserved. No part of this publication may be reproduced, stored or transmitted in any form or by any means, electronic, mechanical, photo copying, recording or otherwise, without the prior permission in writing of the publishers.

All brand names and product names used in this book are trade names, service marks, trademarks or registered trademarks of their respective owners. The publisher is not associated with any product or vendor mentioned in this book.

Medical knowledge and practice change constantly. This book is designed to provide accurate, authoritative information about the subject matter in question. However, readers are advised to check the most current information available on procedures included and check information from the manufacturer of each product to be administered, to verify the recommended dose, formula, method and duration of administration, adverse effects and contra indications. It is the responsibility of the practitioner to take all appropriate safety precautions. Neither the publisher nor the author(s)/editor(s) assume any liability for any injury and/or damage to persons or property arising from or related to use of material in this book.

This book is sold on the understanding that the publisher is not engaged in providing professional medical services. If such advice or services are required, the services of a competent medical professional should be sought.

Every effort has been made where necessary to contact holders of copyright to obtain permission to reproduce copyright material. If any have been inadvertently overlooked, the publisher will be pleased to make the necessary arrangements at the first opportunity.

Inquiries for bulk sales may be solicited at: jaypee@jaypeebrothers.com

Dasgupta's Recent Advances in Obstetrics and Gynecology (Volume 13)

First Edition: **2024**

ISBN: 978-93-5696-498-3

Printed at: Rajkamal Electric Press, Kundli, Haryana.

Dedicated to

Our teachers, mentors, patients, and students

Contributors

Ashok Kumar MD PhD (Maternal Health)
Director Professor and Head
Department of Obstetrics and Gynecology
Atal Bihari Vajpayee Institute
of Medical Sciences and
Dr Ram Manohar Lohia Hospital
New Delhi, India

Atul Ganatra MD DGO
Associate Consultant
Fortis Hospital
Mumbai, Maharashtra, India

B Aruna Suman MD FICOG
Professor and Head
Department of Obstetrics and Gynecology
Government Medical College
Jagtial, Telangana, India

Freni Shah DNB MNAMS
Associate Consultant
Department of Obstetrics and Gynecology
RJ Ganatra Nursing Home
Mumbai, Maharashtra, India

Gaurav S Desai MS FCPS FMAS
Assistant Professor
Department of Obstetrics and Gynecology
Seth Gordhandas Sunderdas
Medical College and King Edward
Memorial Hospital
Mumbai, Maharashtra, India

Girija Wagh
MD FICOG FICS Dip in Endoscopy
Professor and Head
Department of High-Risk Pregnancy
and Perinatology
Bharati Vidyapeeth University Medical
College and Hospital
Pune, Maharashtra, India

Jaydeep Tank MD DNB DGO FOPS FICOG
Obstetrician, Gynecologist, and
IVF Consultant
Department of Obstetrics and Gynecology
Ashwini Maternity and Surgical Hospital
Mumbai, Maharashtra, India
President Elect, FOGSI (2024–2025)

JB Sharma
MD FRCOG (London) FAMS PhD FICOG MFFP
DNB FIMSA
Professor
Department of Obstetrics and Gynecology
All India Institute of Medical Sciences
New Delhi, India
Chairperson (Uro-gynecology)
FOGSI Society (2020–22)

Madhuri Patel MD DGO FICOG
Former Associate Professor
Grant Medical College
Mumbai, Maharashtra, India

Manisha Nandi MS FRM DRM
Fertility Consultant (Reproductive
Medicine)
Bloom IVF
Kolkata, West Bengal, India

Meghana P Reddy MBBS MS
Senior Resident (Obstetrics and
Gynecology)
Atal Bihari Vajpayee Institute
of Medical Sciences and
Dr Ram Manohar Lohia Hospital
New Delhi, India

Mohini Agrawal MS DNB
Fellow
Department of Obstetrics and Gynecology
All India Institute of Medical Sciences
New Delhi, India

Nandita Palshetkar
MD FCPS FICOG FRCOG (UK)
Professor Emeritus in Obstetrics and Gynecology
DY Patil School of Medicine
Navi Mumbai, Maharashtra, India
Infertility Specialist, Lilavati Hospital
IVF Center, Mumbai
Scientific Director and Co-Founder
Bloom IVF
Scientific Director and Co-Founder
BAUFICI Genetics
President, Indian
Society of Assisted Reproduction (2022–2024)
President, Association of Maharashtra Obstetric and Gynaecological Societies (2020–2022)

Narendra Malhotra
MD FICOG FICMCH FRCOG FICS FMAS AFIAP
Consultant
Department of Obstetrics and Gynecology
Ujala Cygnus Rainbow Hospital
Agra, Uttar Pradesh, India

Neerja Bhatla MBBS MD
Professor and Head
Department of Obstetrics and Gynecology
All India Institute of Medical Sciences
New Delhi, India

Niranjan Chavan MD
Professor and Head of Unit
Lokmanya Tilak Municipal Medical College
Director and Consultant
Chavan Maternity and Nursing Home
Mumbai, Maharashtra, India

Niranjana Asokan
MS (Obs & Gyne) DNB MRCOG
Assistant Professor
Department of Obstetrics and Gynecology
Panimalar Medical College Hospital and Research Institute
Chennai, Tamil Nadu, India

Nita Mishra MD
Director
Department of Obstetrics and Gynecology
Nitya Maternity Hospital
Institute of Kidney Disease and Research Centre
Ahmedabad, Gujarat, India

Parikshit Tank
MD DNB FCPS DGO DFP MNAMS FICOG FRCOG
Consultant
Obstetrics and Gynecology, Endoscopy and Assisted Reproduction
Ashwini Maternity and Surgical Hospital
Jupiter Hospital
Mumbai, Maharashtra, India

Pooja Lodha MBBS DNB (Obs & Gyne)
Fellow, Fetal Medicine and Fetal Therapy
Director
Kangaroo Cradle—Fetal Care Centre
Pune, Maharashtra, India
Lead Consultant (Fetal Medicine and Fetal Therapy)
Ruby Hall Clinic and Bharati Vidyapeeth Hospital and Medical College, Pune
Fellowship Guide—Maternal Fetal Medicine, FIGO
Ambassador, Global Library of Women's Medicine (GLOWM), Southeast Asia
Trainer, Ian Donald Ultrasound, India

Poonam Goyal MD FICOG FICMCH
Head, IVF and Infertility
Max Hospital, Vaishali, Uttar Pradesh
Head (Obstetrics and Gynecology) and Director
Panchsheel Hospital, New Delhi, India
ART and Ian Donald Ultrasound Trainer

Pradnya Changede
MBBS MS (Obs & Gyne) FICOG FCPS DGO IBCLC
Associate Professor
Department of Obstetrics and Gynecology
Lokmanya Tilak Municipal General Hospital and Lokmanya
Tilak Municipal Medical College
Mumbai, Maharashtra, India

Contributors

Pratik Tambe MD FICOG
ART Consultant and Gynec Endoscopic Surgeon
Department of Obstetrics and Gynecology
Ashirwad IVF
Mumbai, Maharashtra, India
Chair, AMOGS Endocrinology Committee
Governing Council Member, ICOG
Managing Committee Member, ISAR, MSR, MOGS

Priti Kumar MD (Obs/Gyne)
Professor and Head
Department of Obstetrics and Gynecology
Narayana Institute of Medical Sciences
Kanpur, Uttar Pradesh, India

Rajendra Saraogi MBBS MD DGO FCPS
Consultant
Nanavati Max Super Specialty Hospital
Mumbai, Maharashtra, India
Founder
Saraogi Hospital and IRIS IVF & Endoscopy Centre, Mumbai

Rakhi Singh
MBBS DGO DRM DPE FICOG FIAOG
Obstetrician and Gynecologist
Director of Abalone Clinic and IVF center
Noida, Uttar Pradesh, India
Chairperson of Endocrinology Committee, FOGSI (2020–2022)

Rashmika Gandhi
MBBS MS (Obs & Gyne) DNB Fellowship in Reproductive Medicine Fellowship in Gynae Endoscopy
IVF and Laparoscopy Consultant
Department of IVF & Endoscopy, Obstetrics & Gynecology
Sukhmani Hospital, New Delhi, India

Rohan Palshetkar
MS (Obs & Gyne) FRM ADRME BDRME
Professor
DY Patil School of Medicine
Navi Mumbai, Maharashtra, India
Head of Unit, Bloom IVF, Nerul
Consultant, Sir HN Reliance Foundation Hospital, Surya Hospital, Breach Candy
Palshetkar Patil Nursing Home
Chairperson, FOGSI Young Talent Promotion Committee (2024–2027)
Treasurer, AMOGS; Joint Treasurer, MAGE; Managing Committee Member, MSR & MOGS

Rupal Parekh
MBBS DNB (Obs & Gyne) DGO (Gold Medalist)
Fetal Medicine Fellowship (ICOG)
Fetal Medicine Consultant
Ova Infertility (Vedant Hospital), Thane
Former Clinical Associate (Fetal Medicine)
Surya Mother and Child Hospital
Mumbai, Maharashtra, India

Sanjay Gupte MD DGO FICOG LLB FRCOG
Former Hon Associate Professor
BJ Medical College
Pune, Maharashtra, India
Director, Gupte Hospital and Center for Research in Reproduction
Chairman, FIGO Committee for Ethical and Professional Aspects of Human Reproduction and Women's Health
President, FOGSI 2010
President, DIPSI 2013
National Convener "Save the Mother & Newborn National Initiative"
Secretary, General World Gestosis Organization
Member Central Supervisory Board of PCPNDT Act
Chairman, Ethics Committee of Maharashtra Medical Council
National Coordinator, National Eclampsia Registry
National Consultant, Medicolegal and Ethical Issues in Obstetrics & Gynecology

Shyam V Desai MD DGO MNAMS FMAS
Professor Emeritus and Consultant Gynecologist
Department of Obstetrics and Gynecology
Hinduja Healthcare—Mother Care Nursing Home
Mumbai, Maharashtra, India

Contributors

Sunita Tandulwadkar
MD (Obstetrics and Gynecology) FICS (Gyne-Endoscopy) FICOG
Gynecological Endoscopist and ART IVF Specialist
Chief and Medical Director
Department of Obstetrics and Gynecology
Ruby Hall Clinic, Pune, Maharashtra, India
Chief, Ruby Hall IVF and Endoscopy Center, Pune
Director, Solo Clinic, Center of Excellence Infertility and Endoscopy
Founder and Medical Advisor, Solo Stem Cells, Stem Cells Research and Application Center, Pune
Co-Founder, Solo Research Foundation—Sponsor a Birth
President, IAGE (2019–2020)
Chairperson, Maharashtra Chapter ISAR (2018–2020)
2nd Vice President, Indian Society of Assisted Reproduction (ISAR) (2020–21)

Suvarna Khadilkar
MBBS MD DGO FICOG FIMS CIMP PGDIP (Endocrinology, UK)
Professor and Head
Department of Obstetrics, Gynecology and Endocrinology
University PG Teaching Hospital
Mumbai, Maharashtra, India

Vandana Bansal
MD DNB MNAMS MRCOG (UK) FNB (High Risk Pregnancy and Perinatology)
Director
Department of Fetal Medicine
Consultant (Obstetrics and Gynecology)
Surya Hospitals
Mumbai, Maharashtra, India

Vatsla Vats MBBS MS (Obs & Gyne) DNB
Fellow of Minimal Invasive Gynec Endoscopy
Department of Obstetrics and Gynecology, IVF and Endoscopy
Ruby Hall Clinic
Pune, Maharashtra, India

Vineet Mishra MD PhD
Professor and Head
Department of Obstetrics and Gynecology
Institute of Kidney Diseases and Research Center
BJ Medical College, Civil Hospital
Ahmedabad, Gujarat, India
VP FOGSI West Zone, 2016
Chairperson, Urogynec Committee of FOGSI (2011–2013)

Zeba Pathan
MS (Obs & Gyne) DNB (Obs & Gyne)
Senior Resident
Lokmanya Tilak Municipal General Hospital and Lokmanya Tilak Municipal Medical College
Mumbai, Maharashtra, India

Preface

Respected colleagues and dear friends,

It is with immense pride that we bring to you this 13th volume of *Dasgupta's Recent Advances in Obstetrics and Gynecology* addresses the gaps which may be present in postgraduate teaching.

When it comes to recent advances, not all the advances are available in all the medical colleges. Even though we read and learn about recent advances during clinics, grand rounds, journal clubs, etc., they are far and few between.

> *Small shifts in your thinking, and small changes in your energy, can lead to massive alterations of your end result.*
> –Kevin Micheal

Often students only receive a short period of study leave prior to the examinations during which precious time is lost scouring for resources and locating updated guidelines, research papers, and evidence on topics of thematic interest. Hence, we felt that we should address this paucity with this textbook series which aims to unite seniors, respected, and stalwart postgraduate teachers from all over India who have been mentors and guides to generations of students. Each of the chapters in this book is a crash course on the subject and will serve the reader well by focusing on traditional concepts as well as the most modern updated evidence on the issues at hand.

We hope that this book will be a useful compendium for postgraduate students and readers who wish to keep themselves updated with the latest evidence on the topics we have covered. The chapters have been carefully chosen keeping in mind the current proceedings at national and international meetings while keeping the language used simple, easy to understand, and concise.

We welcome your feedback on this volume and suggestions for future topics which you may wish to see covered.

Yours sincerely,

Nandita Palshetkar
Rohan Palshetkar
Pratik Tambe

Acknowledgments

The editors would like to acknowledge the efforts of all the authors and contributors in the preparation of the manuscript, revision of their chapters, and for reverting back to us within the deadlines.

I am extremely thankful to Shri Jitendar P Vij (Group Chairman), Mr Ankit Vij (Managing Director), Mr MS Mani (Group President), Ms Chetna Malhotra Vohra (Senior Director—Professional Publishing, Marketing, and Business Development), Ms Pooja Bhandari (Director–Production) and Ms Pragati Singh (Development Editor) of M/s Jaypee Brothers Medical Publishers (P) Ltd, New Delhi, India, for giving the go-ahead at the very beginning and helping me in every way possible to bring out this book.

Contents

1. Utility of Color Doppler in Obstetric Practice 1
Narendra Malhotra, Pooja Lodha, Poonam Goyal
- Obstetric Dopplers: Importance *2*
- Obstetric Dopplers: When and Which? *4*
- Obstetric Doppler: Which Indices to Use? *5*
- Obstetric Doppler: General Considerations *5*
- Obstetrical Doppler *7*
- Color Doppler for Fetal Echocardiography *13*

2. Modern Management of Hypertensive Disorders in Pregnancy 16
Girija Wagh, Sanjay Gupte
- Definition and Classification of Hypertensive Disorders in Pregnancy *16*
- Pathogenesis with Gestosis as Focus *18*
- Screening and Risk Assessment of HDP Gestosis *20*
- Prediction of HDP *22*
- Diagnosis of Hypertensive Disorders in Pregnancy *23*
- Management *25*
- Surveillance after Diagnosis *30*
- Postpartum Hypertensive Disorders in Pregnancy *32*

3. Preterm Labor 35
Meghana P Reddy, Ashok Kumar
- Risk Factors *35*
- Management *36*
- Labor and Delivery *42*

4. Pregnancy After Renal Transplantation 44
Vineet Mishra, Nita Mishra
- Sexual Activity *44*
- Pregnancy and Allograft Function *45*
- Risk of Complications during Pregnancy *45*
- Fetal Complications *47*
- Predictors of the Outcomes of Pregnancy *48*
- The Ideal Time to Conceive *48*
- Immunosuppression *48*
- Labor and Delivery *51*

5. Challenges in Screening for Thyroid Disorders 55
Pratik Tambe, B Aruna Suman
- Physiology of the Thyroid Gland   55
- Thyroid-stimulating Hormone   56
- Challenges in Thyroid Function Test Interpretation   59
- Concurrent Medications   60
- Assay Interference   60
- Screening and Interpretation in Clinical Practice   61
- Subclinical Thyroid Disease   61
- Evidence-based Recommendations for Screening   64

6. Postpartum Hemorrhage Care Bundles 67
Madhuri Patel, Pradnya Changede
- Incidence of Postpartum Hemorrhage   67
- Causes of Postpartum Hemorrhage   68
- Need for Postpartum Hemorrhage Bundles   68
- How Bundles were Developed   68
- Need to Develop Three Care Bundles   68
- Postpartum Hemorrhage Care Bundles   69
- Panel Recommendations   73
- Limitations   74
- Advantages of Care Bundles   75

7. Importance of Obstetric Skill Drills 78
Priti Kumar, Niranjana Asokan
- What is an Obstetric Skill Drill?   78
- Purpose   78
- Methodology   79
- Frequency   80
- Advantages   81
- Planning   82
- Obstetric Emergencies   84
- Others   84
- Studies   86

8. Postpartum Collapse 88
Rajendra Saraogi, Rohan Palshetkar, Manisha Nandi
- Introduction and Background   88
- Causes   88
- Approaches in the Event of Maternal Collapse   91

9. Hydrops Fetalis 98
Vandana Bansal, Rupal Parekh
- Epidemiology   98
- Etiopathogenesis   98

- Sonographic Findings in Hydrops Fetalis *102*
- Maternal Effects of Fetal Hydrops *104*
- Investigations in Fetal Hydrops: Role of Individual Tests and Algorithm for Hydrops Fetalis Workup *105*
- Treatment/Fetal Therapy *107*
- Prognosis and Recurrence *110*
- Cases of Hydrops with Potential of Recurrence *112*
- Immune Hydrops *112*
- Serology to Detect Isoimmunization *113*
- Treatment of Immune Hydrops and Fetal Anemia *116*

10. **Social Egg Freezing** 120
    Nandita Palshetkar
    - Terminology *120*
    - Social versus Medical EGG Freezing *121*
    - Procedure *121*
    - Optimal Timing of Oocyte Cryopreservation *123*
    - Optimal Number of Eggs to Freeze *123*
    - Chance of Having a Child *123*
    - Benefits *124*
    - Risks *124*
    - Use of Stored Oocytes *125*
    - Social and Ethical Implications *126*

11. **Ovarian Tissue Cryopreservation** 128
    Rohan Palshetkar, Nandita Palshetkar, Manisha Nandi
    - Patient Selection *128*
    - Special Clinical Considerations for Ovarian Tissue Cryopreservation *130*
    - Key Technical Aspects of Ovarian Tissue Cryopreservation *131*
    - Ovarian Tissue Cryopreservation Procedure *132*
    - Replacing Ovarian Tissue: Safety Issues *133*

12. **Relevance of Magnetic Resonance Imaging in Gynecology** 139
    Atul Ganatra, Freni Shah
    - T1 and T2 Weighted Scans *140*

13. **Modern Management of Endometrial Cancer** 148
    Niranjan Chavan, Zeba Pathan
    - Stage I Cancers *149*
    - Stage II Cancers *152*
    - Stage III Cancers *153*
    - Stage IV Cancers *154*
    - Recurrent Endometrial Cancer *154*

- Understanding the Molecular Biology of Endometrial Cancer *158*
- Immunotherapy in Endometrial Cancer *158*
- Future Directions and Current Clinical Trials *158*

14. Genitourinary Syndrome of Menopause 166
Suvarna Khadilkar

- Genitourinary Syndrome of Menopause: Prevalence *166*
- Genitourinary Syndrome of Menopause: Diagnostic Challenges *166*
- Genitourinary Syndrome of Menopause: Understanding the Condition *167*
- Risk Factors for Genitourinary Syndrome of Menopause *168*
- Clinical Features and Sequelae of Genitourinary Syndrome of Menopause *169*
- Differential Diagnosis of Genitourinary Syndrome of Menopause *170*
- Genitourinary Syndrome of Menopause *173*
- Treatment Modalities for Genitourinary Syndrome of Menopause *173*
- Women with Breast Cancer and Genitourinary Syndrome of Menopause *178*

15. Total Laparoscopic Hysterectomy 180
Sunita Tandulwadkar, Rashmika Gandhi, Vatsla Vats

- Indications *180*
- Contraindications *181*
- Preoperative Evaluation *181*
- Preoperative Preparation *181*
- Surgical Procedure *181*
- Surgical Steps *183*
- Postoperative Care *189*
- Complications *189*

16. Decreased Fetal Movements 195
Parikshit Tank, Jaydeep Tank

- Fetal Movement Physiology *195*
- Factors Affecting Fetal Movement *196*
- Assessing Fetal Movement *197*
- Is there an Evidence Base to Support Formal Fetal Movement Counting? *198*
- Approach to a Woman with Reduced Fetal Movements *198*
- Fetal Cardiotocography in Women with Reduced Fetal Movements *199*
- Assessing Fetal Growth in Women with Reduced Fetal Movement *200*
- Ultrasound in Women with Reduced Fetal Movements *201*
- Special Clinical Situations *201*

17. **Insulin Sensitizers in Polycystic Ovary Syndrome** 204
    Rakhi Singh
    - Insulin Sensitizing Agents   *205*

18. **Vaccination Against Cervical Cancer** 212
    Neerja Bhatla
    - Human Papilloma Virus   *213*
    - Human Papillomavirus Vaccine/Cervical Cancer Vaccine   *214*
    - Features of Human Papillomavirus Vaccine   *215*
    - Barriers for Implementation of Routine HPV Vaccination and Suggested Solutions   *220*

19. **Recurrent Urinary Tract Infections** 225
    JB Sharma, Mohini Agrawal
    - Etiology   *226*
    - Risk Factors   *227*
    - Pathogenesis   *228*
    - Clinical Presentation   *228*
    - Differential Diagnosis   *228*
    - History and Examination   *228*
    - Investigations   *229*
    - Interpretation of Urine Analysis and Approach   *230*
    - Treatment   *231*
    - Prevention   *233*
    - Complications   *233*

20. **Fourth Degree Perineal Tear** 236
    Gaurav S Desai, Shyam V Desai
    - Prevalence   *236*
    - Causes   *237*
    - Prevention   *237*
    - Management   *238*
    - Complications   *238*

Index *241*

CHAPTER 1

Utility of Color Doppler in Obstetric Practice

Narendra Malhotra, Pooja Lodha, Poonam Goyal

■ INTRODUCTION

In developing countries like India, majority of adverse maternal, fetal, and perinatal events occur due to placenta-related disorders. Color Doppler evaluation is an extended armamentarium of the fetal growth examination on ultrasound. It has popularized hugely over the last two decades and has become the third eye of an obstetrician dealing with high risk pregnancy.

Doppler ultrasound provides a unique window into the fetoplacental circulation, allowing assessment of fetal well-being. Umbilical artery Doppler is an integral component of monitoring and managing the small growing fetus and has revolutionized the management of fetal growth restriction.[1]

The middle cerebral artery Doppler has recently gained much importance due to its vital role as a noninvasive means of detecting as well as monitoring fetal anemia and as an integral part of the cerebra-placental ratio, especially toward term.

Ductus venosus Dopplers are important decision makers in early fetal growth-restricted fetuses, especially before 32 weeks.

This chapter aims at the clinical aspects of understanding Obstetric Dopplers and their role in decision making and thus learning to judiciously manage high risk cases to have optimal outcomes.

Doppler ultrasound is a very useful addition to our catalog of tests for antenatal fetal well-being and timely intervention. Based on abnormal Doppler results, obstetrical decision making might improve and prevent intrauterine death because hypoxic cerebral damage may begin before labor and intrapartum asphyxia is probably more damaging when superimposed on underlying hypoxia. Doppler assessment may lead to timely intervention that reduces the risk of fetal brain damage.

With the latest advances in color Doppler such as superb microvascular imaging (SMI), radiant flow, HDlive flow, and HDlive flow silhouette, we can obtain more comprehensive blood flow information over and above the conventional color Doppler.[2] We can also have vascular indices.

■ OBSTETRIC DOPPLERS: IMPORTANCE

- As seen in the **Table 1**, Doppler indices play a crucial role in classification of Dopplers, monitoring, and delivery decision making.[3]
- Doppler is the one parameter which differentiates between constitutionally small fetus and pathologically small baby due to fetal growth restriction **(Figs. 1A and B)**.
- Going a step further, apart from diagnosis of pathological fetal growth restriction, Dopplers also help in decision making regarding frequency of surveillance, and delivery decision making. In fact, the Doppler changes may even guide weather the delivery can take place in a small nursing home or an in a tertiary set up with advanced neonatal ICU facilities. **Flowchart 1** shows monitoring and delivery decision making depending upon umbilical artery Doppler.
- Obstetric Doppler studies have not only changed the management in obstetrics, but have become crucial predictor tools. This prediction can translate into clinical decision making, e.g., starting aspirin to improve placentation in women with high uterine artery pulsatility index (PI) and other predictors of preeclampsia (PE).
- Dopplers are the mainstay for noninvasive diagnosis, monitoring, and post fetal-transfusion follow-up in cases of fetal anemia due to Rh isoimmunization.
- Obstetric Dopplers help in distinguishing causes for a small growing fetus, for example, genetically abnormal fetus, fetal infections, structurally abnormal fetus or uteroplacental insufficiency/fetoplacental insufficiency **(Flowchart 2)**.
- The classification of fetal growth restriction depends upon the Doppler changes. This classification is vital for diagnosis, counseling, further decision making, and prognosis **(Fig. 2)**.[4]

TABLE 1: Early versus late fetal growth restriction (FGR).	
Early onset fetal growth restriction <32 weeks GA	Late onset fetal growth restriction >32 weeks GA
AC/EFW <3rd centile or UA-AEDF OR 1. AC/EFW <10th centile combined with 2. UtA-PI >95th centile and/or 3. UA-PI >95th centile	AC/EFW <3rd centile OR *At least two out of three of the following:* 1. AC/EFW <10th centile 2. AC/EFW crossing centiles >2 quartiles on growth centiles 3. CPR <5th centile or UA-PI >95th centile

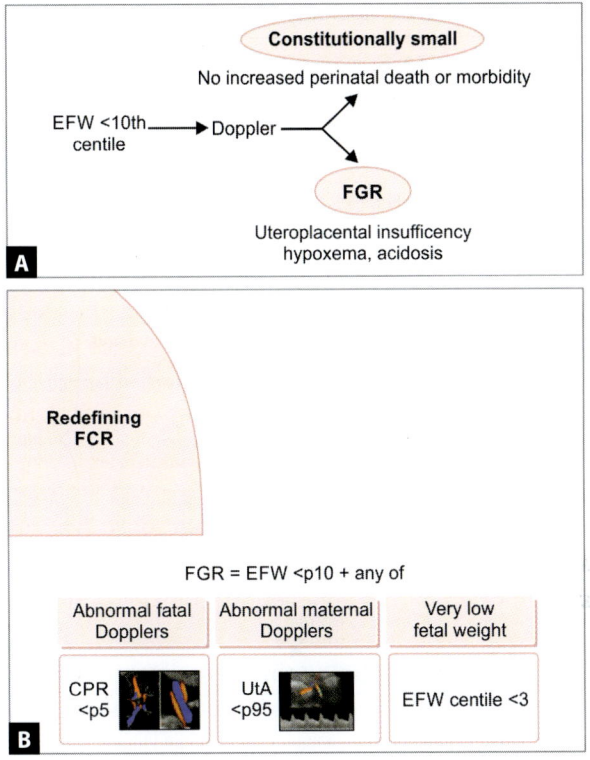

Figs. 1A and B: (A) Defining fetal growth restriction (FGR) using; (B) Redefining FGR using Doppler.

Flowchart 1: Algorithm to monitor and deliver fetal growth restriction (FGR) fetuses on the basis of umbilical artery Doppler.

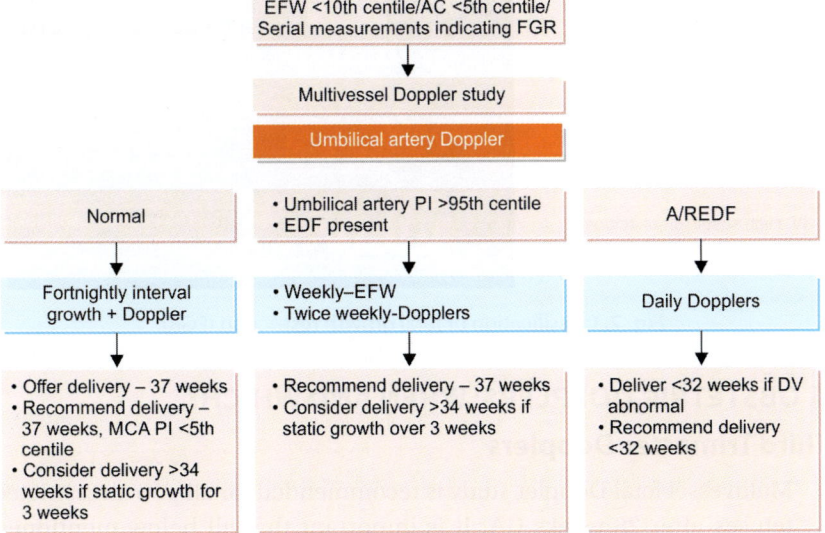

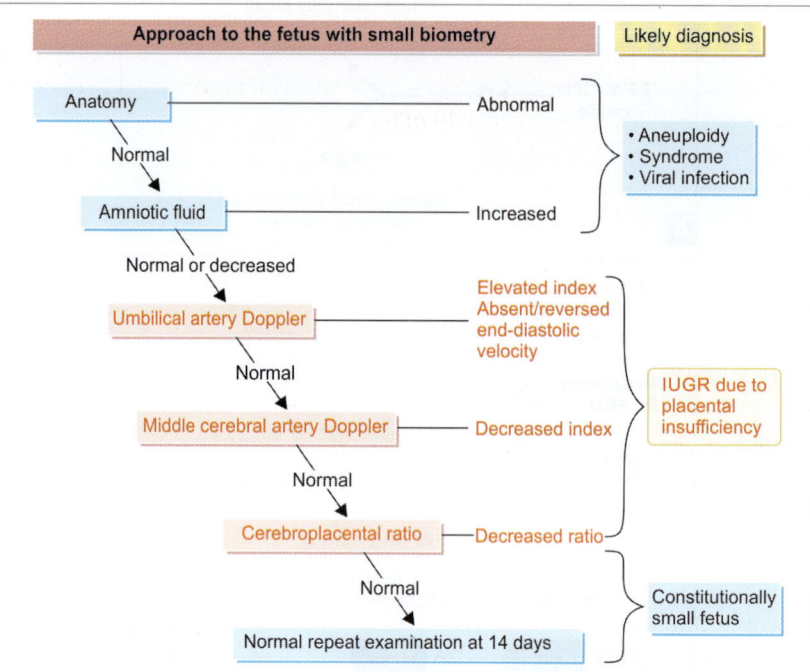

Flowchart 2: Approach toward a small fetus.

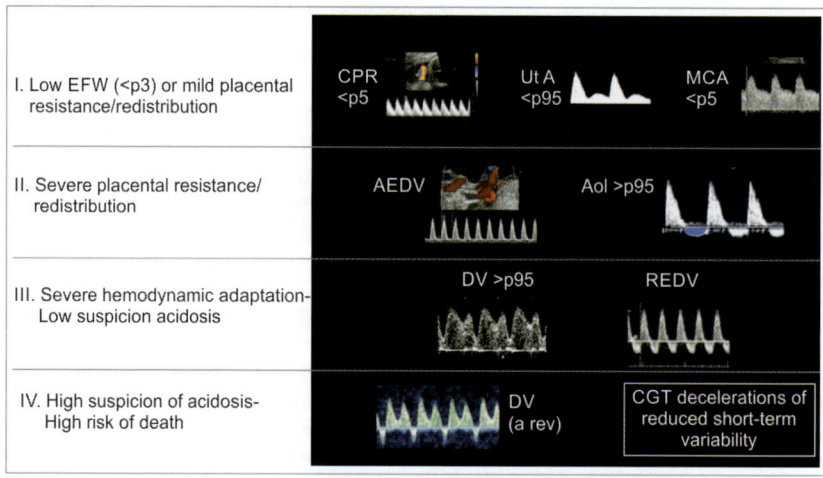

Fig. 2: Classification of fetal growth restriction (FGR).

OBSTETRIC DOPPLERS: WHEN AND WHICH?
Third Trimester Dopplers
- Multivessel fetal Doppler study is recommended for all growth restricted fetuses after 26 weeks GA. It is important that all below mentioned

Dopplers are sampled and not just one Doppler/stepwise Doppler, as there may be a deviation of sequential changes and deterioration of Doppler in different fetuses. Sampling only one Doppler may miss subtle changes in other Dopplers which could be detrimental in decision making. For diagnosis we take PI of blood flow in all vessels.
- *Multivessel Doppler includes:*
  - Umbilical artery
  - Middle cerebral artery
  - Ductus venosus
  - Bilateral (B/L) Uterine arteries
  - Aortic isthmus (not routinely)

First Trimester Dopplers
- *Uterine artery Doppler:* For prediction of PE, fetal growth restriction, it is a marker for uteroplacental circulation. It is done by transabdominal method at the time of NT scan.
- *Ductus venosus Doppler:* Ductus venosus is a minor aneuploidy marker in the first trimester. It is also more commonly found in fetuses with evolving cardiac anomalies.
- Tricuspid regurgitation if present it is a marker for aneuploidy. It is also indication of fetal heart abnormalities.

Second Trimester Dopplers
- Uterine artery B/L
- Fetal renal Doppler can be used to delineate the fetal kidney tissue in obese women/women with suboptimal views.

■ OBSTETRIC DOPPLER: WHICH INDICES TO USE?[5]
- Systolic/diastolic (S/D) ratio, RI and PI are the three well-known indices to describe arterial flow velocity waveforms. All three are highly correlated.
- Most standardized nomograms are published for PI. This is reproducible and easy to use.
- The advantages of using PI for all obstetric Dopplers have been mentioned in **Figure 3**.

■ OBSTETRIC DOPPLER: GENERAL CONSIDERATIONS
All Doppler modalities are based on three fundamental principles.[5]
- Moving structures change the frequency and amplitude of reflected ultrasound signals. Moving structures include not only blood, but also fetal vessels or tissues. This can generate a shift in the backscattered signals.

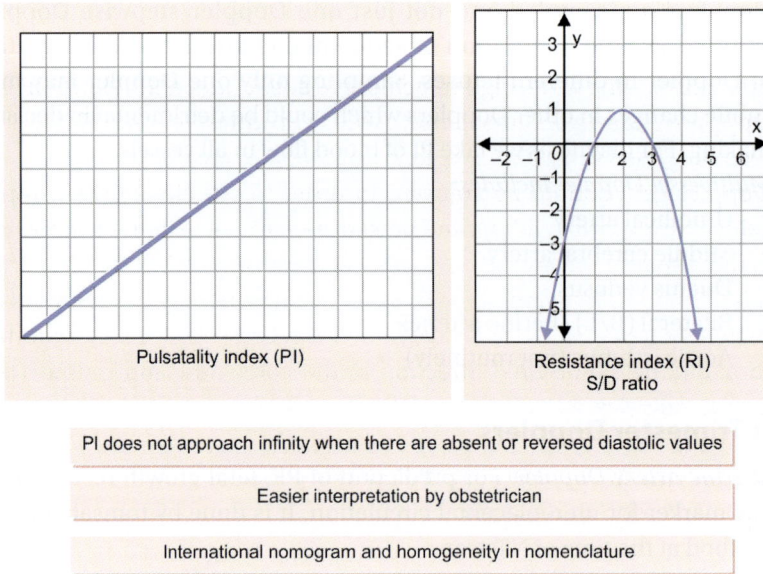

Fig. 3: Which Doppler indices to use in Obstetrics, why?

- Analysis of the components of the reflected signals is utilized for different Doppler modalities—the shift in frequency for directional color and spectral Doppler, and the shift in amplitude for power Doppler ultrasound (PDU).
- All color and power Doppler modalities are pulsed techniques, while spectral Doppler can be pulsed or continuous.

How can the Acquisition of Pulsed Wave Doppler be Optimized?[5]

- Obtain spectral pulsed wave Doppler waveforms in the absence of fetal breathing and body movements.
- Color flow mapping is very helpful in identification of the vessel of interest and in defining the direction of blood flow.
- The optimal insonation is completely aligned with the direction of blood flow angle being not >30°. This ensures the best conditions for assessing absolute velocities and waveforms.
- It is advisable to start with a relatively wide Doppler gate (sample volume) to ensure the recording of maximum velocities during the entire pulse. If interference from other vessels causes problems, the gate can be reduced to refine the recording.
- Pulse repetition frequency (PRF), or scale, is the frequency at which the ultrasound signals (pulses) are emitted. The PRF should be adjusted

according to the vessel studied—a low PRF will enable visualization and accurate measurement of low-velocity flow; however, it will produce aliasing when high velocities are encountered with low PRF.
- Doppler measurements should be reproducible; therefore, it is recommended to obtain more than one Doppler recording.
- Doppler gain should be adjusted in order to see clearly the Doppler velocity waveform, without the presence of artefacts in the background of the display.
- It is advisable not to invert the Doppler display on the ultrasound screen. In the evaluation of the fetal heart and central vessels, it is very important to maintain the original direction of the color flow and pulsed-wave Doppler display.

How can the Acquisition of Color Directional Doppler be Optimized?[5]

- Color Doppler increases the total power emitted. Color Doppler resolution increases when the color box is reduced in size. Care must be taken in assessing the mechanical index (MI) and thermal index (TI) as they change according to the size and depth of the color box.
- The box should be kept as small as possible, to include only the studied area. Increasing the size of the color box also increases the processing time and thus reduces the frame rate.
- The velocity scale or PRF should be adjusted to represent the blood flow velocities of the studied vessel.
- Gain should be adjusted in order to prevent noise and artifacts, seen as a random display of color dots in the background of the screen.
- The angle of insonation affects the color Doppler image; it should be adjusted by optimizing the position of the ultrasound probe.

■ OBSTETRICAL DOPPLER
Technical Aspects and Clinical Implications

- Uterine artery
- Umbilical artery
- Middle cerebral artery
- Ductus venosus.

It is important to understand the fetal circulation in order to interpret the multiverses Doppler study **(Fig. 4)**.

Each vessel which has been included in the obstetric Doppler has its own importance **(Fig. 5)**.

Table 2 states the various modes of fetal surveillance and their clinical implications.

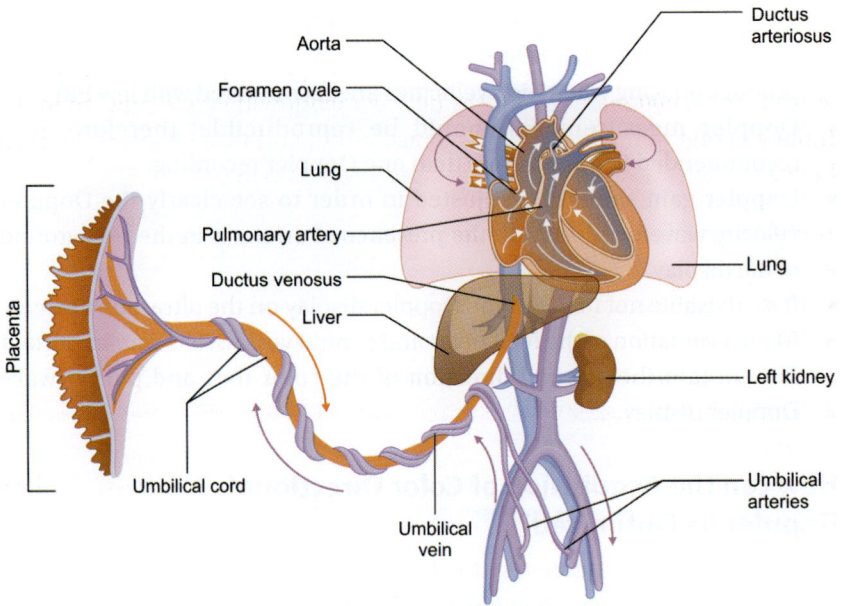

Fig. 4: Fetal circulation.

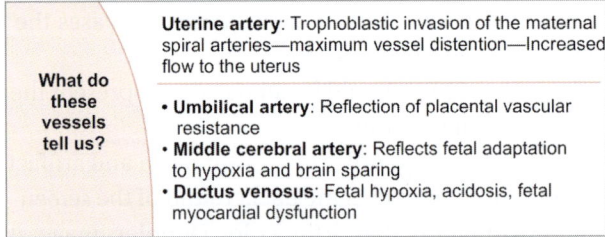

What do these vessels tell us?	**Uterine artery**: Trophoblastic invasion of the maternal spiral arteries—maximum vessel distention—Increased flow to the uterus
	• **Umbilical artery**: Reflection of placental vascular resistance • **Middle cerebral artery**: Reflects fetal adaptation to hypoxia and brain sparing • **Ductus venosus**: Fetal hypoxia, acidosis, fetal myocardial dysfunction

Fig. 5: Obstetric Doppler: Multivessel Doppler and rationale.

TABLE 2: Modes of fetal monitoring.	
Modes of fetal monitoring	**What it measures**
Fetal anatomy	Differential diagnosis
Fetal growth	Placental performance
AFI	Fetal volume status, placental transfer
Uterine Doppler	Maternal side of placenta, trophoblastic
Umbilical Doppler	Fetal side of placenta, villi
MCA Doppler	pCO_2, pO_2, cerebral vasodilatation
Venous Doppler	Acidemia, fetal cardiac function
Dynamic variable (BPP)	Fetal maturation, behavioral state, CNS, PNS

Uterine Artery

Preeclampsia is a major cause of maternal and perinatal death or handicap. More than 50,000 maternal deaths per year worldwide are attributed to PE. India has one of the highest prevalence of PE, and uterine artery Doppler hence becomes a vital tool for screening **(Figs. 6A and B)**.

Uterine artery Doppler: Transabdominal technique
- Obtain a mid-sagittal section of the uterus.
- Identify the cervix.
- Move the probe laterally to visualize the paracervical vascular plexus. Uterine arteries appear coma shape.
- In this first trimester uterine arteries are not insonated as they cross iliac vessels.
- Turn on the color Doppler, identify the uterine artery as it turns cranially to ascent into the uterine body.

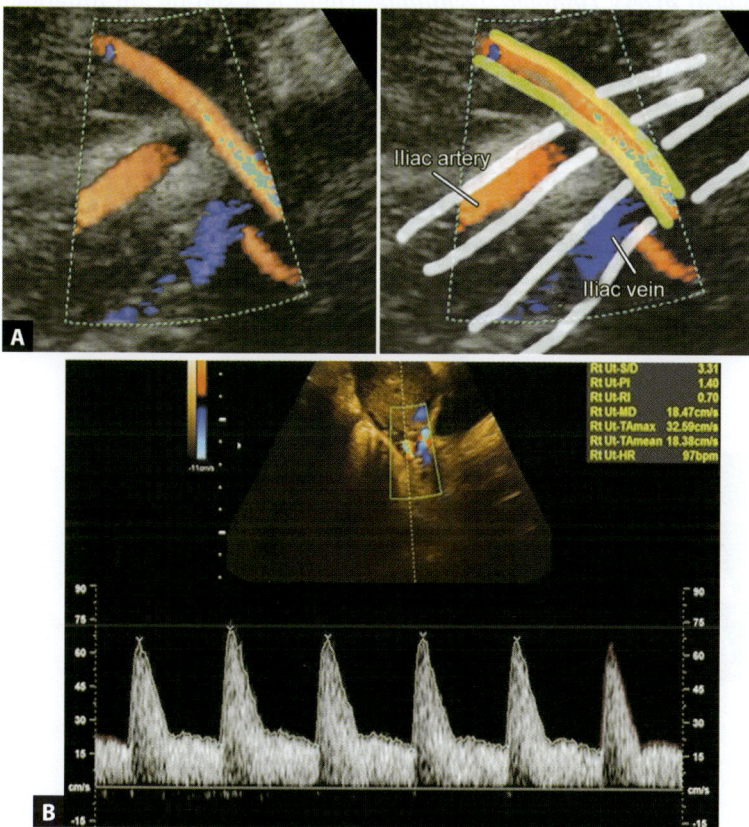

Figs. 6A and B: (A) Uterine artery; (B) Uterine artery waveform at 12 weeks—normal.

- The peak systolic velocity decreases from uterine to the arcuate arteries. PSV >60 cm/second confirms that uterine artery is being sampled.
- The same process is repeated on the contralateral side.

Uterine artery Doppler: Transvaginal technique
- Woman should empty her bladder.
- Transvaginal, the probe is placed in the anterior fornix.
- The same steps are carried out in the same sequence as for the transabdominal technique.

Umbilical Artery Doppler (Fig. 7)

Umbilical arterial (UA) Doppler assessment is used in surveillance of fetal well-being in the third trimester of pregnancy. Abnormal umbilical artery Doppler is a marker of placental insufficiency and consequent intrauterine growth restriction (IUGR) or suspected PE.

Umbilical artery Doppler assessment has been shown to reduce perinatal mortality and morbidity in high-risk obstetric situations.

Umbilical artery Doppler: Technique: There is a significant difference in Doppler indices measured at the fetal end (intra-abdominal), in a free loop and at the placental end of the umbilical cord.

The impedance is highest at the fetal end, and absent/reversed EDV is likely to be seen first at this site. Reference ranges for umbilical artery Doppler indices at each of these sites have been published.

For the sake of simplicity and consistency, by convention, measurements should be made in a free cord loop.

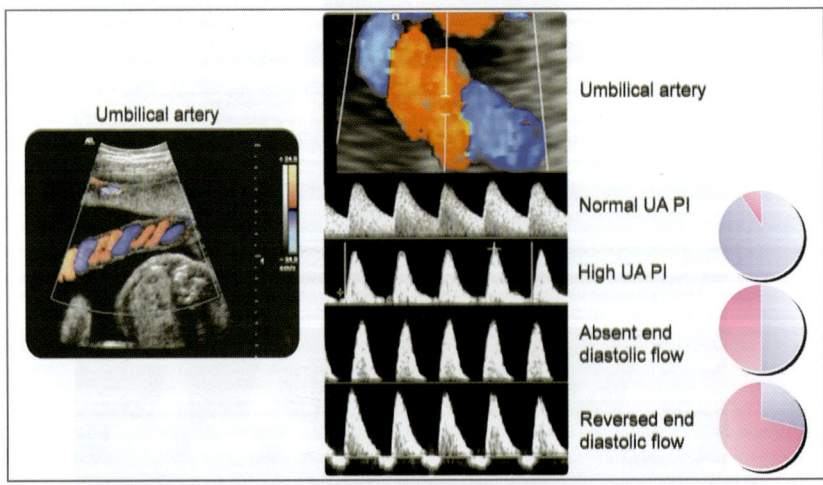

Fig. 7: Umbilical artery waveforms—normal and abnormal. Correlation with severity of placental pathology.

Middle Cerebral Artery

Fetal Doppler of the middle cerebral artery is used in two situations: (a) Noninvasive assessment of fetal anemia and (b) Calculation of the cerebro-placental ratio as a measure of fetal brain sparing in assessing FGR.

Middle cerebral artery Doppler: Technique (Fig. 8)
- Obtain and magnify the axial section of the brain, including the thalami and the sphenoid bone wings.
- Use color flow mapping to identify the circle of Willis and the proximal MCA, just caudal to the transthalamic plane.
- The pulsed-wave Doppler gate should then be placed at the proximal third of the MCA, close to its origin in the internal carotid artery

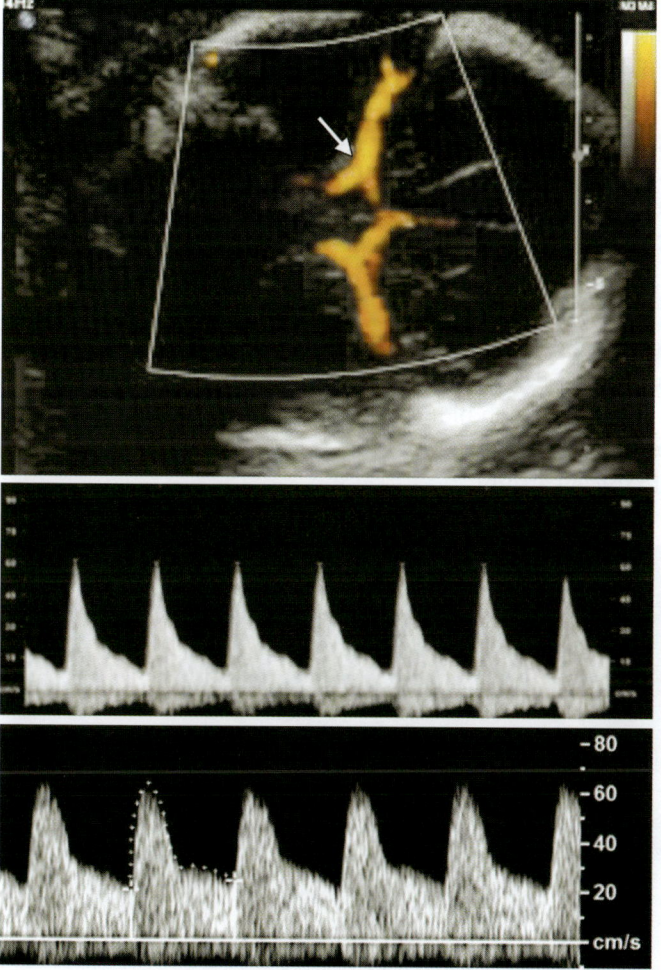

Fig. 8: Middle cerebral artery.

(the systolic velocity decreases with increasing distance from the point of origin of this vessel).
- The angle between the ultrasound beam and the direction of blood flow should be kept as close as possible to 0°.
- Care should be taken to avoid any unnecessary pressure on the fetal head, as this may lead to increased PSV, decreased EDV and increased PI.
- At least three and <10 consecutive waveforms should be recorded. The highest point of the waveform is considered as the PSV (in cm/second).
- Measure the PSV using manual or auto trace methods.
- Appropriate reference ranges should be used for interpretation, and the measurement technique should be the same as that used to construct the reference ranges.

Cerebroplacental Ratio (Fig. 9):
- Cerebroplacental ratio (CPR) reflects the arterial redistribution that occurs during preferential brain perfusion in response to fetal hypoxemia (brain sparing).
- The CPR should be interpreted using gestational age-related reference ranges rather than a single cut-off. Single cut off if used, it is >1.
- The CPR is calculated using umbilical artery PI and middle cerebral artery PI.
- Subtle changes in umbilical and MCA Dopplers can be picked up by CPR.

Ductus Venosus Doppler (Fig. 10)

The ductus venosus is a small trumpet-shaped connection between the umbilical/portal system and the inferior vena cava. Its shape effectively funnels the oxygen-rich blood returning from the placenta directly into the right atrium, with flow dynamics that then facilitate flow across the foramen ovale into the left atrium.

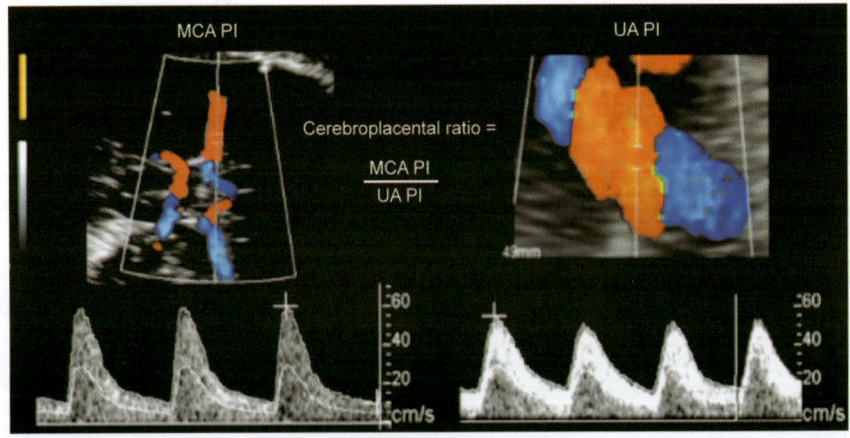

Fig. 9: Cerebroplacental ratio.

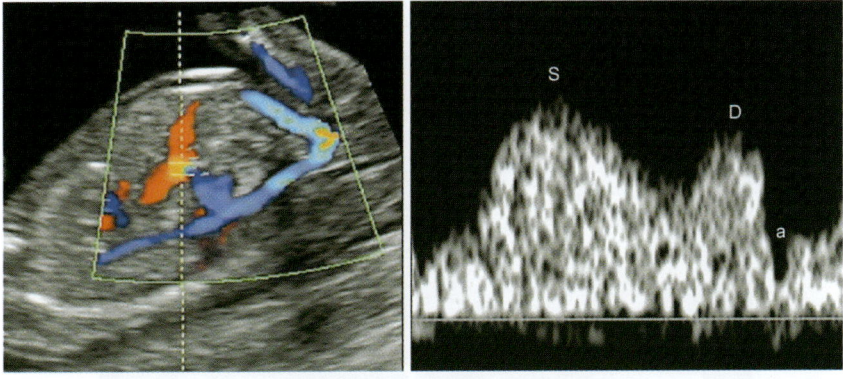

Fig. 10: Ductus venosus Doppler.

Ductus venosus Doppler is used as an aneuploidy marker in the first trimester, and as a vital decision-making tool for early fetal growth restriction prior to 32 weeks.

Ductus venosus Doppler: Technique
- The vessel ductus venosus is identified in a mid-sagittal longitudinal plane of the fetal trunk or in an oblique transverse plane through the upper abdomen.
- It connects the intra-abdominal portion of the umbilical vein to the left portion of the inferior vena cava, just below the diaphragm.
- High velocity flow is seen on color Doppler in the ductus venosus.

COLOR DOPPLER FOR FETAL ECHOCARDIOGRAPHY (FIG. 11)

Adequate imaging of the fetal heart is essential for accurate diagnosis. Color Doppler adds significantly to our ability to diagnose congenital heart disease. Flow patterns across the atrioventricular and semilunar valves can be evaluated by color Doppler and abnormalities suspected on gray-scale imaging can be confirmed.[6]

Over the past few decades, color Doppler has been included as a vital and routine cardiac examination at the anomaly scan. In fact, for women with high risk for fetuses with heart disease, fetal echocardiography has been incorporated into the protocols as early as the first trimester; with excellent resolution via a transvaginal route.

The practice of including color Doppler in most routine fetal heart examination protocols has improved the detection rate of congenital cardiac defects. Color Doppler can give us additional information on blood flow although the canal or vessel is too small to detect morphological changes in the second trimester. It might be a useful tool for screening of defects

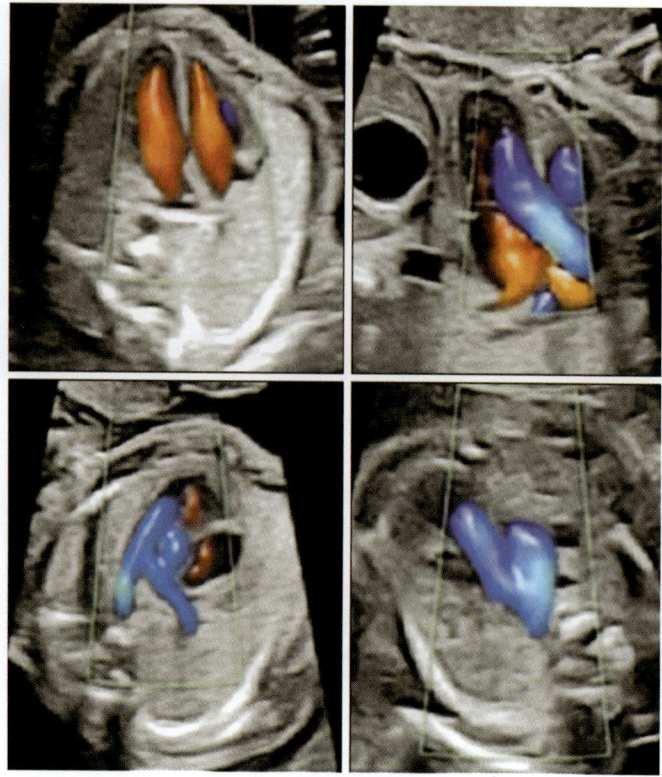

Fig. 11: Color Doppler in fetal echocardiography.

with stenosis, regurgitation, and shunt that are difficult to detect by only the B mode in the second trimester.

The details about utility of Doppler in fetal echocardiography are beyond the scope of this chapter.

■ CONCLUSION

Doppler investigations of the MCA, UA and DV and UAs play an important role in monitoring the compromised fetuses and help to determine the optimal time of delivery. Color Doppler is routinely used for fetal heart examination. Doppler has become an inevitable part of an obstetrician's diagnostic and management protocols.

KEY POINTS

- *Doppler in first trimester:*
  - DV flow
  - Tricuspid regurgitation
  - B/L uterine arteries for PE prediction
  - Check for three-vessel cord
  - Cardiac assessment/axis and crossover of major trunks
- *Doppler in second trimester:*
  - B/L uterine arteries
  - Fetal cardiac assessment/fetal echocardiography
  - Early growth assessment in high-risk pregnancies
  - Renal vessels
- *Doppler in third trimester:*
  - Growth assessment with MCA, DV, UA, UT vessels.
  - Cardiac assessment
  - Renal assessment

■ REFERENCES

1. Kennedy AM, Woodward PJ. A radiologist's guide to the performance and interpretation of obstetric Doppler US. Radiographics. 2019;39(3):893-910.
2. AboEllail MA, Ito M. Advances in color Doppler in obstetrics. J South Asian Feder Obs Gynae. 2019;11(1):1-12.
3. Gordijn SJ, Beune IM, Thilaganathan B, Papageorghiou A, Baschat AA, Baker PN, et al. Consensus definition of fetal growth restriction: a Delphi procedure. Ultrasound Obstet Gynecol. 2016;48(3):333-9.
4. Figueras F, Gratacós E. Update on the diagnosis and classification of fetal growth restriction and proposal of a stage-based management protocol. Fetal Diagn Ther. 2014;36(2):86-98.
5. Bhide A, Acharya G, Baschat A, Bilardo CM, Brezinka C, Cafici D, et al. ISUOG Practice Guidelines (updated): use of Doppler velocimetry in obstetrics. Ultrasound Obstet Gynecol. 2021;58:331-9.
6. Abuhamad A. Color and pulsed Doppler in fetal echocardiography. Ultrasound Obstet Gynecol. 2004;24(1):1-9.

CHAPTER 2

Modern Management of Hypertensive Disorders in Pregnancy

Girija Wagh, Sanjay Gupte

■ INTRODUCTION

Hypertensive disorders in pregnancy (HDP) are responsible for severe adverse perinatal complications as well as future cardiovascular abnormalities in the pregnant woman as well as her offspring with both being at risk of death or deformity. Over the years, many insights have developed in the prediction, diagnosis, and management of this disorder and the approach, therefore, must be modern even if the disorder has been an ancient disease.

In this chapter, we will discuss all the areas of the management of HDPs based on the modern understanding and evidence-based experiences of all the aspects of the disorder such as:
- Definition
- Underlying pathogenesis and gestosis
- Screening with the use of the gestosis score
- Prediction of HDP
- Diagnosis of HDP
- Management protocol
- Our experience

■ DEFINITION AND CLASSIFICATION OF HYPERTENSIVE DISORDERS IN PREGNANCY

Hypertension in pregnancy is defined when the blood pressure records 140/90 mm Hg or more in a pregnant woman during pregnancy or in the immediate puerperium. This definition is now modified by the American Heart Association (AHA) to consider 130/80 mm Hg, while the American College of Obstetricians and Gynecologists (ACOG) continues to prevail on 140/90 mm Hg.[1] Hypertensive disorders of pregnancy include all those conditions associated with hypertension and its occurrence.[2] Hypertension when noted before 20 weeks is called chronic hypertension (CHT) and will continue to persist after 14 days postdelivery. CHT can be due to hypertension after 20 weeks and till 14 days postdelivery is called gestational hypertension (GHT). Women with preexisting hypertension can also conceive to be called pregnant women (PW) with CHT. CHT and GHT associated with proteinuria or severe features is called preeclampsia. Preeclampsia definition was revised in 2014 and reiterated thereafter by several organizations as raised blood pressure (hypertension) of 140 mm Hg or more systolic and 90 mm Hg or more diastolic, developing after completed 20 weeks of gestation associated with any of the following features, namely proteinuria, maternal organ dysfunction, and/or fetal growth restriction. Postpartum hypertension is seen in about 5–10% of PWs as new-onset rise in blood pressure postdelivery up to 6 weeks without antecedent hypertension during pregnancy.[3] They can present with new-onset persistent headaches and visual disturbances[4] **(Fig. 1)**.

Despite this definition in practice, PW presenting with clinical features of preeclampsia without hypertension, laboratory parameters suggestive of HELLP (hemolysis, elevated liver enzymes, low platelet count) or acute fatty liver of pregnancy (AFLP) or have abnormal placental growth factor (PlGF) levels without hypertension are to be labeled as preeclampsia. Women developing intrapartum or postpartum hypertension are defined as transient hypertension if only one such reading is encountered. White coat hypertension when the patient records abnormal blood pressure in the clinical setting and is normotensive at home also needs to be classified under HDP as it has a potential of 25% of converting into GHT or preeclampsia. Masked hypertension is the one which is abnormal

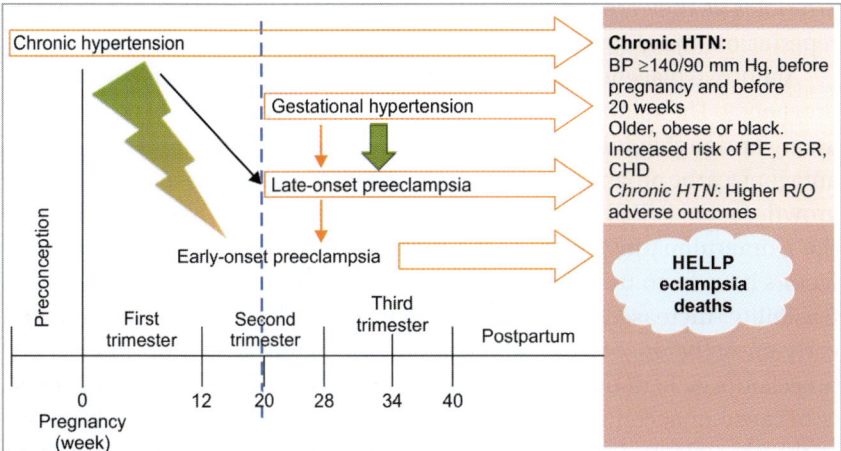

Fig. 1: CHT and GHT have the potential to convert into preeclampsia. (BP: blood pressure; CHD: congenital heart disease; CHT: chronic hypertension; FGR: fetal growth restriction; GHT: gestational hypertension; HELLP: hemolysis, elevated liver enzymes, and low platelet count; PE: Pre-elcampsia; R/O: risk of)

Note: Chronic hypertension has more potential to cause early-onset preeclampsia than late-onset preeclampsia. GHT has more potential of converting into late-onset preeclampsia than early onset. 20-week cut-off is usual but may not always hold true. Postpartum hypertension can be a de novo occurrence.

blood pressure reading at home but normal at the health facility can be wrong method or machine reading but needs to be kept in mind. Delta hypertension is the one when the mean arterial pressure (MAP) is recorded to be abnormal later in pregnancy suddenly and these PWs have a potential to develop seizures and HELLP while still normotensive.

▪ PATHOGENESIS WITH GESTOSIS AS FOCUS

Hypertensive disorders in pregnancy, especially preeclampsia microbiological pathology, is elusive but seems to be combination of factors from the maternal as well as placental pathways, and this also therefore created heterogeneous phenotype of this disorder. Maternal factors such as reproductive history, presence of comorbidities, and genetic and immune factors influence the possibility of developing HDP–gestosis. Reduced uteroplacental perfusion has been demonstrated by Dopplers and magnetic resonance imaging (MRI) studies. This is due to failed spiral arteriole remodeling due to malfunction of the proteases and uterine natural killer cells and leads to ischemia as the spiral arterioles continue to retain the smooth muscle component, leading to narrowed vessels. Rheological consequences such as villous structural alterations are a result of turbulent jets in the intervillous spaces that cause rupture of the anchoring villi, leading to the formation of cystic lesions which are echogenic on ultrasound. Generalized vasoconstriction affects the smooth muscles of the spiral arterioles as they are not lysed and are persistent. This leads to ischemia–reperfusion injury causing oxidative stress.

Abnormal placentation leads to changes in the angiogenic factors in early pregnancy. The soluble fms-like tyrosine kinase 1 (sFlt-1) has been identified as an antiangiogenic factor released by the ischemic placenta which antagonizes the proangiogenic factors—the PlGF and the vascular endothelial growth factor (VEGF). Antiangiogenic action leads to hypertension and the glomerulopathy typical of the maternal syndrome.[5] These angiogenic factors have been used in prediction models and are yet to exhibit clinical feasibility. Increased sFlt-1/PlGF ratio is especially noted in women with early-onset (before 34 weeks of gestation) preeclampsia (EOPET) or placental preeclampsia. Late-onset preeclampsia (LOPET) or maternal preeclampsia is because of accentuation of the prevailing endothelial dysfunction due to the physiological stress of pregnancy. This is commonly seen in women with obesity, diabetes, and hypertension before conception and has less pronounced placental pathology and less fetal complications.

Ischemic placenta increases the inflammatory T-cells and cytokines and decreases the regulatory cells and cytokines, leading to a chronic inflammatory state **(Fig. 2)**. This inflammation is the basis for the development of HDPs and is seen to prevail in all types and classes reiterating the fact that gestosis inflammation is at the core of the pathogenesis of this disorder from which

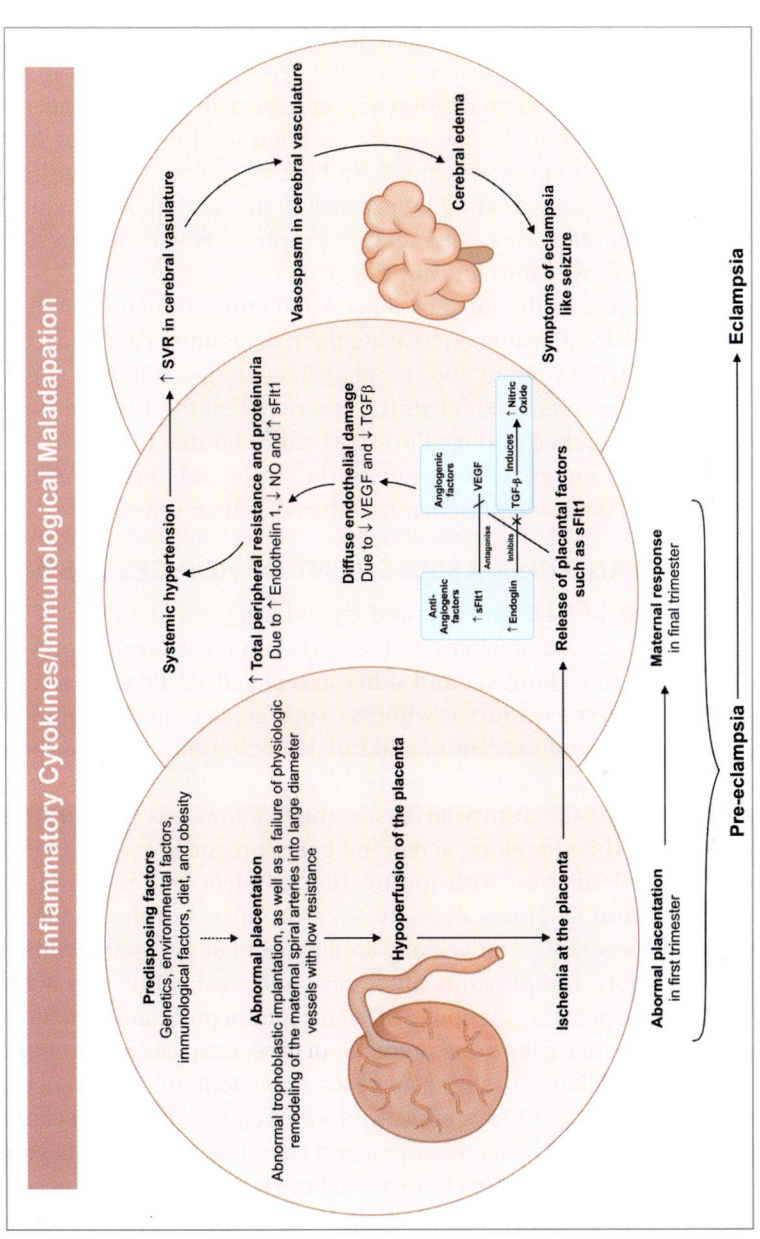

Fig. 2: Pathogenesis of HDP gestosis. (NO: nitric oxide; sFlt-1: soluble fms-like tyrosine kinase 1; SVR: systemic vascular resistance; TGFβ: transforming growth factor β; VEGF: vascular endothelial growth factor)

all the other pathological pathways emerge and exacerbate, giving rise to the plethora of clinical situations and manifestations.

Whatever the pathogenesis, the HDP gestosis disorder is heterogeneous and therefore would present as superimposed preeclampsia in CHT and/or GHT, extreme subtypes such as the EOPET versus LOPET, mild versus severe disease, and presence or absence of fetal restriction and postpartum hypertension. Demarcation between the maternal and placental preeclampsia is not actually clear-cut and each of the subtypes have a potential to evolve into other. Diagnosis and management of HDP gestosis early and management by treating hypertension, prevention of immediate and long-term complications, and seizure prophylaxis with magnesium sulfate are the mainstay of the clinical strategy.

The consequences in the form of generalized endovascular injury and dysfunction can be long-lasting, increasing the risk of future cardiovascular diseases in the affected women and has plausible intergenerational effects. PW with preeclampsia have podocyturia, where the glomerular epithelial cells (podocyturia) are shed through the urine before and after the occurrence of preeclampsia characterized by proteinuria.[6] Impaired angiogenesis of Pre-elcampsia (PE) is a result of ischemia-induced cellular senescence.

■ SCREENING AND RISK ASSESSMENT OF HDP GESTOSIS

Every PW is at risk of HDP gestosis and considering the quantum of the disorder and its grave consequences, all measures should be taken to prevent the occurrence of preeclampsia and other associated HDPs with serious outcomes. History over a century is witness to the fact that quality antenatal care, early suspicion and detection, and quick ameliorating interventions can reduce the disease burden considerably. In recent times, lowering the threshold to start the antihypertensive medications has proved to be protective and for this therefore, screening every pregnancy will ensure a better outcome.[7] Prediction with multivariate models and combination with biomarkers and Dopplers have shown a promise, but the challenge with these is they cannot be universally applicable to all pregnant women. Maternal risk factors and previous obstetrical and medical history act as good grounds to suspect the possibility of occurrence of preeclampsia. Blood pressure of 140/90 mm Hg is a good predictor of preeclampsia and therefore, blood pressure surveillance itself is a good screening tool. In the absence of hypertension, any evidence of systemic involvement must make one suspect HDP gestosis. Vigilant clinical assessment and surveillance can act as good screening tools for HDP screening tools are to have a clarity of their objective and here it is HDPs. The greatest value of a screening strategy is enabling the identification of the PW at risk of developing HDP or having already developed one. Thus, the tool should be applied at the onset of the pregnancy and closer to the occurrence of the disorder in those at-risk mothers and this precisely is what the gestosis HDP score has to offer.

The Gestosis India Association has proposed the gestosis HDP score, a clinical score which acts as a basic, first contact tool to identify at-risk mothers, to educate them, and ensure they get optimum antenatal care and guidance with nutrition, aspirin and calcium prophylaxis, exercise, regular blood pressure surveillance, and stepped-up screening with biomarkers or Dopplers only if found necessary. The score is validated prospectively and has proved its utility with 83.1% sensitivity, 97.51% specificity, positive predictive value (PPV) 85.51%, and negative predictive value (NPV) of 95.35%.[8] The maternal risk factors are awarded grading based on their potential of causing gestosis and also considers some evolving factors such as the MAP and weight gain[9] **(Table 1)**.

TABLE 1: HDP gestosis score for screening and early detection and planning antenatal strategy.

Maternal clinical factors	Score allocated	Maternal clinical factors	Score allocated
Maternal anemia	1	GDM	2
BMI >30 kg/m²	1	Obesity grade III (BMI >40 kg/m²)	2
Primigravida	1	Multifetal pregnancy	2
Short duration of sperm exposure (cohabitation)	1	HTN in previous pregnancy	2
Women born as SGA	1	Pregnancy with ART (OD/surrogacy)	3
Family history of cardiovascular disease	1	Chronic hypertension	3
Maternal hypothyroidism	1	Mental disorders	3
PCOS	1	Pregestational diabetes	3
Interpregnancy interval >7 years	1	Inherited/acquired thrombophilia	3
IVF/ICSI pregnancy	1	Maternal chronic kidney disease	3
MAP >85 mm Hg	1	Autoimmune disease (SLE/ALPA/RA)	3
Chronic vascular disease (Dyslipidemia)	1		
Excessive weight gain in pregnancy	1		

(ALPA: antiphospholipid syndrome; ART: antiretroviral therapy; BMI: body mass index; GDM: gestational diabetes mellitus; HDP: hypertensive disorders in pregnancy; HTN: hypertension; ICSI: intracytoplasmic sperm injection; IVF: in vitro fertilization; MAP: mean arterial pressure; PCOS: polycystic ovary syndrome; RA: rheumatoid arthritis; SGA: small for gestational age; SLE: systemic lupus erythematosus)

Flowchart 1: Gestosis score application in every pregnant woman.

```
                    Pregnant woman confirmed IU pregnancy
                                    │
                            Gestosis score
                           ┌────────┴────────┐
                         <3                  >3
                          │                   │
```

- **<3 branch:**
  - Vigilant ANC correct BP/Weight measurement
  - DIPSI 12–14 W and 24–28 W/34
  - Anemia/TSH surveillance 1/trimester L/F FGR
  - Nutritional guidance for all

- **>3 branch:**
  - Aspirin 75–150 mg/day
  - Early warning signs headache/excessive vomiting/epigastric pain/excessive edema/acute pain/vision changes/feeling of ill being/respiratory difficulties/giddiness/syncope/seizures

Side panel:
- Correct BP checking MAP desired 130/80: be on guard 140/90: Antihypertensives
- Weight gain >1 kg/m vigilant Obesity: Structured weight gain
- Lifestyle: High protein and fiber diet; Stress management; Walk twice daily
- Supplements: Calcium/Iron/D/DHA/Folic acid

(ANC: antenatal care BP: blood pressure; DIPSI: Diabetes in Pregnancy Study Group of India DHA: docosahexaenoic acid; FGR: fetal growth restriction; MAP: mean arterial pressure; TSH: thyroid-stimulating hormone)

Note: Gestosis score applied universally helps in early detection of at-risk women and selectively offers interventions. Thus, appropriate predictive approaches can be offered in women with risk factors. It also guides toward structured antenatal care. This strategy can definitely prevent preeclampsia up to 95%.

The gestosis score offers an objective way of assessing the plausible maternal factors which can award the woman the risk of developing gestosis. It also acts as a checklist to ensure that every factor is accounted for and noted and helps guide the clinician to explain to the PW as well as guide the antenatal care. The stepwise algorithmic approach can be adapted to thus plan the clinical course of care for the mother.

The gestosis score helps not to miss out on risk factors and educate the patient as well as her family about optimum antenatal care and early warning signs **(Flowchart 1)**. Any abnormal features such as hypertension, hypothyroidism, edema, excessive weight gain, or fetal growth restriction (FGR)—care must be escalated based on each condition. Thus, first-time assessment and ongoing surveillance both can be achieved by the gestosis score.

■ PREDICTION OF HDP

Predictive biomarkers have created interest for prediction of preeclampsia, especially preterm preeclampsia or EOPET. Effective predictor is the one which will facilitate early diagnosis (before 16 weeks being ideal), targeted surveillance, and timely delivery. Before 16 weeks, prediction can help use antiplatelet agents to ameliorate the disorder effectively.[10] Late-onset disease

TABLE 2: UAPI during pregnancy to predict preeclampsia and FGR.

Trimester	TAS mean PI 95th centile	TVS mean PI 95th centile
First: 11–13 weeks	2.35	3.10
Second: At 23 weeks	1.44	1.58
Third: 30–34 weeks	1.17	–

(FGR: fetal growth restriction; TAS: transabdominal sonography; TVS: transvaginal sonography; UAPI: uterine artery pulsatility index)

continues to necessitate careful vigilance and timed delivery.[11] Angiogenic markers such as sFlt-1 and PlGF singularly and in ratio have been identified to be good predictors as well as for triaging in an ambiguous clinical situation to avoid unnecessary intervention. Combining these with maternal factors and uterine artery Dopplers has increased the predictive performance of the strategy. Doppler studies using the uterine artery pulsatility index (UAPI) at 11–13 + 6 weeks help to identify the spiral arteriole resistance and offer a window of opportunity to use low-dose aspirin to overcome this. Moreover, surveillance with UAPI **(Table 2)** can be done throughout pregnancy in the at-risk PWs.[12]

All the current screening approaches and predictive tools are summarized further **(Table 3)** for quick reference and overview.

DIAGNOSIS OF HYPERTENSIVE DISORDERS IN PREGNANCY

Hypertensive disorders in pregnancy may be diagnosed as a part of regular prenatal care of measuring blood pressure, occurrence of edema, or sudden weight gain. It can be an acute diagnosis made in a moderately or a critically ill patient when presenting either with hypertension with severe features of the disease. Clinical symptoms that mandate attention are unusual vomiting, right upper abdominal pain, photophobia, state of confusion, unable to see cell phone numbers properly, sudden weight gain—sometimes 5 kg in 48 hours, reduced urine output, complaints of "I just do not feel right," shortness of breath, seizures, unconsciousness, acute abdominal pain, or prevaginal bleeding. All these symptoms look nonspecific and create ambiguity, but astute and careful attention can help pick up PWs with these presentations.

Even a single reading of abnormal blood pressure puts the PW at 40% risk of developing preeclampsia.[13] Blood pressure assessment in the hospital setting has to be appropriate technique with the use of Korotkoff sounds I and V to denote the systolic blood pressure (SBP) and diastolic blood pressure (DBP), respectively. Some PWs (5%) have an exaggerated gap between the IV (muffling) and V (disappearance) Korotkoff sounds, with the fifth sound

TABLE 3: Summarized predictive tools for HDPs especially preeclampsia.

Test	Clinical scores ACOG/RCOG/gestosis score	First trimester combined test	sFlt:PlGF ratio	PlGF
Features	Maternal factors are quantified and graded and are a clinical test	MF + MAP + UAPI + PlGF	Screen positive is >38	Screen positive <100 pg/mL represents
Advantages	• Only clinical factors therefore feasible • Universally applicable to all • No need of specific tests or sonography • No additional cost	• Sensitivity for preterm preeclampsia (~82%) • Better compliance with prophylactic LDA	• If sFlt1:PlGF is 38 or less, there is 99.3% NPV for PE within a week—a strong "rule-out" test • Reduces admissions for women with ambiguity	• Screen positive in women with suspected PE at <35 W: 96% sensitivity and 98% NPV for PE developing within 2 weeks • Reduces the time for diagnosis, adverse outcomes, and costs of repeat visits
Disadvantages	Only 41% sensitivity for ACOG/RCOG scores but 83% for the gestosis score. Compliance to LDA is poor	• Additional cost for PlGF and USG • Does not predict term PE with high sensitivity • Detects only 42.5% of all PE • Its use (combined with LDA prophylaxis) cannot reduce rates of PE occurring at >37 W, which is most of the disease	• Only suspects PE at <37 W—not applicable universally to all • Unable to accurately predict ("rule-in") PE: Low sensitivity and PPVs	• Only for suspected PE at <35 W—not applicable universally • Unable to accurately predict ("rule-in") PE at term

ACOG: American College of Obstetricians and Gynecologists; LDA: low-dose aspirin; MAP: mean arterial pressure; MF: maternal factors; NPV: negative predictive value; PE: preeclampsia; PlGF: placental growth factor; PPV: positive predictive value; RCOG: Royal College of Obstetricians and Gynaecologists; sFlt-1: soluble fms-like tyrosine kinase 1; UAPI: uterine artery pulsatility index; USG: ultrasonography; W: weeks) approaching zero. In such a situation, both the fourth and fifth sounds should be recorded (e.g., 120/80/40, with sound I: 120, sound IV: 80, and sound V: 40), fourth sound will more closely approximate the true DBP. The PW should be in a sitting position, comfortable with loose clothes, and rested or in a semirecumbent position if in bed and with an appropriate-sized cuff.

Mean arterial pressure is a sensitive marker of HDP in screening for PE.[14] But MAP in isolation would act as a proxy for other risk factors, including maternal weight and CHT.[15] MAP is assessed with the use of two machines and appropriate cuff size simultaneously in both the arms, supported at the level of the heart with the PW in sitting position. Mean arterial blood pressure was derived by using the formula (2DBP + SBP)/3. The cut-off of mid-pregnancy (12-24 weeks) MAP >89.7 mm Hg is a useful parameter to predict the development of GHT and can be used for triaging, while MAP <89.7 mm Hg can be used as a negative predictor for the development of GHT or PE.[16] MAP has been found to be a low performer to predict preeclampsia on its own.

In the recent times, CHT is more prevalent and has a potential of contributing to adverse outcomes such as congenital heart diseases in the fetus, miscarriages, stroke, cardiomyopathy, and superimposed preeclampsia. When diagnosed before, during, or after the course of the pregnancy, it has to be evaluated in detail to identify the probable cause, the level of chronicity by fundoscopy, and cardiac and renal evaluations and a switch to appropriate medications is to be done to maintain effective blood pressure to avoid complications. It is best to engage in a multidisciplinary consultation for the same.

Severe features of the disease are identified by careful systemic evaluation and any evidence of pulmonary edema, altered sensorium, stroke, or nephropathy cardiomyopathy has to be thoroughly evaluated. Laboratory evaluations are essential to diagnose the occurrence of nephropathy and HELLP and to differentiate from hemolytic–uremic syndrome (HUS) and acute fatty liver of pregnancy (AFLP). Evaluation of the placental function and the fetal parameters such as gestational age, biometry, and Doppler studies are needed to guide management as well to assess the severity and to decide the delivery effectively.

■ MANAGEMENT

The mainstay of management is antihypertensive treatment. This has three components as follows: (1) Shift to an appropriate antihypertensive in PW with CHT, preferably to nifedipine or labetalol, (2) initiating antihypertensive therapy during pregnancy for the first time, and (3) management of acute hypertensive crisis. The goal of all the three situations is to maintain the BP below 130/80 mm Hg as this way, optimum placental perfusion is maintained as well as the PW is protected from complications. The antihypertensive strategy has been depicted in **Table 4**.

- *Hypertensive crisis* is seen to affect 1–2% of PWs with HDP and especially so with underlying CHT, while sudden onset can also occur with preeclampsia. It includes urgency as well as emergency and is characterized by persistent, acute-onset severe hypertension with 160 mm Hg SBP, and/or 110 mm Hg DBP. PW have a low threshold for organ damage than nonpregnant women, quick and thorough assessment of maternal condition with history, risk factors, and course of prenatal period along with fetal assessment with biometry and Dopplers to evaluate FGR is necessary. Quick reference management of hypertensive crisis to reduce the blood pressure and avert seizures is essential **(Table 5)**. Immediate management is rapid reduction of blood pressure and **Table 4** shows the medications and dosages used for this. Women with CHT are more at risk of developing stroke (can be attributed to microaneurysms in the cerebral vasculature) or cardiac complications, while those with preeclampsia are at risk of seizures. Hypertensive crisis may present postpartum or during puerperium and same management approach is essential.

TABLE 4: Antihypertensive medication doses and contraindications summary.

HTN drug	Starting dose	Step-up dose	High dose	Maximum dose
Labetalol	100 mg bid/tid/qid	200 mg bid/tid/qid	300 mg tid/qid	1,200 mg/day
Nifedipine	10 mg bid or tid Or Slow release 10 mg SR bid	20 mg bid/tid Or 20 mg sustained release (SR) bid	30 mg tid/qid	120 mg/day
Methyldopa	250 mg tid/qid	500 mg tid/qid	750 mg tid/qid	2,250 mg/day

Notes:
- Labetalol is contraindicated in uncontrolled asthma. It causes neonatal bradycardia and hypoglycemia, necessitating newborn screening for the same.
- Nifedipine is contraindicated in aortic stenosis.
- Methyldopa can cause decreased variability on electronic fetal monitoring (EFM) and postpartum depression.
- Appropriate drug therapy is essential and the mother has to be encouraged for home BP monitoring and timely referral.
- Clinical surveillance for looking out for adverse effects of the medications has to be done.
- Pregnant woman with proteinuria and/or severe features should be delivered in time. Undue prolongation of pregnancy should not be undertaken. Compliance of the patient and education about early warning signs is essential.
- If BP control is not optimum switch from starting to step-up dose. Before high dose of the same medication, consider using another drug in combination. Need of three or more drugs mandates delivery.

TABLE 5: Management of hypertensive crisis.	
Trigger for initiating this checklist is SBP >160 mm Hg or DBP >110 mm Hg	
Contradictions: Pulmonary edema, renal failure, and myasthenia gravis	
[ ]	Initiate magnesium sulfate for seizure prophylaxis (if not already initiated)
[ ]	Load 4–6 g of magnesium sulfate in 100 mL solution IV over 20 minutes
[ ]	Magnesium sulfate on infusion pump
[ ]	Magnesium sulfate and pump labeled
[ ]	Magnesium sulfate 10 g of 50% solution IM (5 g in each buttock), if no IV access
[ ]	Magnesium sulfate maintenance 1–2 g/h, continuous infusion
Antihypertensive medications:	
Labetalol	20, 40, 60, and 80 mg, IV* over 2 minutes, escalating doses—repeat every 10 minutes, or 200 mg orally if no IV access; avoid in asthma or heart failure—can cause neonatal bradycardia
Nifedipine	10 mg orally followed by 20 mg SR

*Maximum cumulative IV administered doses should not exceed 25 mg hydralazine; 220 mg labetalol in 24 hours.

(IM: intramuscular; IV: intravenous; DBP: diastolic blood pressure; SBP: systolic blood pressure; SR: sustained release)

Notes:
- Repeat blood pressure every 10 minutes during administration
- If first-line agents are unsuccessful, recommend emergency consultation with a specialist, e.g., MFM, Internal Medicine, OB Anesthesiology, Critical Care for second-line management decisions such as sodium nitroprusside (risk of fetal cyanide toxicity)

- *Seizure prevention and control* are important components of management of HDP as eclampsia can escalate the morbidity and increase possibility of death and serious complications. Magnesium sulfate has been proved to be a safe and an effective drug for seizure prophylaxis as well as prevention and additionally awards a neuroprotection effect as well as stabilization in HELLP syndrome. There are many regimens of magnesium sulfate and modern ways of delivering the drug for convenient and safe delivery **(Table 6)**.

Magnesium sulfate regimens or dosing for prevention or severe preeclampsia have not been determined and the same dosing as for eclampsia is practiced and recommended by most bodies. Magnesium sulfate has been proven to be a safe drug, necessitating close clinical monitoring as the levels achieving a therapeutic level and the ones which can cause adverse effects are narrow. It therefore is essential that every clinician is well aware about the pharmacokinetics of this life-saving medicine and uses it with confidence. Magnesium sulfate after administration binds to the protein (40%) and the

TABLE 6: Magnesium sulfate regimens for eclampsia and modern way of dose delivery.

Name of the regimen	Loading dose	Maintenance dose	Comment
Pritchard	4 g IV diluted to a 20 mL solution [50% × 4: 2 mL] amps diluted with 12 mL DW/RL: Given over 5–10 minutes slowly + 5 g (50% × 5 amp) delivered in each buttock (gluteal muscle) IM—total of 14 g	5 g IM every 4 hours in alternate buttock for 24 hours after the occurrence of the last seizure or birth, whichever is last	• Recommended by the WHO as any HCP can deliver • Painful • High-loading dose • Easy to deliver • Needs less monitoring • Gluteal abscess due to muscle necrosis • CI in thrombocytopenia
Zuspan regimen	4 g IV diluted to a 20 mL solution (50% × 4: 2 mL] amps diluted with 12 mL DW/RL: Given over 5–10 minutes slowly	1–2 g IV infusion (5 g added to 500 mL RL/NS at 20–25 drops/min) for 24 hours after the occurrence of the last seizure or birth, whichever is last	• Pain-free • Monitoring necessary to ensure the right drop rate • IV, so it can be stopped in case of overdose • Fluid overload is a possibility
Sibai regimen	6 g IV diluted to a 20 mL solution [50% × 6: 2 mL] amps diluted with 10 mL DW/RL: Given over 20 minutes slowly	2 g IV infusion for 24 hours after the occurrence of the last seizure or birth, whichever is last	• Pain-free • Monitoring necessary to ensure the right drop rate • IV, so it can be stopped in case of overdose • Fluid overload is a possibility
Our practice (modern approach)	4 g [50% × 4: 2 mL] amps diluted added to 100 mL NS over 10 minutes slowly	1–2 g IV infusion attached to the syringe pump with 24 g (24 amps of 50% amps attached loaded in the 25 mL syringe) for 24 hours after the occurrence of the last seizure or birth, whichever is last	• Pain-free • Automated delivery rate ensuring right dose for the stipulated time • No fluid overload

(CI: confidence interval; HCP: healthcare personnel; IM: intramuscular; IV: intravenous; NS: normal saline; RL: Ringer's lactate; SR: sustained release; WHO: World Health Organization)

Important tips:
- Give 2 g MgSO$_4$ (50% solution) IV over 5 minutes
- Take one 10 mL syringe
- Draw two 50% ampules of MgSO$_4$ (4 mL = 2 g) into syringe
- Give IV slowly over 5 minutes
- Always give the loading IV 4 g dose slowly over 5–10 minutes as sudden fast injection can cause severe flushing, discomfort, and neurogenic response.

ionic unbound form spreads into the interstitial spaces, bones, placenta, fetus, and amniotic fluid. After 3-4 hours of administration, magnesium reaches a stable level of 0.250-0.442 L/kg.[18] Magnesium is excreted only in the urine and with 90% of the dose is being eliminated within 24 hours of IV administration. After IV dosing, there are two separate ways of distribution and elimination. Quick distribution is the rapid alpha phase, while slow elimination is the beta phase. Magnesium sulfate can be clinically monitored effectively as the therapeutic concentrations and overdosing can be identified with close surveillance. For treatment of seizures, concentration of 1.8-3.0 mmol/L is effective.[18] Loss of patellar reflex implies plasma concentrations between 3.5 and 5 mmol/L and further monitoring has to be followed and acted upon as shown in **Table 7**.

TABLE 7: Monitoring of magnesium sulfate is essentially clinical.

Clinical parameter	Magnesium level	Action	Comment
Seizure control	1.8–3.0 mmol/L	Continue the same concertation and surveillance	Immediate fit—give 2 g and step up to 2 g/h for effective control
Loss of patellar reflex	3.5 and 5 mmol/L	Withhold further dose and restart after reflexes appear at a lower dose	Most important clinical parameter when appears calls for vigilance
Urine output <100 mL/4 h or 25 mL/h	Can occur at any level if nephropathy	Next, IM dose to be reduced to 2.5 g or the IV infusion to 0.5 g/h	• *Inadequate hydration nephropathy:* Serum creatine >1.1 mg/L • Magnesium sulfate is not nephrotoxic
Respiratory rate <16/min	5–6.5 mmol/L (respiratory paralysis)	Stop magnesium sulfate or give calcium gluconate or consider intubation and PPV	
Altered cardiac conduction	>7.5 mmol/L	ICU/CCU	Rarely seen
Cardiac arrest	>12.5 mmol/L	ICU/CCU	Rarely seen

(CCU: critical care unit; ICU: intensive care unit; IM: intramuscular; IV: intravenous; PPV: positive predictive value)

Notes:
- Serum monitoring of magnesium levels has been advocated but has not been shown to be superior to clinical monitoring.
- The maintenance dose of magnesium sulfate is given only after assuring that patellar reflex is present. Respiration is not depressed: [respiratory rate (RR) >16/min]. Urine output during previous 4 hours exceeded 100 mL (25 mL/h)

TABLE 8: Eclampsia management algorithm.

Time	Action
0–5 minutes	• Airway, lateral decubitus, suction, oxygenation, restrain with care, and protection • Secure IV line (18–20 g intracath), deliver 4 g magnesium sulfate over 5–6 minutes 4 amps of 50% w/v + 12 mL DW = 20 mL • Foley's catheter/assess PO_2/RBSL/Dipstick proteinuria/attach a multipara monitor
10–15 minutes	• Samples for blood and urine for testing • *Antihypertensive treatment:* If conscious—oral nifedipine 10 mg SR or labetalol 200 mg unconscious—labetalol drip • *Magnesium sulfate infusion:* 24 amps of 50% withdrawn in 50 mL syringe—attached to the syringe pump 1 g/h • *Pritchard's IM regimen of loading dose:* 5 g in each buttock • *Assess history/obstetric parameters:* GA/fetal status (Doppler/NST)/Bishop's score • Order for sonography with Doppler
15–20 minutes	• Procure the laboratory reports fetal assessment • Plan delivery • *Stable:* Consider delivery—obstetric parameters • Consider transfer to HDU/ICU facility

(HDU: high-dependency unit; ICU: intensive care unit; IM: intramuscular; NST: nonstress test; PO_2: partial pressure of oxygen; RBSL: risk-based screening level; SR: sustained release)

Notes:
- *Recurrent seizures:* Repeat the 2 g bolus after the primary 4 g dose
- *Refractory seizures:* Lorazepam mg
- *Deeply unconscious:* Consider intubation

Eclampsia Management

The overview of management of eclampsia is represented in the algorithm in **Table 8**.

In the modern approach to HDPs, focus has to shift to CHT with more women presenting with this condition. Optimum screening for their cardiac health, obesity-related issues, and tight blood pressure control have proven to reduce the adverse outcomes.

■ SURVEILLANCE AFTER DIAGNOSIS

Preeclampsia is a pregnancy-specific disorder and of placental origin. Surveillance after diagnosis has to be meticulous, balancing to avoid maternal complications and avoid fetal jeopardy either due to prematurity or IUFD. The management algorithm is depicted in **Flowcharts 2 and 3**.

Flowchart 2: Assessment after the diagnosis of preeclampsia.

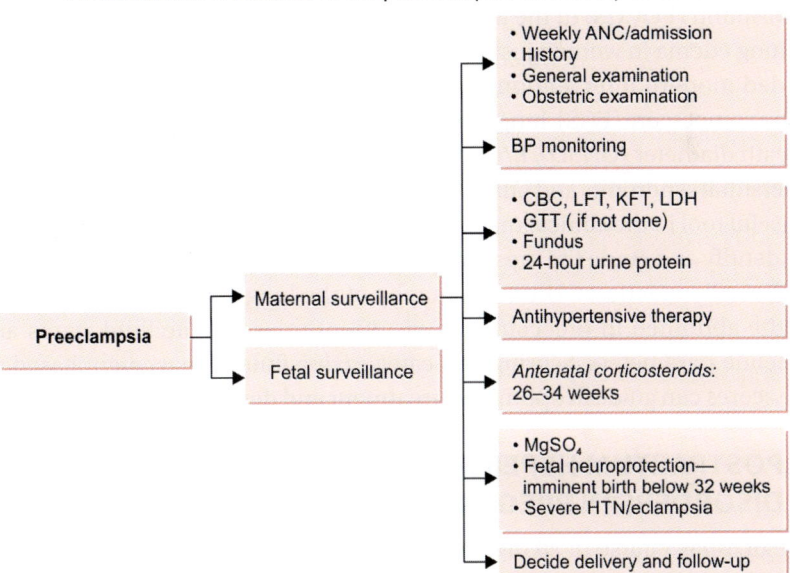

(BPP: biophysical profile; EFW: estimation of fetal weight; NST: nonstress test)

Flowchart 3: Surveillance of the preeclampsia till delivery decision.

(ANC: absolute neutrophil count; BP: blood pressure; CBC: complete blood count; GTT: glucose tolerance test; HTN: hypertension; KFT: kidney function test; LDH: Lactate dehydrogenase; LFT: liver function test; MgSO$_4$: magnesium sulfate)

Ambulatory management at home has been proposed as an option for patients with PE without severe features. This is done for a well-informed PW with access to serial and frequent surveillance, laboratory assessments, scans, and blood pressure monitoring.[19]

Delivery Decision

Pregnant woman showing any severe features should be delivered without delay with optimum stabilization, antenatal steroids and magnesium sulphate for neuroprotection as well as seizure prevention. PW without severe features at or beyond 38 weeks of gestation, delivery rather than expectant management upon diagnosis is recommended with severe features if diagnosed at or beyond 34 weeks of gestation, after maternal stabilization, or with labor or pre-labor rupture of membranes. Delivery should not be delayed for the administration of steroids. Labor induction before 39 weeks will prevent deterioration in maternal condition and minimize the risks for the neonates.

Additional Surveillance in the Modern Management

It has been observed that volume assessment and fluid management can prevent maternal deaths in the PW with severe hypertension. A systematic review and meta-analysis (MA) to evaluate the role and ability of point-of-care ultrasound (POCUS) in the assessment of volume status and early detection of lung edema in women just before delivery or intrapartum is assuring. The added modern interventions such as POCUS-derived parameters such as echo comet score (ECS), lung ultrasound (LUS) scores, β-patterns, optic nerve sheath diameter (ONSD), E/e' ratio, presence of pleural effusion, pulmonary interstitial syndrome, and pulmonary congestion were studied. POCUS can be a useful tool in the clinical management of the PWs with severe hypertension to identify and grade the presence of extravascular lung water (EVLW) before it clinically manifests. Ultrasonography of the lung should accompany that of the abdomen in preeclamptic parturient to assess the fluid status and baseline parameters. Scoring and categorizing fluid management based on the scores can guide in optimizing treatment and decreasing complications.[20]

POSTPARTUM HYPERTENSIVE DISORDERS IN PREGNANCY

Use of 5-day course of 20 mg furosemide daily caused 60% reduction in the prevalence of persistently elevated blood pressure at 7 days, thus was shown to expediate postpartum BP recovery in HDP.

CONCLUSION

Hypertensive disorders in pregnancy are a conglomerate of disorders where hypertension is the important segregating parameter; however, an intense clinical surveillance for any other signs of HDPs even in the absence of hypertension should be attended to and investigated. Gestosis score provides a baseline checklist to guide the clinician to offer focused care and surveillance to the PWs scored 3 or more than 3. Aspirin has helped in reducing 60% of preeclampsia. With the liberal use of magnesium sulfate and tight BP control, more complications can be averted. Magnesium sulfate is a safe drug and has to be delivered in a modern way and maternal surveillance can evolve to POCUS and the cardiological expertise to deliver safe maternal care.

■ REFERENCES

1. Sisti G, Williams B. Body of evidence in favor of adopting 130/80 mm Hg as new Blood pressure cut-off for all the hypertensive disorders of pregnancy. Medicina (Kaunas). 2019;55(10):703.
2. Roberts JM, August PA, Bakris G, Barton JR, Bernstein IM, Druzin ML, et al. Hypertension in pregnancy: report of the American College of Obstetricians and Gynecologists' Task Force on Hypertension in Pregnancy. Obstet Gynecol. 2013;122:1122-31.
3. Matthys LA, Coppage KH, Lambers DS, Barton JR, Sibai BM. Delayed postpartum preeclampsia: an experience of 151 cases. Am J Obstet Gynecol. 2004;190:1464-6.
4. Sibai BM. Etiology and management of postpartum hypertension–preeclampsia. Am J Obstet Gynecol. 2012;206:470-5.
5. Rana S, Lemoine E, Granger JP, Karumanchi SA. Preeclampsia: pathophysiology, challenges, and perspectives. Circ Res. 2019;124:1094-112.
6. Garovic VD. The role of the podocyte in preeclampsia. Clin J Am Soc Nephrol. 2014;9:1337-40.
7. Gupta M, Yadav P, Yaqoob F. A Prospective Study to Determine the Predictive Ability of HDP-Gestosis Score for the Development of Pre-eclampsia. J Obstet Gynaecol India. 2022;72(6):485-91.
8. FOGSI-GESTOSIS-ICOG. (2019). Hypertensive Disorders in Pregnancy (HDP) Good Clinical Practice Recommendations 2019. [online] Available from: https://www.fogsi.org/wp-content/uploads/gcpr/hdp-fogsi-gestosis-icog-gcpr-2019.pdf [Last accessed December, 2023].
9. Rolnik DL, Wright D, Poon LC, O'Gorman N, Syngelaki A, de Paco Matallana C, et al. Aspirin versus placebo in pregnancies at high risk for preterm preeclampsia. N Engl J Med. 2017;377:613-22.
10. Chappell LC, Brocklehurst P, Green ME, Hunter R, Hardy P, Juszczak E, et al. Planned early delivery or expectant management for late preterm pre-eclampsia (PHOENIX): a randomized controlled trial. Lancet. 2019;394:1181-90.
11. ISUOG Guidelines, Ultrasound Obstet Gynecol 2018;52:128-139.
12. Barton JR, Sibai BM. Prediction and prevention of recurrent preeclampsia. Obstet Gynecol. 2008;112(2 PART 1):359-72.
13. Walsh CA, Baxi LV. Mean arterial pressure and prediction of pre-eclampsia. BMJ. 2008;336(7653):1079-80.
14. Wright A, Wright D, Ispas CA, Poon LC, Nicolaides KH. Mean arterial pressure in the three trimesters of pregnancy: effects of maternal characteristics and medical history. Ultrasound Obstet Gynecol. 2015;45:698-706.
15. Shanker O, Gupta M. Role of mean arterial pressure in mid-trimester pregnancy for the prediction of gestational hypertension and pre-eclampsia. J South Asian Feder Obstet Gynaecol. 2021;13(3):151-5.
16. Mayrink J, Souza RT, Feitosa FE, Rocha Filho EA, Leite DF, Vettorazzi J, et al. Mean arterial blood pressure: potential predictive tool for preeclampsia in a cohort of healthy nulliparous pregnant women. BMC Pregnancy Childbirth. 2019;19(1):460.

17. Lu JF, Nightingale CH. Magnesium sulfate in eclampsia and pre-eclampsia: pharmacokinetic principles. Clin Pharmacokinet. 2000;38(4):305-14.
18. Gestational Hypertension and Preeclampsia: ACOG Practice Bulletin, Number 222. Obstet Gynecol. 2020;135:e237-60.
19. Bajwa SJS, Kurdi MS, Sutagatti JG, Bajwa SK, Theerth KA. Point-of-care ultrasound (POCUS) for the assessment of volume status and fluid management in patients with severe pre-eclampsia: a systematic review and meta-analysis. Indian J Anaesth. 2021;65(10):716-30.
20. Perdigao JL, Lewey J, Hirshberg A, Koelper N, Srinivas SK, Elovitz MA, et al. Furosemide for accelerated recovery of blood pressure postpartum in women with a hypertensive disorder of pregnancy: a randomized controlled trial. Hypertension. 2021;77(5):1517-24.

CHAPTER 3

Preterm Labor

Meghana P Reddy, Ashok Kumar

■ INTRODUCTION

Preterm labor is defined as delivery occurring before 37 weeks of gestation but after 20 weeks of gestation.[1] American College of Obstetricians and Gynecologists (ACOG) refines it by defining preterm labor as having regular uterine contractions accompanied by cervical changes of effacement or dilatation of at least 2 cm or both.[2] Preterm births are associated with neonatal complications such as low birth weight, prematurity and neonatal death. The preterm babies that however survive are at an increased risk of infections, neurological impairment, psychiatric or behavioral issues and risk of noncommunicable diseases at adulthood. Preterm births are a major contributor to the global burden of diseases by adding 15 million preterm babies every year. The rate of preterm birth ranges from 5 to 18% across 184 countries.[1] As per 2015 WHO statistics India ranks top among these countries. The lower the gestational age at birth, higher are the complications. The classification of preterm births into extremely preterm, very preterm, and late preterm is given in **Table 1**.

■ RISK FACTORS

Preterm birth is precipitated due to numerous factors, both preconceptional and conceptional factors. Many times, there are multiple factors which act in combination. They are listed in **Table 2**. The main risk factor is previous preterm birth as it has a recurrence rate of 14.3% after one and the risk almost doubles to 28% after two previous preterm births.[3]

TABLE 1: WHO classification of preterm births and their incidence.[1]

Type of preterm	Completed weeks of gestation	Incidence
Extremely preterm	<28 weeks	5%
Very preterm	28–32 weeks	10%
Moderate-to-late preterm	32 to < 37 weeks	85%

TABLE 2: Risk factors for preterm birth.

Preconceptional risk factors	Risk factors in present pregnancy
Prior preterm birth	Uterus over distension—multifetal gestation, polyhydramnios
History of recurrent midtrimester abortions, repeated evacuations	Antepartum hemorrhage
Genetic factors: • Collagen vascular disorders • Susceptible TNF	Birth defect in fetus
Uterine abnormalities: • Septate/subseptate uterus • Bicornuate uterus	Cervical injury especially during pregnancy (odd ratio-6.5)
Lifestyle factors: • Cigarette smoking • Illicit drug abuse • Extremes of BMI • Low socioeconomic status • Excessive physical activity	*Maternal infections:* • Bacterial vaginosis and susceptible-alpha genotype, increases PTB chance by nine-fold • Asymptomatic bacteriuria • Periodontal infection • Group B streptococcal infection—vaginal-urinary • Intrauterine infection— *Ureaplasma urealyticum* (U. urealyticum), *Fusobacterium*, *Mycoplasma hominis* (M. hominis)
Interpregnancy interval <18 months or >59 months	*Maternal medical conditions:* Hypertensive disorders of pregnancy, diabetes mellitus, anemia, chronic kidney disease, and systemic lupus erythematous (SLE)
History of cervical procedures—cervical amputation	Minimal or no prenatal care

■ MANAGEMENT

Management of a preterm labor aims to provide appropriate care so as to optimize the neonatal outcome. Management depends on the gestational age and the neonatal resuscitation facilities available at the given center. Approximately 30% of preterm labor spontaneously resolves and 50% of patients hospitalized for preterm labor actually give birth at term.[4]

The management of an established preterm labor is different than that of a threatened preterm labor and is thus very important to distinguish these two.

1. *Established preterm labor:* A woman is in established preterm labor if she has progressive cervical dilatation from 4 cm with regular contractions before 37 weeks of gestation

2. *Threatened preterm labor:* Uterine contractions in the absence of cervical changes.

Management strategies can be employed in accordance to the NICE guidelines 2015[5] on the management of preterm labor.

Corticosteroids

Corticosteroids when administered to the pregnant woman antenatally cross the placenta and reach the fetal lung and stimulate surfactant synthesis and maturation of other systems. Corticosteroids therapy is effective in lowering the incidence of respiratory distress syndrome (RDS), intraventricular hemorrhage (IVH), necrotizing enterocolitis, and neonatal mortality rates if birth was delayed for at least 24 hours after initiation of corticosteroid. Betamethasone and dexamethasone are widely studied and used worldwide for this indication **(Table 3)**.

- *Betamethasone* is available in two different forms: Both are often used in combination to maximize the drug's efficiency
    1. Betamethasone sodium phosphate, a solution with a short biological half-life of 36–72 hours
    2. Betamethasone acetate, a suspension with a relatively long half-life.
- *Dexamethasone:* It is available as dexamethasone sodium phosphate, a solution with a short biological half-life of 36–72 hours.

In India, as part of INAP (India Newborn Action Plan), the auxiliary nurse midwives are authorized to administer prereferral doses of corticosteroids to women in preterm labor to improve the survival of the preterm neonate. This step has been taken to bring neonatal mortality rates to below 10 per 1,000 live births. To achieve this, the corticosteroid coverage (at least single dose) to women in preterm labor should be 75% by 2017, 90% by 2020, and 100% by 2030.[6,7]

Despite the proven beneficial effects of the corticosteroids on the fetal lung maturity, they are not routinely prescribed for the general population because of the various short-term and long-term effects on the neonate as well as the mothers.

Fetal Side Effects

- Short-term impairment of growth with reductions in head circumference, weight, and stature at birth, neonatal sepsis, and hypoglycemia.

TABLE 3: Dosing schedules of the antenatal corticosteroid for fetal lung maturity.

Drug	Dosing		Total dose
Betamethasone	12 mg intramuscular 24 hours apart	2 doses	24 mg
Dexamethasone	6 mg intramuscular 12 hours apart	4 doses	24 mg

- Long-term impairment of cerebral myelination, neurological anomalies, alterations of pulmonary tissue, growth, and developmental disorders of the hypothalamic-pituitary-adrenal (HPA) axis
- A single course of corticosteroid is not associated with increased risk of short-term or long-term side effects.

Maternal Side Effects
- Steep variation in the blood sugar level—so close blood sugar monitoring is advised specially in diabetic mothers.
- Preterm premature rupture of membranes (PPROM) and prelabor rupture of membranes (PROM) mothers without overt chorioamnionitis do not exhibit increased chances of sepsis after single course of steroid administration.

Magnesium Sulfate

The preterm infants are at an increased risk of brain injury and cerebral palsy. This is because of the oligodendrocyte injury in the periventricular white matter. The N-methyl D-aspartate (NMDA) receptors present on these oligodendrocytes are thought to be important in the glial injury process. NMDA receptor antagonists are potent neuroprotective agents in several animal models of perinatal brain injury.

Several studies have demonstrated the neuroprotective effect of magnesium sulfate. The recommendations for its use are given in **Table 4**.

Mechanism of action:[8] The exact mechanism is not clearly understood. There are several proposed theories for its neuroprotective effect.
- Fetal cerebral vessel vasodilator—mitigating the ischemic effects
- Anti-inflammatory action prevents generation of proinflammatory cytokines interleukin-6 and tumor necrosis factor-α.

TABLE 4: Recommendations on magnesium sulfate in preterm birth.

	Level of recommendation	Completed weeks of gestation	Remarks
ACOG[2]	Recommended	24–34 weeks POG	• Only when delivery is imminent • For a short duration <48 hours
RCOG NICE 2015[5]	Should be offered	24 + 0 to 29 + 6 weeks POG	In established labor and delivery within 24 hours
FIGO GCPR 2021[9]	• Recommended • Consider	• Viability—30 weeks POG • <32–34 weeks POG	

- Downregulation of NMDA receptors → decreasing calcium influx into oligodendrocytes → stabilizes membrane potential (prevents excitotoxic calcium-induced injury).
- Antiapoptotic action, also by blocking calcium channels.

Tocolysis

Tocolytic (acute) therapy may offer some short-term benefit in the management of preterm labor by buying time to:
- Administer corticosteroids to enhance pulmonary maturity in fetus
- Facilitate transfer of patient to a tertiary care center

The tocolytic agents have several maternal and fetal side effects and are not routinely offered **(Tables 5 and 6)**.

Indications for tocolysis:
- Regular uterine contractions of at least 30 seconds duration at a rate of 4 per 30 minutes
- *Cervical changes:*
  - With effacement of ≥50%
  - Cervical dilation of 1–3 cm (0–3 for nullipara)
- Gestational age from 24 to 33 completed weeks
- With normal fetal heart rate.

Contraindications for tocolytic therapy:
- Intrauterine fetal demise
- Lethal fetal anomaly
- Non-reassuring fetal heart rate status
- Severe preeclampsia or eclampsia
- Maternal bleeding with hemodynamic instability
- Chorioamnionitis
- Preterm premature rupture of membranes with signs of infection.
- Maternal contraindications to tocolysis (agent specific)

Antibiotics

Routine antibiotic administration is not recommended by WHO for women in preterm labor with intact membranes and no clinical signs of infection. However, antibiotic administration is recommended in women with P-PROM.

Bed Rest

Although bed rest is frequently prescribed during management of preterm labor, it is rarely indicated, and ambulation should be considered in most cases. Available data do not show improved neonatal outcomes with bed rest; however, maternal thromboembolic events have been reported with decreased ambulation in pregnancy.

TABLE 5: Tocolytic agents and their profile.

Agent or class	Drugs	Dosage	Maternal side effects	Fetal or neonatal side effects	Contraindications
Calcium channel blockers	Nifedipine	• 30 mg PO • Followed by 10–20 mg every 4–6 hourly	Dizziness, flushing, and hypotension	Not known	Hypotension and preload dependent cardiac lesions (aortic insufficiency)
NSAIDs	Indomethacin	• 50–100 mg PO (or) 50 mg per rectally • Followed by 25–50 mg PO 4–6 hourly for 48 hours	Nausea, esophageal reflux, gastritis, and platelet dysfunction	• Constriction of ductus arteriosus in utero and patent ductus arteriosus in neonate • Oligohydramnios, necrotizing enterocolitis in preterm newborn	• Platelet dysfunction and bleeding disorder • Hepatic dysfunction, peptic ulcer disease, renal dysfunction, asthma
Beta-agonists	Isoxsuprine	• *IV:* Four ampoules in 500 mL 5% dextrose/RL @ 8–10 drops/minute, dose titrated according to response and not exceeding 40 drops/minute • *IM:* Used if IV facilities not available at the onset of labor *Dose:* 10 mg, 1–2 hourly • *Oral tablets:* Substitution for parenteral route once uterine activity has subsided *Dose:* 60–80 mg in divided doses	Tachycardia, hypotension, tremors, palpitations, shortness of breath, chest discomfort, pulmonary edema, hypokalemia, hypoglycemia, and fetal tachycardia		• Poorly controlled diabetes mellitus • Tachycardia sensitive maternal cardiac lesions

Contd...

Contd...

Agent or class	Drugs	Dosage	Maternal side effects	Fetal or neonatal side effects	Contraindications
	Terbutaline	• 0.25 mg SC every 20 minutes—3 hours Or • Continuous infusion gradually increased to 17.5 to 30 µg/minute			
Oxytocin receptor antagonists	Atosiban	• IV bolus: 6.75 mg – 0.9 mL, over 1 minute • IV infusion: 18 mg/hour. @24 mL/hour—3 hours • Subsequent IV infusion: 6 mg/hour @8 mL/hour—up to 45 hours	Hypersensitivity reactions at injection site	–	None
Miscellaneous	Magnesium sulfate	• 4–6 g IV bolus • Followed by IV infusion @1 g/hour	• Flushing, diaphoresis, nausea, loss of deep tendon reflexes, respiratory depression, and cardiac arrest • Neuromuscular blockade when used along with calcium channel blockers	Neonatal depression	Myasthenia gravis

TABLE 6: Recommendations on tocolysis in preterm birth.

	Level of recommendation	Completed weeks of gestation	Remarks
NICE[5]	Consider	24+0 to 25+6	Nifedipine, oxytocin antagonists
	Offer	26 to 33+6	No beta agonists
ACOG[2]	Not recommended	Before viability	*Exception:* Surgery on a mother with previable fetus
	Recommended for short-term use (48 hours) Maintenance therapy—not recommended.	Viability—34 weeks	First-line treatment with beta-agonists, calcium channel blockers, and NSAIDs

■ LABOR AND DELIVERY

Delivery must be conducted at a facility equipped with skilled neonatologists to resuscitate preterm babies. Specialized personnel in resuscitative techniques corresponding to gestational age and fully oriented to specific problems should be present at delivery. Vaginal delivery is preferred, and cesarean delivery must be limited to obstetric indications. However, it is recommended to consider cesarean delivery in women with established preterm labor with breech presentation presenting between 26 and 36 weeks of gestation.[5] If instrumental delivery is needed, then ventouse delivery is avoided. Obstetric forceps are used when indicated. In absence of relaxed vaginal outlet, an episiotomy for delivery may be necessary, but perinatal outcome data do not support routine episiotomy or forceps delivery to protect "fragile" preterm fetal head.

Timing of cord clamping for preterm babies born vaginally or by cesarean section (NICE 2015)[5]:
- Wait at least 30 seconds, but no longer than 3 minutes, before clamping the cord of preterm babies if the mother and baby are stable.
- Position the baby at or below the level of the placenta before clamping the cord.
- If a preterm baby needs to be moved away from the mother for resuscitation, or there is significant maternal bleeding, then, consider milking the cord and clamping the cord as soon as possible.

■ CONCLUSION

Preterm labour is one of the 5 'P' of the problems of pregnancy. Despite understanding the problem, the prevalence is still static even in developed countries. It is a multifactorial problem which needs to be screened and caught at the earliest to reduce neonatal morbidity and mortality. Antenatal corticosteroids (for lung maturity), magnesium sulfate (for neuroprotection) and tocolytics are the mainstay of treatment for preterm labour. The main aim is to ensure that we are able to catch it and deliver a preterm baby with adequate coverage and at a tertiary care center where NICU facilities are available.

■ REFERENCES

1. World Health Organization. (2023). Preterm birth. [online] Available from https://www.who.int/news-room/fact-sheets/detail/preterm-birth [Last accessed December, 2023].
2. American College of Obstetricians and Gynecologists' Committee on Practice Bulletins—Obstetrics. Practice Bulletin No. 171: Management of Preterm Labor. Obstet Gynecol. 2016;128(4):e155-64.
3. Bakketeig LS, Hoffman HJ, Harley EE. The tendency to repeat gestational age and birth weight in successive births. Am J Obstet Gynecol. 1979;135(8):1086-103.
4. Lewit EM, Baker LS, Corman H, Shiono PH. The direct cost of low birth weight. Future Child. 1995;5(1):35-56.
5. NICE. (2022). Overview: preterm labour and birth: guidance. [online] Available from https://www.nice.org.uk/guidance/ng25 [Last accessed December, 2023].
6. NRHMORISSA. (2023). Mission: National Health. [online] Available from http://www.nrhmorissa.gov.in/ [Last accessed December, 2023].
7. Ministry of Health and Family Welfare, Government of India. (2014). New born baby. [online] Available from https://www.newbornwhocc.org/INAP_Final.pdf [Last accessed December, 2023].
8. Bachnas MA, Akbar MIA, Dachlan EG, Dekker G. The role of magnesium sulfate ($MgSO_4$) in fetal neuroprotection. J Matern Fetal Neonatal Med. 2021;34(6):966-78.
9. Shennan A, Suff N, Jacobsson B. FIGO good practice recommendations on magnesium sulfate administration for preterm fetal neuroprotection. Int J Gynecol Obstet. 2021;155:31-3.

CHAPTER 4

Pregnancy After Renal Transplantation

Vineet Mishra, Nita Mishra

■ INTRODUCTION

After receiving a kidney donation from her identical twin sister in 1956, 23-year-old Edith Helm became pregnant for the first time in 1958. She gave birth to a healthy, full-term child weighing 3,300 g through cesarean section. Wanda Foster, her twin sister, also had four healthy pregnancies after receiving the kidney.[1] Since then, several healthy pregnancies among kidney transplant patients have been documented, giving hope to women who have long-wanted children. The only active registry is the National Transplantation Pregnancy Registry in the United States, which was founded in 1991. Other voluntary registries include the National Transplant Pregnancy Registry in the United Kingdom, which was founded in 1997, the European Dialysis and Transplant Association Registry, and the Australian and New Zealand Dialysis and Transplant Association Registry. All of these registries are constrained by small patient populations and inevitable reporting bias.[2-5] We must keep in mind that these retrospective studies are the primary source of the majority of our present information that directs the management of pregnancy in kidney transplant patients.

■ SEXUAL ACTIVITY

As a result of aberrant hypothalamus-pituitary-ovarian axis, women with chronic kidney disease (CKD) experience irregular menstrual cycles, anovulation, diminished libido, and poor fertility. Women with CKD often experience menopause onset 5 years sooner than the general population.[6,7] A total of 74% of hemodialysis female patients experience menstrual abnormalities, and amenorrhea affects 50% of them.[8] Due to poor renal clearance, elevated levels of luteinizing hormone (LH) and follicular stimulating hormone (FSH), and decreased levels of estradiol and progesterone, women with end-stage renal disease (ESRD), particularly those with amenorrhea, have high blood prolactin levels. Anovulation is caused by chronically increased gonadotropins brought on by the lack of the LH surge and the loss of the negative feedback on the hypothalamic and pituitary centers.[6,8,9] As a result, pregnancy is uncommon among women receiving dialysis, with conception rates as low as 1–7%. Even after a successful conception, about 25–38% of pregnancies result in viable fetuses.[10] However, after a successful kidney transplant, the transient transition to hypogonadotropic hypogonadism can occur as fast as 2–3 weeks, and within 6 months, circulating sex hormones recover to normal range.[11] It is crucial that women with the ability to get pregnant begin using contraception as soon as possible following transplant since the hypothalamic-pituitary-gonadal axis returns quickly.[12]

■ PREGNANCY AND ALLOGRAFT FUNCTION

Normal pregnancy results in hyperfiltration, intrarenal vasodilation, and a surge in effective plasma flow without a corresponding rise in intraglomerular pressure. With a drop in the serum concentration of urea and creatinine, the glomerular filtration rate increases by roughly 50%.[13] The ability of the renal allograft to adjust to the physiological changes of pregnancy is demonstrated by a rise in creatinine clearance of about 30% in the first trimester, which is sustained with a slight decline in the second trimester, and recovers to prepregnancy level during the third trimester.[14] According to Davison, healthy women's increases in 24-hour creatinine clearance were equivalent to those of allograft patients at 39% against 35% of gestation at 11 weeks. Additionally, compared to healthy women, allograft recipients have a higher 24-hour protein excretion, which rises throughout pregnancy, triples by the third trimester and regularly exceeds 500 mg (vs. 200 mg in healthy women), and then returns to prepregnancy levels at 3 months after delivery.[15] Never ascribe proteinuria in pregnancy to typical pregnancy-related changes; instead, screen out common comorbidities such as urinary tract infection (UTIs) and preeclampsia.

■ RISK OF COMPLICATIONS DURING PREGNANCY

Preeclampsia and Hypertension

It has been observed that 51–70% of kidney transplant patients had hypertension. Preeclampsia is six times more common in kidney transplant patients than the general population and ranges from 24 to 38% of the time.[4,16-18] Because preeclampsia frequently raises blood pressure beyond 20 weeks in previously normotensive women and hyperfiltration-related worsening of preexisting proteinuria, it can be challenging to differentiate it from hypertension in renal transplant patients. Since kidney transplant recipients frequently take calcineurin inhibitors, which raise uric acid levels, hyperuricemia becomes a less useful indicator for identifying preeclampsia.[19] Acute rejection is also accompanied by a considerable rise in proteinuria and a rapid worsening of hypertension, which further complicates the diagnosis of preeclampsia. Preterm birth, intrauterine development retardation, and the likelihood of graft loss are all made more likely by hypertension during pregnancy.[18] If the blood pressure is continuously >140/90 mm Hg, antihypertensives should be started. The conventional medications that have been used safely to regulate blood pressure during pregnancy include hydralazine and alpha-methyldopa. Beta-blockers and calcium channel blockers are additional antihypertensives that are safe to take during pregnancy. The link between angiotensinogen converting enzyme inhibitors and pulmonary hypoplasia and oligohydramnios in fetuses makes them contraindicated. All recipients of kidney transplants should take low dosage aspirin since it lowers the incidence of preeclampsia in high-risk populations.[20]

Allograft Function

Without risk factors, pregnancy does not enhance the rate of graft loss. At a follow-up of 10 years, there was no difference in the graft failure rate between pregnant women and nonpregnant allograft patients (19% vs. 21%).[14] History of drug-treated hypertension, prepregnancy creatinine 1.4 mg/dL, and proteinuria are risk factors for graft loss. Out of 133 female renal transplant recipients, 20 lost their grafts within 5 years, and it was shown in the National Transplantation Pregnancy Registry (NTPR) registry that these patients had higher serum creatinine levels before pregnancy (1.6 mg/dL vs. 1.1 mg/dL), higher serum creatinine levels after pregnancy (2.2 mg/dL vs. 1.3 mg/dL), and higher rejection rates during or within 3 months of pregnancy (45% vs. 4.6%). Pregnancy creatinine levels >1.4 mg/dL and >1.7 mg/dL were associated with 3.5-fold and 7.6-fold greater risks, respectively, of allograft failure at 5 years.[4] In all seven of the women who experienced graft loss within 2 years after delivery, prepregnancy creatinine was >1.5 mg/dL, according to Keitel et al.[21] In a case-control research, Sibanda et al. found no indication of increased renal allograft loss during pregnancy; nevertheless, the 2-year post-pregnancy graft survival was poorer in transplant recipients with hypertension than in those without (100% vs. 87%). It is advised that proteinuria in renal transplant patients be <500 mg prior to conception because nephrotic range proteinuria increases the risk of spontaneous abortion, intrauterine growth retardation, and preterm in pregnant women.[22]

Rejection Risk and its Management

It is possible that the antigenic stimulation produced by the fetus may also cause graft rejection. Pregnancy is a condition of immunological tolerance linked with immunodepressant activity of lymphocytes, which builds tolerance to the fetus and may help the kidney allograft. Additionally, due to the restoration to normal immunosurveillance state during the postpartum period, acute rejection may be more common.[23] High blood creatinine levels, rejection prior to pregnancy, and fluctuating doses of immunosuppressive medications are risk factors that raise the likelihood of rejection, but varied immunosuppression regimens do not.[24] The diagnosis of rejection is challenging since the condition is typically accompanied by a little increase in creatinine and may be confused by the pregnancy-related reduction in creatinine owing to hyperfiltration. To detect rejection in an allograft during pregnancy, ultrasonography guided renal biopsy is safe.[25] High dosage steroids continue to be the primary line of therapy for allograft rejection during pregnancy. There are few studies and no concrete recommendations about the use of additional medications for treating pregnancy-related rejection, such as antithymocyte globulin and rituximab.[26]

Infections

Due to the use of immunosuppressive drugs, pregnant kidney transplant recipients are more susceptible to infections, particularly bacterial UTIs and severe pyelonephritis. Up to 30% of women get UTI because of reflux, moderate hydronephrosis following transplant, and pregnancy-related dilatation of the ureters and renal collecting ducts. Every visit should include a urine dipstick screening for UTIs, and every 4 weeks, urine cultures should be taken. Antibiotics should be administered to asymptomatic bacteria for 2 weeks, after which prophylaxis should be continued the entire pregnancy. Nitrofurantoin and cephalexin are two antibiotics that are used to treat UTIs.[22] While secondary infection has a lesser chance of harming fetuses (2%), primary cytomegalovirus (CMV) infection leads in 45-50% transmission to fetus with 6-19% of them being symptomatic at birth. The amniotic fluid is cultured to determine the presence of fetal CMV. It has not been proven that treating the mother with ganciclovir or CMV hyperimmunoglobulin will stop fetal CMV illness.[27] Herpes simplex infection in the mother is linked to a higher risk of miscarriage and can be passed from mother to child during delivery. Acyclovir is used as a form of treatment, and cesarean sections are favored since they reduce the risk of newborn herpes. Hepatitis B immunoglobulin and the hepatitis B vaccination should be administered to infants whose mothers have the virus in order to avoid neonatal infection, which protects >90% of newborns.

■ FETAL COMPLICATIONS

In allograft patients, the live birth rate varies from 72 to 80%, which is equivalent to the general population.[4,18] According to reports, preterm birth happens more frequently as a result of maternal or fetal impairment than from spontaneous preterm labor, with rates as high as 45 to 55% compared to 6 to 20% in the general population.[4] Preterm birth is predisposed by maternal hypertension and a high blood creatinine level of 1.6 mg/dL.[18] They also frequently have preterm delivery (52-53%), low birth weight (42-46%), and intrauterine growth restriction (IUGR) (30-50%).[4,23,28] According to a research by Bramham et al.,[17] receivers of renal allografts have a 12-fold greater risk of preterm births, a 10-fold higher risk of low birth weight newborns, and a 7-fold higher risk of small for gestation babies compared to the general population. A newborn's gestational age is 34.5 weeks on average, and their birth weight is 2,270 g on average.[16] Although there is a greater risk of perinatal death in the absence of risk factors such as hypertension, proteinuria, and poor allograft functioning, the miscarriage incidence varies from 10 to 27% (compared to 9 to 10% in the general population).[4,17,18]

■ PREDICTORS OF THE OUTCOMES OF PREGNANCY

Hypertension, high prenatal creatinine >1.4 mg/dL, proteinuria, and history of >2 renal transplants are risk factors linked to poor pregnancy outcomes. According to a study by Bramham et al.,[17] there was an approximately 6-fold increased risk of adverse fetal outcomes (stillbirth, miscarriage, neonatal death, birth 32 weeks, and congenital anomalies) in women with high prenatal creatinine and high diastolic pressure during the second and third trimesters. Pregnant women who have nephrotic range proteinuria have an increased risk of spontaneous abortion, intrauterine growth restriction, and preterm.[22] Therefore, a favorable pregnancy outcome is connected with prenatal creatinine 1.4 mg/dL, the absence of hypertension, and low proteinuria 500 mg.

■ THE IDEAL TIME TO CONCEIVE

The best period of time to get pregnant following a kidney transplant is still up for debate. According to recommendations made by the American Society of Transplantation, women who have had a kidney transplant should wait between 1 and 2 years before trying to get pregnant. Following transplantation, deferring pregnancy for 2 years is advised by European best practice standards.[22,29] However, as long as the graft function is steady and the women are not using teratogenic drugs, it is safe to get pregnant even 6 months after receiving a kidney transplant. Conception within 2 years after receiving a transplant increases the chance of a viable fetal outcome.[16] Waiting longer may potentially cause postpartum renal dysfunction that is worsened and may not recover, along with already deteriorating renal function as a result of chronic allograft nephropathy. A recent research found that while pregnancy in the third post-transplant year was not linked to a higher risk of mortality censored graft loss, it was linked to an increased risk of allograft failure in the first and second post-transplant years.[30]

■ IMMUNOSUPPRESSION

Due to the possible teratogenic risk and side effects, managing immunosuppression in pregnant kidney transplant patients is crucial.

All immunosuppressive medications pass the maternal-fetal circulation and have been found in fetal circulation to varying degrees.[31] A (no human danger), B (animal studies suggesting risk but no evidence of human risk), C (human risk not ruled out), D (evidence of human risk), and X (completely prohibited) are the medication classifications used by the Food and Drug Administration (FDA) to determine how safe they are during pregnancy. Most medications come under category C, where risk and benefits must be balanced. **Table 1**[32] provides a summary of the most popular immunosuppressive medications used by kidney transplant patients as well as information on their pregnancies.

Calcineurin Inhibitors

Tacrolimus and cyclosporine are two examples of calcineurin inhibitors that are regarded as safe to use while pregnant. The blood levels of calcineurin inhibitors found in the fetus are roughly half those of the mother because they cross the placenta and enter the fetal circulation.[33] About 4-5% of women on calcineurin inhibitors had significant congenital structural malformations, which is equivalent to the reported frequency of 3-4% in the general population.[4,34] Cyclosporine has been demonstrated to promote thromboxane and endothelin production, increasing vascular bed resistance and contributing to the pathophysiology of preeclampsia.

TABLE 1: Immunosuppressant drugs used in transplantation.	
Induction	*FDA category*
Basiliximab	B
Alemtuzumab	C
Antithymocyte globulin	C
Methylprednisolone	C
Maintenance	
Azathioprine	D
Cyclosporine	C
Tacrolimus	C
Mycophenolate mofetil	D
Sirolimus, rapamycin	C
Prednisone	B
Belatacept	C
Leflunomide	X
Treatment of rejection	
Antithymocyte globulin	C
Basiliximab	B

In prenatal treatment to calcineurin inhibitors results in immature T-cells, deformed peripheral lymphatic organs, and ineffective T-cell reactivity, according to animal studies.[35] Cyclosporine may generate immature T-cells and a deficiency in B-cells in newborn humans, which may eventually result in the emergence of autoimmunity.[36] Children who were exposed to cyclosporine in utero and had a mean age of 4.4 years had developmental impairments in 16% of cases.[37] The long-term effects of calcineurin inhibitor exposure in utero are still poorly understood, and there are little data on pediatric neurodevelopmental follow-up.[38,39] First trimester, second trimester, and third trimester cyclosporine trough levels typically decline by 23%, 39%, and 29%, respectively.[40] We advise more regular monitoring of the whole blood trough level during pregnancy, with measurements taking place every 2 weeks during the first and second trimesters, once a week during the third trimester, and once more within a week after delivery.

Azathioprine

Even though the FDA has classified azathioprine as a class D medicine, it is safe to use as immunosuppressive during pregnancy since it quickly breaks down into 6-mercaptopurine. Although 6-mercaptopurine enters the fetal blood, the fetus is spared from its harmful effects because the fetal liver lacks the enzyme inosinate pyrophosphorylase needed to convert it to the active metabolite thioinosinic acid.[41] If the mother's white cell count is >7,500/mm^3, it is also linked to dose-related myelosuppression in the baby, Albeit newborn leukopenia is often uncommon.[42]

Corticosteroids

Prednisone (category B) and methylprednisolone (category C) are two steroids that are often administered to kidney transplant recipients.[16,22,32] 90% of the maternal dosage of corticosteroids is efficiently broken down in the placenta before it reaches the fetus. The ratio of maternal to cord blood is around 10:1.[43] At dosages >20 g/day, sporadic occurrences of fetal adrenal immunosuppression, thymic hypoplasia, and cleft palate have been documented.[44]

Mycophenolate Mofetil

The category D medicine mycophenolate mofetil is linked to an increased risk of spontaneous abortion and congenital deformity. The most frequent congenital abnormalities are limb and facial anomalies, which include microtia, hypoplastic nails, short fifth fingers, cleft lips and palates, congenital diaphragmatic hernias, and congenital heart problems.[45] Mycophenolate mofetil should be stopped 6 weeks before conception as it is not recommended during pregnancy. Mycophenolate-using transplant patients do not increase the risk of abnormalities in their offspring.[46]

Sirolimus

A category C medication is sirolimus. In animal investigations, it has been linked to higher fetal mortality, lower fetal weights, and delayed ossification of skeletal structure, although no teratogenicity has been shown.[26] Human exposure data are few, however sirolimus should be stopped 6 weeks before conception because it is not recommended for use during pregnancy.[22,47]

■ LABOR AND DELIVERY

The ideal method of birth is vaginal delivery, and obstetric reasons are the only times a cesarean section is recommended. The false pelvis, where the renal allograft is situated, is not obstructing the course of the fetus' delivery. If there are no obstetrical difficulties, spontaneous labor may continue up to 38–40 weeks. High-risk obstetricians, neonatologists, and transplant nephrologists should be part of a multidisciplinary team to treat pregnancies in renal transplant recipients.[22] We advise close follow-up visits every 2 weeks with a transplant nephrologist during prenatal care.

■ CONCLUSION

A successful pregnancy requires meticulous preparation and a renal transplant to restore fertility. Primary care physicians and nephrologists should exert more effort to discuss menstruation and reproductive difficulties with kidney transplant recipients. The transplant team should provide thorough information and counseling to women of reproductive age who are considering pregnancy.

The criteria for kidney transplant recipients who are contemplating about pregnancy are summarized as follows:[29,32]
- At least 6 months following transplant
- Allograft stability and a creatinine level under 1.4 mg/dL
- No current instances of severe rejection
- 140/90 mm Hg or lower blood pressure
- No or little proteinuria, <500 mg/day
- <15 mg of prednisone every day
- <2 mg/kg/day of azathioprine
- 6 weeks before pregnancy, stop taking sirolimus and mycophenolate mofetil

Throughout pregnancy, a multidisciplinary approach by the transplant nephrologist and maternal-fetal medicine is crucial and can provide positive outcomes for mother and child.

■ REFERENCES

1. Murray JE, Reid DE, Harrison JH, Merrill JP. Successful pregnancies after human renal transplantation. N Engl J Med. 1963;269:341-3.
2. Davison JM, Redman CW. Pregnancy post-transplant: the establishment of a UK registry. Br J Obstet Gynaecol. 1997;104(10):1106-7.
3. Rizzoni G, Ehrich JH, Broyer M, Brunner FP, Brynger H, Fassbinder W, et al. Successful pregnancies in women on renal replacement therapy: report from the EDTA Registry. Nephrol Dial Transplant. 1992;7(4):279-87.
4. Coscia LA, Constantinescu S, Moritz MJ, Frank AM, Ramirez CB, Maley WR, et al. Report from the National Transplantation Pregnancy Registry (NTPR): outcomes of pregnancy after transplantation. Clin Transpl. 2010:65-85.
5. Levidiotis V, Chang S, McDonald S. Pregnancy and maternal outcomes among kidney transplant recipients. J Am Soc Nephrol. 2009;20(11):2433-40.
6. Holley JL, Schmidt RJ, Bender FH, Dumler F, Schiff M. Gynecologic and reproductive issues in women on dialysis. Am J Kidney Dis. 1997;29(5):685-90.
7. Weisinger JR, Bellorin-Font E. Outcomes associated with hypogonadism in women with chronic kidney disease. Adv Chronic Kidney Dis. 2004;11(4):361-70.
8. Matuszkiewicz-Rowinska J, Skórzewska K, Radowicki S, Niemczyk S, Sokalski A, Przedlacki J, et al. Endometrial morphology and pituitary-gonadal axis dysfunction in women of reproductive age undergoing chronic haemodialysis: a multicentre study. Nephrol Dial Transplant. 2004;19(8):2074-7.
9. Matuszkiewicz-Rowińska J, Skórzewska K, Radowicki S, Niemczyk S, Przedlacki J, Sokalski A, et al. Menstrual disturbances and alternations in hypophyseal gonadal axis in end-stage premenopausal women undergoing hemodialysis: a multi-center study. Pol Arch Med Wewn. 2003;109(6):609-15.
10. Giatras I, Levy DP, Malone FD, Carlson JA, Jungers P. Pregnancy during dialysis: case report and management guidelines. Nephrol Dial Transplant. 1998;13(12):3266-72.
11. Saha MT, Saha HHT, Niskanen LK, Salmela KT, Pasternack AI. Time course of serum prolactin and sex hormones following successful renal transplantation. Nephron. 2002;92(3):735-7.
12. Guazzelli CAF, Torloni MR, Sanches TF, Barbieri M, Pestana JOMA. Contraceptive counseling and use among 197 female kidney transplant recipients. Transplantation. 2008;86(5):669-72.
13. Davison JM, Dunlop W. Renal hemodynamics and tubular function in normal human pregnancy. Kidney Int. 1980;18(2):152-61.
14. Kim HW, Seok HJ, Kim TH, Han DJ, Yang WS, Park SK. The experience of pregnancy after renal transplantation: pregnancies even within postoperative 1 year may be tolerable. Transplantation. 2008;85(10):1412-9.
15. Davison JM. The effect of pregnancy on kidney function in renal allograft recipients. Kidney Int. 1985;27(1):74-9.
16. Deshpande NA, James NT, Kucirka LM, Boyarsky BJ, Garonzik-Wang JM, Montgomery RA, et al. Pregnancy outcomes in kidney transplant recipients: a systematic review and meta-analysis. Am J Transplant. 2011;11(11):2388-404.
17. Bramham K, Nelson-Piercy C, Gao H, Pierce M, Bush N, Spark P, et al. Pregnancy in renal transplant recipients: a UK national cohort study. Clin J Am Soc Nephrol. 2013;8(2):290-8.

18. Sibanda N, Briggs JD, Davison JM, Johnson RJ, Rudge CJ. Pregnancy after organ transplantation: a report from the UK Transplant pregnancy registry. Transplantation. 2007;83(10):1301-7.
19. Morales JM, Hernandez Poblete G, Andres A, Prieto C, Hernandez E, Rodicio JL. Uric acid handling, pregnancy and cyclosporin in renal transplant women. Nephron. 1990;56(1):97-8.
20. Duley L, Henderson-Smart DJ, Meher S, King JF. Antiplatelet agents for preventing pre-eclampsia and its complications. Cochrane Database Syst Rev. 2007;(2)CD004659.
21. Keitel E, Bruno RM, Duarte M, Santos AF, Bittar AE, Bianco PD, et al. Pregnancy outcome after renal transplantation. Transplant Proc. 2004;36(4):870-1.
22. European best practice guidelines for renal transplantation. Section IV: long-term management of the transplant recipient. IV.10. Pregnancy in renal transplant recipients. Nephrol Dial Transplant. 2002;17(suppl 4):50-5.
23. Stratta P, Canavese C, Giacchino F, Mesiano P, Quaglia M, Rossetti M. Pregnancy in kidney transplantation: satisfactory outcomes and harsh realities. J Nephrol. 2003;16(6):792-806.
24. Armenti VT, McGrory CH, Cater JR, Radomski JS, Moritz MJ. Pregnancy outcomes in female renal transplant recipients. Transplant Proc. 1998;30(5):1732-4.
25. Davidson JM, Lindheimer MD. Maternal-Fetal Medicine: Principles and Practice. Philadelphia, USA: Saunders; 2004.
26. Armenti VT, Moritz MJ, Cardonick EH, Davison JM. Immunosuppression in pregnancy: choices for infant and maternal health. Drugs. 2002;62(16):2361-75.
27. Gibbs RS, Sweet RL, Duff P. Maternal Fetal Medicine: Principles and Practice. Saunders; 2004.
28. del Mar Colon M, Hibbard JU. Obstetric considerations in the management of pregnancy in kidney transplant recipients. Adv Chronic Kidney Dis. 2007;14(2):168-77.
29. McKay DB, Josephson MA, Armenti VT, August P, Coscia LA, Davis CL, et al. Reproduction and transplantation: report on the AST consensus conference on reproductive issues and transplantation. Am J Transplant. 2005;5(7):1592-9.
30. Rose C, Gill J, Zalunardo N, Johnston O, Mehrotra A, Gill JS. Timing of pregnancy after kidney transplantation and risk of allograft failure. Am J Transplant. 2016;16(8):2360-7.
31. Chambers CD, Braddock SR, Briggs GG, Einarson A, Johnson YR, Miller RK, et al. Postmarketing surveillance for human teratogenicity: a model approach. Teratology. 2001;64(5):252-61.
32. Coscia LA, Constantinescu S, Davison JM, Moritz MJ, Armenti VT. Immunosuppressive drugs and fetal outcome. Best Pract Res Clin Obstet Gynaecol. 2014;28(8):1174-87.
33. Venkataramanan R, Koneru B, Wang CCP, Burckart GJ, Caritis SN, Starzl TE. Cyclosporine and its metabolites in mother and baby. Transplantation. 1988;46(3):468-9.
34. Finnell RH. Teratology: general considerations and principles. J Allergy Clin Immunol. 1999;103(2):S337-42.
35. Heeg K, Bendigs S, Wagner H. Cyclosporine A prevents the generation of single positive (Lyt2$^+$ L3T4$^-$, Lyt2$^-$ L3T4$^+$) mature T-cells, but not single positive

(Lyt2⁺ T3⁻) immature thymocytes, in newborn mice. Scand J Immunol. 1989;30(6):703-10.
36. Schen FP, Stallone G, Schena A, Manfredi G, Derosa C, Procino A, et al. Pregnancy in renal transplantation: immunologic evaluation of neonates from mothers with transplanted kidney. Transplant Immunol. 2001;9(2-4):161-4.
37. Stanley CW, Gottlieb R, Zager R, Eisenberg J, Richmond R, Moritz MJ, et al. Developmental well-being in offspring of women receiving cyclosporine post-renal transplant. Transplantat Proc. 1999;31(1-2):241-2.
38. Avramut M, Zeevi A, Achim CL. The immunosuppressant drug FK506 is a potent trophic agent for human fetal neurons. Dev Brain Res. 2001;132(2):151-7.
39. Victor RG, Thomas GD, Marban E, O'Rourke B. Presynaptic modulation of cortical synaptic activity by calcineurin. Proc Natl Acad Sci USA. 1995;92(14):6269-73.
40. Kim H, Jeong JC, Yang J, Yang WS, Ahn C, Han DJ, et al. The optimal therapy of calcineurin inhibitors for pregnancy in kidney transplantation. Clin Transplant. 2015;29(2):142-8.
41. Saarikoski S, Seppälä M. Immunosuppression during pregnancy: transmission of azathioprine and its metabolites from the mother to the fetus. Am J Obstet Gynecol. 1973;115(8):1100-6.
42. Davison JM, Dellagrammatikas H, Parkin JM. Maternal azathioprine therapy and depressed haemopoiesis in the babies of renal allograft patients. Br J Obstet Gynaecol. 1985;92(3):233-9.
43. Beitins IZ, Bayard F, Ances IG, Kowarski A, Migeon CJ. The transplacental passage of prednisone and prednisolone in pregnancy near term. J Pediatr. 1972;81(5):936-45.
44. Chhabria S. Aicardi's syndrome: are corticosteroids teratogens? Arch Neurol. 1981;38:70.
45. Sifontis NM, Coscia LA, Constantinescu S, Lavelanet AF, Moritz MJ, Armenti VT. Pregnancy outcomes in solid organ transplant recipients with exposure to mycophenolate mofetil or sirolimus. Transplantation. 2006;82(12):1698-702.
46. Jones A, Clary MJ, McDermott E, Coscia LA, Constantinescu S, Moritz MJ, et al. Outcomes of pregnancies fathered by solid-organ transplant recipients exposed to mycophenolic acid products. Prog Transplant. 2013;23(2):153-7.
47. McKay DB, Josephson MA. Pregnancy after kidney transplantation. Clin J Am Soc Nephrol. 2008;3(Suppl 2):S117-25.

CHAPTER 5

Challenges in Screening for Thyroid Disorders

Pratik Tambe, B Aruna Suman

■ INTRODUCTION

Thyroid problems impact around 11% of the Indian population, and laboratory tests play a crucial role in the timely identification and subsequent treatment of these conditions. Typical blood tests measure levels of various substances including thyroid-stimulating hormone (TSH), free thyroxine, free tri-iodothyronine, thyroglobulin (Tg), thyroglobulin antibodies (Tg-Ab), thyroid peroxidase antibodies (TPO-Ab), TSH receptor antibodies (TRAb), and calcitonin. Thyroid function tests (TFTs) are frequently requested endocrine tests in both hospital and outpatient settings. TFTs account for over 60% of all endocrine investigations.

The serum TSH and thyroid hormone levels are commonly employed in these examinations. Antibody levels, specifically TPO-Ab, and TRAb are utilized for the diagnosis of Hashimoto's thyroiditis and Graves' disease respectively. Tg, calcitonin, and procalcitonin serve as significant biomarkers for differentiated thyroid cancer and medullary thyroid carcinoma (MTC) respectively. In addition to laboratory examinations, thyroid ultrasonography or radionuclide scans may be necessary for the management of the disease. In 2013, the United States conducted 77 million annual tests to measure TSH and free T4 levels, with a total cost of $1.6 billion.[1]

A fundamental comprehension—understanding the typical functioning of the thyroid gland is crucial when analyzing the test outcomes. It is crucial to be cognizant of the potential drawbacks associated with the utilization of these examinations. When the results are inconsistent, doctors must take into account assay interferences and the impact of concurrent drugs. Thyroid function can appear aberrant even when there is no true malfunction of the thyroid during pregnancy.[2]

■ PHYSIOLOGY OF THE THYROID GLAND

The synthesis of thyroid hormone is regulated by the hypothalamus-pituitary-thyroid axis. The hypothalamus releases thyrotropin-releasing hormone (TRH), which triggers the anterior pituitary gland to secrete TSH. TSH then stimulates the thyroid gland to produce thyroxine (T4) and tri-iodothyronine (T3), with T4 accounting for 85–90% and T3 accounting for 10–15% of the total production. The bioactive form of thyroid hormone, T3, is mostly produced through the peripheral conversion of T4 to T3 by deiodinase enzymes.

The vast majority of T4 and T3 hormones in the bloodstream are strongly attached to carrier proteins, specifically thyroid-binding globulin (TBG), transthyretin, and albumin. Only a minute fraction is in circulation as unbound hormone. The unbound hormone exerts its effects on target tissues throughout the body by attaching to specific receptors located within the nucleus of target cells. A negative feedback loop operates between the hypothalamus and the pituitary gland to regulate the synthesis of thyroid hormones. The release of TSH is highly responsive to even small changes in thyroid hormone levels, as evidenced by a study including >13,000 participants, which showed an inverse log-linear relationship. Aberrant TSH levels are thus linked to early thyroid dysfunction, before the occurrence of genuine problems in thyroid hormone levels. Therefore, TSH levels serve as the most reliable indicator for investigating thyroid disorders.[3]

■ THYROID-STIMULATING HORMONE

Thyroid-stimulating hormone is a glycoprotein composed of two subunits, known as a D-dimer. It consists of an alpha chain that contains 92 amino acids, which is the same as the alpha chain found in human chorionic gonadotrophin (hCG), follicle-stimulating hormone (FSH), and luteinizing hormone (LH). Additionally, it has a distinctive beta subunit consisting of 118 amino acids. Most hormones follow a circadian pattern, with the lowest point occurring in the late afternoon and the highest point between midnight and 4 am.

As previously mentioned, TSH values are strongly advised as the initial screening tests for thyroid dysfunction. Currently, there is widespread usage of highly sensitive third generation immunometric sandwich or noncompetitive assays that can detect TSH levels below 0.01 mIU/L. The identification of obvious hypo- and hyperthyroidism can be easily detected by these tests. Exercise caution when utilizing TSH tests to detect subclinical hypothyroidism and secondary hypothyroidism in hospitalized patients, as this could lead to an inaccurate diagnosis. In these clinical settings, it is advisable to include testing for free thyroid hormones as well. Due to the delayed response of TSH levels to improvements in free thyroid hormone levels, it is advisable to monitor them during the early treatment of thyroid diseases in order to make required adjustments to drug doses.[4]

T3 and T4

Traditionally, the evaluation of thyroid hormone levels encompassed the entirety. Nevertheless, due to the predominant binding of the hormone to carrier proteins like TBG in the peripheral system, situations such as pregnancy and sudden onset sickness that impact TBG levels can lead to aberrant total thyroid hormone levels, even in the absence of genuine thyroid malfunction. Concurrent medicines such as estrogen, tamoxifen, androgens, and glucocorticoids can also modify TBG levels. Currently, the measurement of free thyroid hormone has taken the position of total thyroid hormone testing. FT3 and FT4 levels are measured in picomoles, while TT3 and TT4 levels are assessed in nanomoles. Therefore, precisely measuring FT4 is more challenging.[1]

Free thyroid hormone levels were previously estimated by the resin uptake test, FT4 index, and the T4/TBG ratio a few decades ago. Equilibrium dialysis and ultrafiltration are necessary prior to direct measurements of FT3 and FT4 in order to enhance accuracy. Regrettably, the intricate technical nature and exorbitant expenses associated with these technologies render them suitable solely for research purposes, rather than for implementation in a large-scale screening program.

Competitive immunoassays are the predominant method used for indirect measures in testing. The current utilization of the two-step FT4 assay format is as follows:

The extraction of free thyroid hormone from the serum is performed using particular high-affinity antibodies. The thyroid hormones that are attached to antibodies are placed in a controlled environment with a thyroid hormone probe that has been marked with a label. The number of vacant antibody-binding sites is inversely related to the concentration of unbound thyroid hormone. Due to FT4 levels being 2–3 times greater than FT3 levels, the accuracy of FT4 readings surpasses that of FT3.[5]

Thyroglobulin

Thyroglobulin is a glycoprotein generated in the thyroid follicular cells. It exists as a homodimer with a molecular weight of 660 kilodaltons (kDa). Its clinical use is in its use as a biomarker for differentiated thyroid cancer (DTC) following complete thyroidectomy and radioablation.

The majority of laboratories utilize immunometric assays for the quantification of serum Tg levels. Nevertheless, high Tg-Ab can erroneously result in decreased levels of serum Tg. These can be identified in as many as 25% of survivors of DTC. Therefore, it is advisable to detect both Tg and Tg-Ab in these individuals. Imaging studies such as thyroid ultrasound, I-131 (iodine-131) whole body scan, and positron emission tomography and computed tomography (PET-CT) scan are considered to be more dependable.[6,7]

Thyroglobulin Antibodies

Thyroglobulin antibodies serve as an indicator of autoimmune thyroid conditions and are found to be increased in approximately 10% of the overall population, particularly among women. Nevertheless, when compared to TPO-Ab or TRAb, it lacks the same level of sensitivity and specificity as a thyroid biomarker. The primary clinical application of this is as previously stated in DTC.

Thyroid Peroxidase Antibodies

The presence of TPO-Ab is observed in 5–20% of the overall population and is consistently elevated in individuals with Hashimoto's thyroiditis. It has a significant impact on the therapy of subclinical hypothyroidism. According to the latest guidelines published in 2019 by the Indian Thyroid Society (ITS) and the Federation of Obstetric and Gynaecological Societies of India (FOGSI), patients with subclinical hypothyroidism and high levels of TPO-Ab are advised to undergo levothyroxine treatment. This sentiment is also reiterated by the guidelines set forward by the American Thyroid Association.[8,9]

Thyroid Receptor Antibodies

Thyroid receptor antibodies can be classified into three categories based on their mode of action: stimulating, blocking, or neutral. Two commonly seen types of antibodies are thyroid-stimulating antibodies. These can be quantified using either competitive TSH-binding inhibition (TBI) or thyroid-stimulating immunoglobulin (TSI) assays. TBI lacks the ability to differentiate between the various forms of TRAb. Conversely, TSI tests are capable of identifying only the TRAb that stimulate.

Thyroid receptor antibody is not commonly found in the general population and is only associated with Graves' illness. Therefore, their assessment can be utilized to detect hyperthyroidism that is not caused by Graves' disease, during the treatment of Graves' illness, prediction of thyrotoxicosis in fetuses and newborns, and Graves' ophthalmopathy.[10]

Calcitonin

This is a peptide hormone consisting of 32 amino acids that is synthesized by the parafollicular C cells located in the thyroid gland. The precursor peptides pre-procalcitonin and procalcitonin (PCT, consisting of 116 amino acids) are cleaved to produce the active version of the hormone. The main purpose of calcitonin estimation utility is to serve as a tumor marker for medullary thyroid carcinoma (MTC), as mentioned earlier.

Elevated levels of this substance can also be observed in other illnesses such as autoimmune thyroiditis, hypercalcemia, chronic renal failure, bacterial infections, pregnancy, breastfeeding, and malignancies affecting the lung, breast, pancreas, and leukemia. Elevated levels are attributed to medications such as proton pump inhibitors and glucagon-like peptide-1 agonists. Calcitonin assays have various technical obstacles, including as sample stability, biphasic half-life, and the existence of calcitonin isoforms. Precalcitonin is devoid of such issues and circulates at levels that are 100 times higher, making its measurement more accurate.[11]

CHALLENGES IN THYROID FUNCTION TEST INTERPRETATION

A comprehensive understanding of fundamental thyroid physiology and the various types of available testing is essential for accurately interpreting their results. Additionally, it is important to consider assay interference, concurrent drugs, pregnancy, and non-thyroid disease when interpreting TFT data.

Pregnancy

It is crucial to have a fundamental comprehension of the typical alterations in thyroid function that occurs during pregnancy and the period after giving birth in order to effectively manage patients. Without expertise, it is difficult to interpret TFT during pregnancy. Elevated concentrations of hCG in the early stages of pregnancy, due to the presence of a similar alpha subunit, activate TSH receptors, resulting in a 10–20% expansion of the thyroid gland, a 30% rise in thyroid hormone production, and reduced TSH levels.

Pregnancy, characterized by excessive estrogen levels, results in elevated production of hepatic TBG (thyroxine-binding globulin) and higher overall levels of thyroid hormones. The levels of thyroid hormone typically stabilize at the conclusion of the initial trimester. Simultaneously, the levels of hCG decline, leading to a drop in free thyroid hormone and an increase in TSH. The level of TBG remains elevated till the end of the pregnancy.

Therefore, it is necessary to establish trimester-specific reference ranges for TFTs in order to accurately evaluate thyroid condition during pregnancy. In India, the ITS-FOGSI Guidelines suggest using cut-off ranges of 2.5, 3.0, and 3.0 for the first, second, and third trimesters, respectively, instead of population-specific reference ranges.[8]

Research has shown that when a pregnant woman has an underactive thyroid gland in the early stages of pregnancy, it can lead to negative effects on both the mother's pregnancy experience and the cognitive development of the fetus. Given the ease of diagnosing maternal thyroid dysfunction using trimester-specific ranges and the widespread availability of inexpensive, safe, and successful medication, it is highly advised to conduct universal thyroid screening during pregnancy by measuring serum TSH levels.[12,13]

Postpartum thyroiditis may occur in around 5.4% of women with autoimmune diseases or autoimmune thyroid diseases. The typical progression begins with temporary hyperthyroidism occurring a few months after childbirth, followed by temporary hypothyroidism, and ultimately leading to a restoration of normal thyroid function. Treatment is unnecessary in the majority of situations. Hyperthyroid individuals may necessitate the administration of beta-blockers if they have symptoms, while hypothyroid women may require levothyroxine if they experience symptoms or are breastfeeding.

■ CONCURRENT MEDICATIONS

Medications that are often taken can have an impact on thyroid function in ways that are different from the ones previously mentioned. Dopamine agonists, glucocorticoids, somatostatin analogs, and metformin induce a reduction in the release of TSH by the pituitary gland. Frusemide, salicylates, phenytoin, and heparin all vie for thyroid hormone-binding sites on carrier proteins, particularly at high doses. The administration of lithium and tyrosine kinase inhibitors can result in the development of primary hypothyroidism. In patients at the first stages of treatment or following alterations in medication dosages, as previously mentioned, incongruous outcomes may also arise.

Amiodarone is a pharmaceutical agent that hinders the activity of type 1 deiodinases. The frequent use of it often leads to a slight increase in FT4 levels, a drop in FT3 levels, and an elevation in TSH levels. Although residing in areas with adequate iodine levels, individuals may nevertheless get amiodarone-induced hypothyroidism (AIH). Amiodarone-induced thyrotoxicosis (AIT) is more prevalent than AIH in areas with iodine deficiency.[14]

■ ASSAY INTERFERENCE

Human anti-animal antibodies in the patient's serum can disrupt the detection of TSH. These antibodies have the ability to hinder the binding of TSH to capture or detection antibodies during the measurement process, resulting in inaccurately low TSH levels. False elevation of TSH levels may occur if the antibodies form cross-links with the capture and detection antibodies. Rheumatoid factor also causes assay interferences. There have been reports of auto-antibodies targeting T4, and as a result, most manufacturers now include blocking agents in their assays to prevent these problems.

High-dose biotin might also result in interference. It is frequently present in supplements designed to promote the health of nails and hair. Biotin is frequently used in immunoassay platforms to immobilize antigens (such as TSH and FT4) or antibodies (such as TRAb). Elevated biotin levels in the serum sample can lead to an inaccurately high FT4 result.

In sandwich tests for TSH, the serum sample is subjected to incubation with a TSH-Ab that has been labeled with biotin. Elevated levels of biotin in the sample lead to a diminished or nonexistent signal. This will yield an inaccurately low TSH outcome. The presence of low TSH and high FT4 levels in these people creates a misleading perception of hyperthyroidism. The perplexing influence of biotin is much more pronounced when combined with an erroneously elevated TRAb outcome. Prior knowledge about the use of vitamins and biotin as supplements would greatly aid in understanding these matters.[15]

SCREENING AND INTERPRETATION IN CLINICAL PRACTICE

Given that the symptoms of thyroid illness can be mild and a physical examination may not provide any useful information in the early stages of the disease, it is crucial to prioritize the use of TFTs in patient evaluation. While TSH alone may be adequate for screening the general population, both FT4 and TSH assays are necessary for detecting subclinical hypothyroidism, central hypothyroidism, medication therapy, and hospitalized patients. Additionally, these assays are essential for accurately monitoring the progress of treated patients **(Flowchart 1)**.

SUBCLINICAL THYROID DISEASE

Due to the increased accessibility of precise diagnostic tests, there is currently a growing number of people being diagnosed with subclinical thyroid conditions. Subclinical hyperthyroidism is characterized by a low level of TSH and a normal range of FT4. Treatment should be explored for patients with subclinical hyperthyroidism who are elderly and/or at risk for atrial fibrillation and osteoporosis. Subclinical hypothyroidism is characterized by an increased level of TSH and a normal range of FT4. Initiate levothyroxine treatment if there is an elevation in TPO-Ab levels.

Overt Hypothyroidism

Patients exhibit symptoms of increased body weight, lack of energy, and difficulty passing stool. Primary hypothyroidism TFTs reveal decreased levels of FT4 and increased levels of TSH. Iodine shortage is the primary cause, although in places where iodine levels are sufficient, Hashimoto's thyroiditis is the prevailing cause. It is advisable to conduct TPO-Ab testing in such cases. Additional factors encompass prior cervical surgery, radioiodine therapy, and excessive administration of antithyroid drugs.

Individuals suffering from secondary hypothyroidism will exhibit decreased levels of FT4 and either decreased or abnormally normal levels of TSH. Past medical records may indicate a history of brain or pituitary surgery or radiotherapy. To exclude the possibility of panhypopituitarism, it is necessary to analyze the levels of the remaining anterior pituitary hormones. The pituitary panel should consist of morning measurements of adrenocorticotrophic hormone and cortisol, follicle-stimulating hormone, luteinizing hormone, estradiol, growth hormone, prolactin, and insulin-like growth factor-1.

Challenges in Screening for Thyroid Disorders

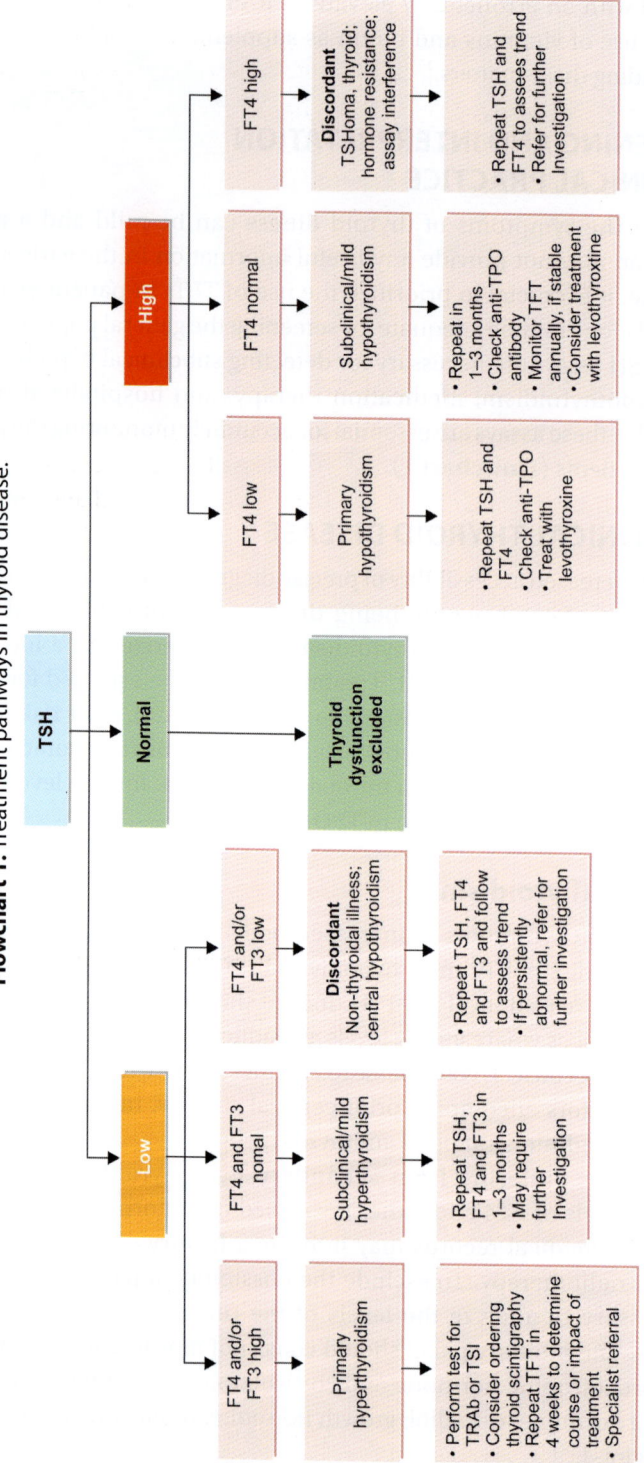

Flowchart 1: Treatment pathways in thyroid disease.

(TFT: thyroid function test; TPO: thyroid peroxidase; TSH: thyroid-stimulating hormone)

Due to the physiological alterations that occur during pregnancy, it is necessary for pregnant women with preexisting hypothyroidism to augment their levothyroxine dosage by 30%. It is important to properly evaluate thyroid function every 4 weeks throughout pregnancy because maternal hypothyroidism is linked to less than optimum obstetric outcomes and impaired fetal neurocognitive development.

Following administration of levothyroxine, there is an improvement in FT4 levels prior to TSH levels. Secondary hypothyroidism is characterized by persistently low or low-normal levels of TSH even after therapy. Therefore, it is necessary to monitor the levels of FT4.[16]

Overt Hyperthyroidism

Patients exhibit symptoms of weight loss, heightened sensitivity to heat, and palpitations. The majority of individuals with thyrotoxicosis experience primary hyperthyroidism, characterized by a high FT4 level and suppressed TSH. The TRAb test is used to definitively diagnose Graves' disease, the most prevalent cause of primary hyperthyroidism. TRAb levels can potentially function as a prognostic indication of remission.

Thyroid receptor antibodies is evaluated in pregnant women with Graves' disease or a previous medical history to determine the likelihood of fetal/neonatal thyrotoxicosis during the later stages of pregnancy. Regular monitoring of FT4 and TSH levels is necessary during the treatment phase. The FT4 often exhibits a more rapid response compared to TSH following treatment. The recovery of TSH may be delayed by many months compared to the recovery of FT4. Therefore, the dosage of medicine should be adjusted based on FT4 levels rather than TSH.[17]

Some patients may experience secondary hyperthyroidism due to a TSH-secreting pituitary adenoma (TSHoma) or resistance to thyroid hormone-β (RTH-β), if they have elevated FT4 levels and raised or inappropriately normal TSH levels. Patients diagnosed with TSHoma should undergo magnetic resonance imaging (MRI) of the pituitary gland to detect the presence of a macroadenoma. These exhibit a favorable response to somatostatin analogs.

Thyroid Nodules and Multinodular Goiter

Patients presenting with a thyroid nodule or a multinodular goiter should have TFTs in order to evaluate the functional status of the thyroid nodule. Typically, hyperfunctioning thyroid nodules are benign. Elevated TSH levels and levels within the upper range of normal are linked to a higher likelihood of developing cancer. For such patients, it is advisable to undergo radionuclide scanning to verify the diagnosis of toxic adenoma or multinodular goiter. Patients who have normal thyroid function or are experiencing an underactive thyroid should be evaluated for a fine-needle aspiration cytology/biopsy (FNAC) in order to exclude the possibility of thyroid cancer.[18]

■ EVIDENCE-BASED RECOMMENDATIONS FOR SCREENING

For the general population, a basic TSH assay is the most effective initial test to exclude the possibility of thyroid malfunction. The sensitivity and specificity of this screening test are optimal and surpass those of FT3 and FT4. FT4 testing is beneficial when the level of TSH is <0.05 mIU/L.[19]

With the aim of alleviating the workload on laboratories and pathology departments and enhancing cost-efficiency, institutions have chosen to provide a TSH assay as the primary test, unless it is deemed necessary to do otherwise. The measurement of FT4 level is limited to cases where the TSH level is abnormal and is used to evaluate the effectiveness of treatment.[20]

During pregnancy, it is advised to conduct universal screening using serum TSH, and the exact cut-off values for each trimester have already been mentioned earlier. It is important to exercise caution when interpreting TFTs, taking into account factors such as pharmacological therapy, other illnesses, concurrent drugs, and potential difficulties with the assays themselves.

The Indian government has implemented a comprehensive screening program for thyroid problems during pregnancy in all public hospitals. A routine TSH assay is conducted during the initial appointment, and additional evaluation is conducted according on the specific clinical circumstances. In rural or primary health centers, this could involve directing the patient to a hospital at the district level or to specialized medical care at a university teaching hospital.

Implementing awareness initiatives targeting primary health center personnel, ASHA workers, and the general public can significantly contribute to the timely detection of thyroid problems during pregnancy. Similarly, it is recommended to conduct TSH screening on the initial appointment in private practice. If abnormal TSH readings are identified, the pregnant lady should be directed to an appropriate endocrinologist to prevent difficulties during pregnancy and childbirth.

■ CONCLUSION

Investigations play a crucial role in identifying and managing thyroid problems. Thyroid screening presents unique difficulties in diagnosing, interpreting, and managing both obvious and subtle cases of underactive and overactive thyroid function, thyroid growths, and the presence of multiple nodules in the thyroid gland. The tests must be interpreted in accordance with clinical findings and are subject to their own limitations. When the results are incongruous, it is necessary to consider potential complications or interference with the assays or the impact of concurrent drugs and interpret the data accordingly. Regular and ongoing communication with a team of healthcare professionals from different fields is crucial for promptly diagnosing and treating patients with thyroid problems.

■ REFERENCES

1. Thienpont LM, Uytfanghe KV, Poppe K, Velkeniers B. Determination of free thyroid hormones. Best Pract Res Clin Endocrinol Metab. 2013;27:689-700.
2. Soh SB, Aw TC. Laboratory testing in thyroid conditions: pitfalls and clinical utility. Ann Lab Med. 2019;39(1):3-14.
3. Rothacker KM, Brown SJ, Hadlow NC, Wardrop R, Walsh JP. Reconciling the log-linear and non-log-linear nature of the TSH-free T4 relationship: intra-individual analysis of a large population. J Clin Endocrinol Metab. 2016;101:1151-8.
4. Li H, Yuan X, Liu L, Zhou J, Li C, Yang P, et al. Clinical evaluation of various thyroid hormones on thyroid function. Int J Endocrinol. 2014;2014:618572.
5. Saw S, Sethi S, Aw TC. Technical evaluation of thyroid assays on the Vitros ECi. Clin Chem. 1999;45:578-80.
6. Haugen BR, Alexander EK, Bible KC, Doherty GM, Mandel SJ, Nikiforov YE, et al. 2015 American Thyroid Association Management Guidelines for adult patients with thyroid nodules and differentiated thyroid cancer: The American Thyroid Association Guidelines Task Force on Thyroid Nodules and Differentiated Thyroid Cancer. Thyroid. 2016;26:1-133.
7. Spencer CA. Clinical review: clinical utility of thyroglobulin antibody (TgAb) measurements for patients with differentiated thyroid cancers (DTC). J Clin Endocrinol Metab. 2011;96:3615-27.
8. Indian Thyroid Society and Federation of Obstetrics and Gynaecological Societies of India (ITS-FOGSI). (2019). Recommendations for the Management of Thyroid Dysfunction in Pregnancy. [online] Available from: www.fogsi.org. [Last accessed December, 2023].
9. Alexander EK, Pearce EN, Brent GA, Brown RS, Chen H, Dosiou C, et al. 2017 Guidelines of the American Thyroid Association for the diagnosis and management of the thyroid disease during pregnancy and postpartum. Thyroid. 2017;27:315-89.
10. Barbesino G, Tomer Y. Clinical review: clinical utility of TSH receptor antibodies. J Clin Endocrinol Metab. 2013;98:2247-55.
11. Trimboli P, Seregni E, Treglia G, Alevizaki M, Giovanella L. Procalcitonin for detecting medullary thyroid carcinoma: a systematic review. Endocr Relat Cancer. 2015;22:R157-64.
12. Vila L, Velasco I, González S, Morales F, Sánchez E, Torrejón S, et al. Controversies in endocrinology: on the need for universal thyroid screening in pregnant women. Eur J Endocrinol. 2014;170:R17-30.
13. Ong GS, Hadlow NC, Brown SJ, Lim EM, Walsh JP. Does the thyroid-stimulating hormone measured concurrently with first trimester biochemical screening tests predict adverse pregnancy outcomes occurring after 20 weeks gestation? J Clin Endocrinol Metab. 2014;99(12):E2668-72.
14. Bogazzi F, Bartalena L, Martino E. Approach to the patient with amiodarone-induced thyrotoxicosis. J Clin Endocrinol Metab. 2010;95:2529-35.

15. Piketty ML, Prie D, Sedel F, Bernard D, Hercend C, Chanson P, et al. High-dose biotin therapy leading to false biochemical endocrine profiles: validation of a simple method to overcome biotin interference. Clin Chem Lab Med. 2017;55:817-25.
16. Soh SB, Topliss DJ. Thyroid dysfunction in pregnancy: optimising obstetric outcomes. Endocrinology Today. 2013;4:8-16.
17. Ross DS, Burch HB, Cooper DS, Greenlee MC, Laurberg P, Maia AL, et al. 2016 American Thyroid Association guidelines for diagnosis and management of hyperthyroidism and other causes of thyrotoxicosis. Thyroid. 2016;26:1343-421.
18. Boelaert K, Horacek J, Holder RL, Watkinson JC, Sheppard MC, Franklyn JA. Serum thyrotropin concentration as a novel predictor of malignancy in thyroid nodules investigated by fine-needle aspiration. J Clin Endocrinol Metab. 2006;91:4295-301.
19. Sheehan MT. Biochemical testing of the thyroid: TSH is the best and, often times, only test needed—a review for primary care. Clin Med Res. 2016;14:83-92.
20. Zhelev Z, Abbott R, Rogers M, Fleming S, Patterson A, Hamilton WT, et al. Effectiveness of interventions to reduce ordering of thyroid function tests: a systematic review. BMJ Open. 2016;6:e010065.

CHAPTER 6: Postpartum Hemorrhage Care Bundles

Madhuri Patel, Pradnya Changede

■ INTRODUCTION

Postpartum hemorrhage (PPH) is one of the major contributors to maternal morbidity and mortality. According to the World Health Organization (WHO), 95% of all maternal deaths occurred in low- and middle-income countries (LMIC) in 2020.[1] Timely diagnosis and treatment can prevent most maternal deaths.

The definition of PPH is mentioned in **Table 1**.[2]

■ INCIDENCE OF POSTPARTUM HEMORRHAGE

The incidence of PPH is 5% of deliveries (when blood loss is not correctly assessed) and 10% when blood loss is correctly assessed.[3]

TABLE 1: Definition of postpartum hemorrhage (PPH).

Name of the organization	Definition
• World Health Organization • French College of Gynecologists and Obstetricians	Blood loss >500 mL, irrespective of route of delivery
• International Federation of Gynecology and Obstetrics • Chinese Ministry of Health and Queensland Health Authority • German Society of Gynecology and Obstetrics	Blood loss of 500 mL or more during vaginal birth or blood loss of 1,000 mL or more during cesarean birth
The American College of Obstetrics and Gynecologists	Cumulative blood loss of at least 1,000 mL of blood or any amount of blood loss accompanied by signs and symptoms of hypovolemia within 24 hours of birth
Royal College of Obstetricians and Gynecologists	• Blood loss of >500 mL irrespective of route of delivery • (Mild PPH blood loss of 500–1,000 mL, major PPH blood loss of >1,000 mL) • Major PPH is subdivided as moderate PPH • Blood loss of 1,001–2,000 mL and severe PPH as blood loss of >2000 mL)

■ CAUSES OF POSTPARTUM HEMORRHAGE

The causes of postpartum hemorrhage are 4 Ts—tone, tissue, trauma, and thrombin.[4]
1. *Tone:* Atonic uterus (80%)
2. *Tissue:* Retained placental bits (tissue)
3. *Trauma:* Genital tract trauma
4. *Thrombin:* Abnormalities of coagulation.

■ NEED FOR POSTPARTUM HEMORRHAGE BUNDLES[5]

Implementation of effective interventions can prevent PPH-related morbidity and deaths. Inconsistent or delay in use of interventions required for effective management of PPH results in increased maternal deaths. The Institute for Healthcare Improvement (IHI) has defined bundle as "a limited set of evidence-based interventions for a defined patient population and care setting, procedure, or treatment." Bundles are a small number of interventions implemented together for a definite patient population and setting of care. These interventions when applied together result in better outcomes as compared to individual implementation of interventions. Bundles are unique as they include limited number (3-5) of interventions. Use of all interventions is a must to measure compliance of bundle implementation.

In 2017, the WHO studied whether current evidenced-based interventions for PPH recommended by the WHO if used as bundle approach increased adherence to PPH guidelines.

■ HOW BUNDLES WERE DEVELOPED

International experts in maternal health were consulted for the process of development of care bundles between October 2017 and December 2017. Three-stage modified Delphi method (including questionnaires and in-person technical consultation) was used. The definition of care bundles and their characteristics were finalized by an expert panel. Types of bundles and included interventions were finalized after systematic literature search.

The interventions considered for inclusion in the PPH bundles were obtained from 2012 and 2017 WHO recommendations for postpartum hemorrhage.[5]

■ NEED TO DEVELOP THREE CARE BUNDLES

The need to develop three care bundles for PPH was noted as follows:[5]
1. Care bundle for prevention and recognition of PPH (rejected later)
2. Care bundle for first response to PPH
3. Care bundle for response to refractory PPH

The care bundle on recognition and prevention of PPH was rejected later and the bundles on first response and refractory PPH were made.
1. *Prevention and recognition of postpartum hemorrhage bundle:* The use of uterotonics, controlled cord traction (CCT) for placenta removal, and assessment of uterine tone was considered for bundle approach for prevention and recognition of PPH. This proposed bundle of interventions had a lot of similarity to the Active Management of the Third Stage of Labor (AMTSL). Expert panel felt that a bundle was *not required to be developed* for PPH prevention. Independent interventions should be carried out for PPH prevention as CCT was recommended only in the presence of skilled birth attendant.
2. *PPH first response bundle:* It consisted of the use of uterotonics, crystalloid intravenous (IV) fluids (isotonic), massage of uterus, and tranexamic acid (TXA).
3. *Response to refractory PPH bundle:* It included maneuvers such as uterine compression (bimanual), aortic compression, intrauterine balloon tamponade (IBT), and nonpneumatic antishock garment (NASG).

The use of IV fluids, uterotonics, and TXA is continued in refractory PPH bundle.

POSTPARTUM HEMORRHAGE CARE BUNDLES (FIG. 1 AND BOX 1)

The *"first response to PPH bundle:"* It comprises of use of uterotonics, crystalloid IV fluids (isotonic fluids), injection of TXA, and use of uterine massage.

"MOTIV8" or "MOTIVate" is the acronym used for usage of massage, oxytocics (uterotonic agents), TXA, and IV fluids.

Fluid resuscitation is started initially along with IV uterotonics such as oxytocin. If IV uterotonics are unavailable, initial fluid resuscitation is done in addition to use of misoprostol (sublingual route) or other uterotonics (parenteral administration). If placenta is retained, it should be extracted. Antibiotics (single dose recommended) should be used in case of retained placenta.

Isotonic Crystalloids

It is recommended to administer 500 mL of isotonic crystalloids intravenously in 30 minutes to prevent hypotension. In the continuation phase, 500 mL of isotonic crystalloids is administered for a time duration of 60 minutes.

Uterotonics

- *Oxytocin:* It is the gold standard drug for PPH prevention and treatment. It is administered routinely for active management of third stage of labor.

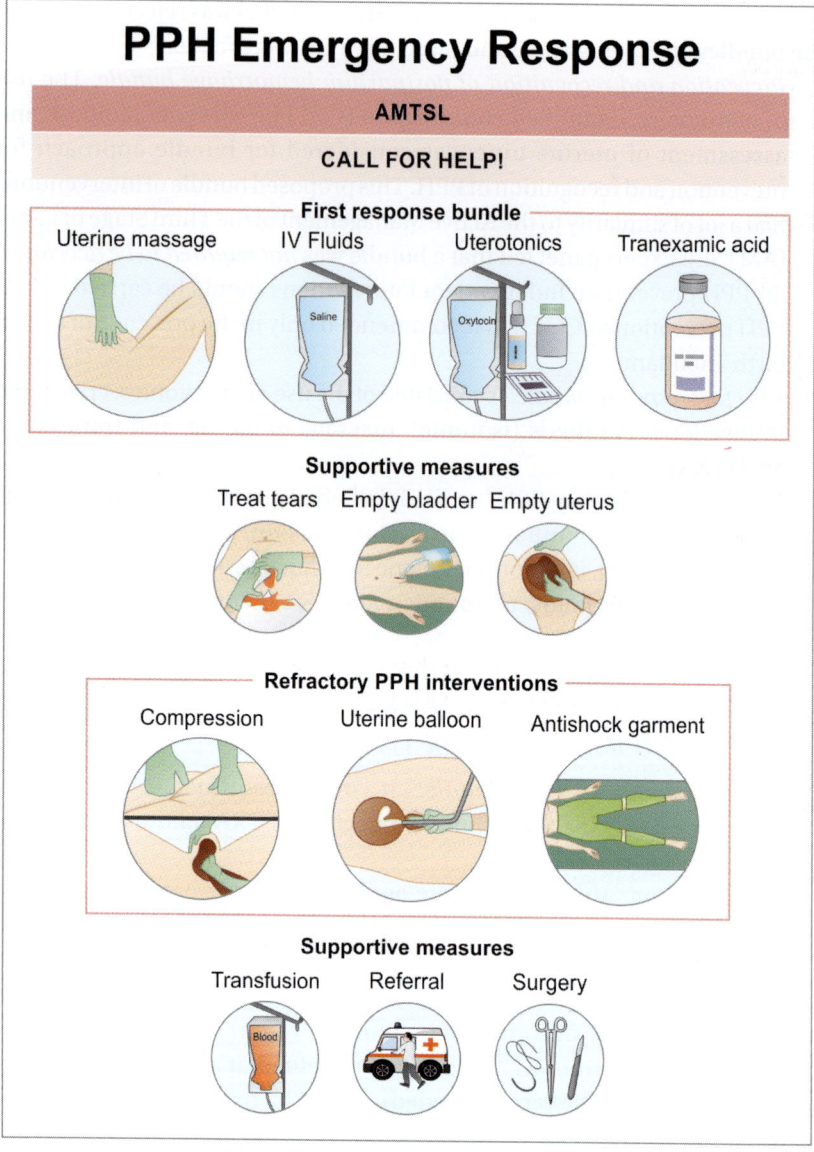

Fig. 1: PPH bundles.[10] (AMTSL: Active management of the third stage of labor; IV: intravenous; PPH: postpartum hemorrhage)

The WHO recommends use of 10 international units (IU) of oxytocin IV or intramuscular (IM) for PPH prevention. Use of oxytocin is recommended for all births (vaginal as well as cesarean deliveries). IV oxytocin is recommended for the treatment of PPH.

For treatment, parenteral route (intravenous route preferred or intramuscular) or intravenous (infusion)

> **BOX 1:** PPH care bundles.[5]
>
> *Care bundle for first response to PPH includes:*
> - Use of uterotonic drugs
> - Resuscitation with intravenous isotonic crystalloids
> - Administration of tranexamic acid
> - Massage of uterus
>
> *Care bundle for response to refractory PPH includes:*
> - Use of compression such as aortic compression or bimanual uterine compression
> - Use of IBT
> - Use of NASG
>
> (IBT: intrauterine balloon tamponade; NASG: nonpneumatic antishock garment; PPH: postpartum hemorrhage)

The drug is administered by:
- Initial dose: 20 U in 500 mL normal saline (NS) over 1 hour (can be increased to 40 units)
- Maintenance dose: 2.5 units per hour
  (20 U in 1 liter NS over 8 hours solution 125 mL per hour)
  The WHO recommends use of carbetocin in *PPH prevention* when:
    - Its cost is comparable to other uterotonics
    - Unavailability of oxytocin
    - No guarantee of quality of oxytocin.

Other uterotonics such as ergometrine, fixed-dose combination of oxytocin, and ergometrine or misoprostol 800 microgram (sublingual) are recommended when oxytocin is unavailable or if bleeding persists despite use of oxytocin[6,7] **(Table 2)**.

- *Uterine massage:* It is done manually per abdomen by circular motion along the fundus of uterus. Massage is continued till uterus contracts.
- *TXA:* In 2009, the WOMAN [World WOMAN (World Maternal Antifibrinolytic)] trial was launched.[8] It was a double-blind, randomized, placebo-controlled, multicenter trial conducted to study the effect of TXA. 1 g of TXA IV was administered within 3 hours of the time of delivery. If bleeding persisted, second dose of 1 g was repeated 30 minutes after the first dose. It was noted that deaths due to PPH reduced significantly with use of TXA. The rate of thromboembolic events or complications was not increased. Decreased mortality due to PPH was noted when TXA was administered within 3 hours of childbirth. Such reduction in deaths due to bleeding was not noted when TXA was given after a duration of 3 hours.

Refractory hemorrhage is defined as bleeding that does not respond to first-response measures and results in worsening of maternal condition.
- The "*response to refractory PPH bundle*" comprises compressive measures such as use of aortic compression or bimanual uterine compression, use of the NASG, and IBT.

TABLE 2: Comparison of various uterotonic drugs.[6,7,9]

	Oxytocin	Carbetocin	Misoprostol	Ergometrine	Carboprost
Dose	• Prevention of PPH 10 IU IM or IV • Treatment 40 units IV	• Only for prevention 100 μg • IM or IV (Single dose)	• Prevention 600 μg PO • Treatment 800 μg	• 0.2 mg IM • Fixed dose 5 U oxytocin with 0.5 U ergometrine	250 μg every 15 minutes (maximum 8 doses 2 mg)
Onset of action	• IV within 1 minute • IM route within 3–7 minutes	• IV within 2 minutes • IM within 11 minutes	• Within 10–15 minutes • Oral, sublingual rapid onset	Within 2–5 minutes	• IM 15–60 minutes • Can be given intramyometrial
Duration of action	• IV up to 3–5 minutes • Peak after 30 minutes • IM effect lasts longer for more than 1 hour	• IV 60 minutes • IM 120 minutes • (4–10 times longer than oxytocin)	• Rectal route • Prolonged duration • Oral peak 30 minutes • Vaginal 70–80 minutes	3 hours	• Peak after 20 minutes in IM • Declines slowly
Half-life	1–6 minutes	40 minutes	20–40 minutes	30–120 minutes	3 hours
Side effects	Uterine hyperstimulation, flushing, antidiuretic, hypotension	• Flushing • Hypotension • Caution in epilepsy, asthma, and hypertension	Shivering, fever	• Nausea • Vomiting, rise in BP • C/I hypertension and preeclampsia and heart disease	• GI side effects, bronchospasm, C/I asthma, active cardiac, renal, and hepatic disease, acute PID

(BP: blood pressure; GI: gastrointestinal; IM: intramuscular; IV: intravenous; PID: pelvic inflammatory disease; PPH: postpartum hemorrhage)

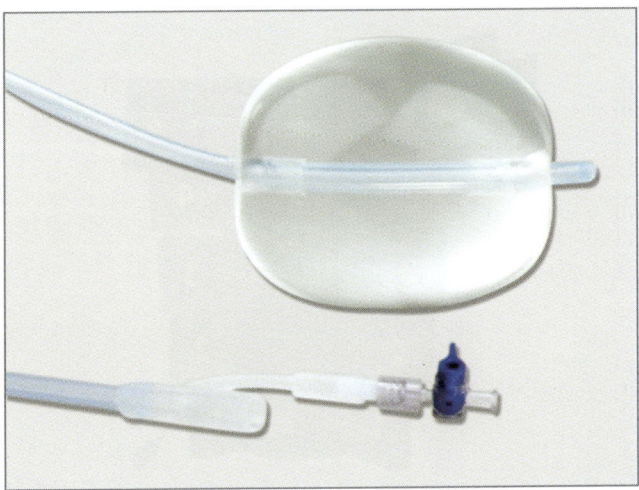

Fig. 2: Intrauterine balloon tamponade (IBT) using Bakri balloon.[11]

Use of uterotonics such as oxytocin and TXA (second dose) should be continued while using this bundle.

- *External aortic compression:* A closed fist is used to give pressure on abdominal aorta by applying external pressure on abdomen at the level of the umbilicus (slightly to the woman's left) to reduce vaginal bleeding.
- *IBT:* Uterine balloon tamponade is recommended by FIGO (International Federation of Gynecology and Obstetrics) in cases of refractory PPH. It is an effective nonsurgical technique which can help treat PPH.
  Types—Shivkar's pack, Bakri balloon **(Fig. 2)**, Ellavi balloon
- *Nonpneumatic antishock garment (NASG):* The WHO recommends NASG as a temporary measure to stop bleeding until appropriate care is available. It is a compression device made of stretch neoprene. It comprises six fastener segments which can close tightly with velcro **(Fig. 3)**. Hook-and-loop segments are applied rapidly, starting at the ankles. Counterpressure is provided by lower body, which improves cardiac output and blood pressure. It is recommended for transfer of patient to the tertiary center.
  IBT or NASG may not be available in some settings.

■ PANEL RECOMMENDATIONS[5]
- Interventions such as uterotonics, crystalloids, and TXA, which are elements of first response bundle should not be included in refractory bundle.

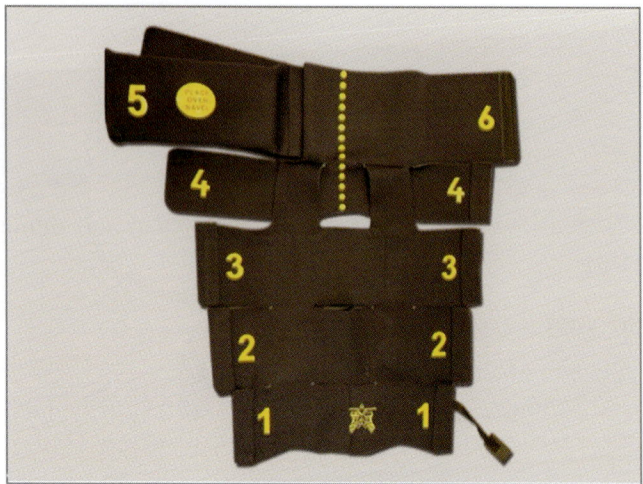

Fig. 3: Nonpneumatic antishock garment (NASG).[12]
Source: UNICEF. Nonpneumatic antishock garment (NASG). [online] Available from: https://www.unicef.org/innovation/non-pneumatic-anti-shock-garment-nasg [Last accessed December, 2023].

- The WHO would reconsider all these interventions for inclusion in future WHO recommendations.

The panel acknowledges that the full bundle comprising maneuvers such as aortic compression or bimanual uterine compression and use of devices such as IBT and NASG may not be used by healthcare providers if some of these interventions have controlled bleeding. However, interventions were included in a bundle because care bundle approach has been recommended by the WHO as it improves compliance of strategies.

Supporting elements of PPH care bundles are training, teamwork, advocacy, communication, and use of best clinical practices.

■ LIMITATIONS[5]

- A modified approach may be required for postcesarean bleeding.
  - Uterine massage may be less effective for women undergoing cesarean section as compared to those undergoing vaginal birth.
  - IV fluids and uterotonics have been used during cesarean section; thus, these two components of the first response bundle (IV fluids and uterotonics) are of limited use.
- Restricted definition of refractory PPH may generate difficulty for clinicians to diagnose PPH in women whose condition was stable initially.
- Bundle approach may be of limited clinical use if large number of women such as those with PPH refractory to standard treatment are ineligible for bundle application.

- There is potential to "overtreat" some women if all interventions are used.
- If PPH responds to one measure, all interventions in the bundle may not be used.
- Single healthcare worker may find it difficult to perform all the interventions mentioned in bundle.
- Variable clinical presentation may require a more tailor-made, individualized approach rather than the approach of care bundle.
- Implementation strategy is yet to be developed for bundles.

■ ADVANTAGES OF CARE BUNDLES[5]

- When adherence is high, improved patient outcomes are associated with use of care bundles.
- The concept of care bundles ensures standardized and expedited treatment.
- Care bundles helpcare providers remember the sequence of packaged effective interventions.
- Compliance of bundle is achieved only after completing and recording all bundled interventions.
- Compliance for the whole bundle implies higher compliance rate for its individual elements.
- Importance of qualities such as teamwork, good communication, and cooperation are emphasized.
- Quality and sustainability are assured.
- Adherence to PPH guidelines is ensured with the use of bundle approach.

In addition to the abovementioned PPH care bundle, an obstetric hemorrhage safety bundle was developed in the United States by a workgroup of the Partnership for Maternal Safety Council on Patient Safety in Women's Health Care.[13] Partnership of professional organizations was developed so that this safety bundle is adopted by all birthing facilities in the United States. This bundle has four domains:

1. *Readiness domain—every unit:*
    - Hemorrhage cart
    - Hemorrhage medication accessible immediately
    - A response team should be established.
    - Massive transfusion protocols for immediate release of blood products
    - Drills for units
2. *Recognition and Prevention domain—every patient:*
    - Risk of hemorrhage should be assessed at all times
    - Cumulative blood loss should be measured.
    - Protocol for active management of the third stage of labor
3. *Response domain—every hemorrhage:*
    - Emergency plan for obstetric hemorrhage
    - Support program

4. *Domain of reporting and systems learning—every unit:*
   - A culture of huddles for at-risk patients; debriefs after event to identify gaps
   - Serious hemorrhages should undergo multidisciplinary review
   - Outcomes to be monitored in perinatal quality improvement committee.

■ CONCLUSION

Postpartum hemorrhage care bundles have been suggested for use to reduce morbidity and mortality due to PPH. With the use of these bundles, improved quality of care for patients has been ensured due to adherence to evidence-based guidelines. Implementation of these PPH care bundles in practice is a topic for further research. Thorough research will determine the effectiveness of bundle care approach to prevent maternal deaths due to PPH. These PPH bundles should be continuously assessed (living bundles) as new evidence emerges from the WHO recommendations and guidelines.

■ REFERENCES

1. World Health Organization. Maternal health. [online] Available from: https://www.who.int/health-topics/maternal-health#tab=tab_1 [Last accessed December, 2023].
2. Belfort MA. (2023). Overview of postpartum hemorrhage. [online] Available from: https://www.uptodate.com/contents/overview-of-postpartum-hemorrhage [Last accessed December, 2023].
3. ACOG Committee Opinion. (2019). Quantitative Blood Loss in Obstetric Hemorrhage. [online] Available from: https://www.acog.org/clinical/clinical-guidance/committee-opinion/articles/2019/12/quantitative-blood-loss-in-obstetric-hemorrhage# [Last accessed December, 2023].
4. Anderson JM, Etches D. Prevention and Management of Postpartum Hemorrhage. Am Fam Physician. 2007;75(6):875-82.
5. Althabe F, Therrien MNS, Pingray V, Hermida J, Gülmezoglu AM, Armbruster D, et al. Postpartum hemorrhage care bundles to improve adherence to guidelines: A WHO technical consultation. Int J Gynaecol Obstet. 2020;148(3):290-9.
6. World Health Organization. WHO recommendations: Uterotonics for the prevention of postpartum haemorrhage. [online] Available from: https://apps.who.int/iris/bitstream/handle/10665/277276/9789241550420-eng.pdf [Last accessed December, 2023].
7. World Health Organization. WHO recommendations for the prevention and treatment of postpartum haemorrhage. [online] Available from: https://apps.who.int/iris/bitstream/handle/10665/75411/9789241548502_eng.pdf [Last accessed December, 2023].
8. Picetti R, Miller L, Shakur-Still H, Pepple T, Beaumont D, Balogun E, et al. The WOMAN trial: clinical and contextual factors surrounding the deaths of 483 women following post-partum haemorrhage in developing countries. BMC Pregnancy Childbirth. 2020;20(1):409.

9. Escobar MF, Nassar AH, Theron G, Barnea ER, Nicholson W, Ramasauskaite D, et al. FIGO recommendations on the management of postpartum hemorrhage 2022. Int J Gynecol Obstet. 2022;157(Suppl 1):3-50.
10. FIGO. PPH Emergency Care Using a Bundle Approach (PPH EmC). [online] Available from: https://www.jhpiego.org/wp-content/uploads/2020/07/MGH-PPH-EmC-Executive-Summary_July-2020.pdf [Last accessed December, 2023].
11. Cook Medical. Bakri® Postpartum Balloon with Rapid Instillation Components. [online] Available from: https://www.cookmedical.com/products/wh_sosr_webds/ [Last accessed December, 2023].
12. UNICEF. Nonpneumatic antishock garment (NASG). [online] Available from: https://www.unicef.org/innovation/non-pneumatic-anti-shock-garment-nasg [Last accessed December, 2023].
13. Main EK, Goffman D, Scavone BM, Low LK, Bingham D, Fontaine PL, et al. National Partnership for Maternal Safety: Consensus Bundle on Obstetric Hemorrhage. J Midwifery Womens Health. 2015;60(4):458-64.

CHAPTER 7

Importance of Obstetric Skill Drills

Priti Kumar, Niranjana Asokan

■ INTRODUCTION

Obstetrics is a field where emergencies can occur unanticipated. An uncomplicated low-risk pregnancy can develop cord prolapse during delivery and create complete chaos in the labor room. There are times when we can anticipate obstetric emergencies and times when they occur all of a sudden. Traditional methods such as incident reporting and analysis have been useful, but they are correct deficiencies after it has occurred. There is a need for methods for better training that will prevent the deficiency from occurring. Skill drills are very useful in that aspect as they are proactive and reduce risk in handling obstetric emergencies.

■ WHAT IS AN OBSTETRIC SKILL DRILL?

Obstetric skill drill is a method where one can practice managing obstetric emergency in a mock scenario. The team experiences duplication of real-life scenario that allows them to practice, learn, evaluate, and understand the management. In a skill drill, there is no real emergency. Hence, mistakes can be corrected without harm to patient. It allows the team to build skills and obtain knowledge in managing the emergency situation. Drills are a follow-up for training. During the theory sessions, personnel are educated on the skill. When performing the drill, they understand and incorporate that skill. Skill drills allow us to have an effective response to the emergency.

■ PURPOSE

Skill drills are a means of quality improvement in obstetrics department. Running a skill drill allows us to teach the obstetric team as well as evaluate, correct, and improve the management protocol. Frequent skill drills can improve the knowledge, teamwork, and communication methods among doctors, nurses, and other allied staff in handling an emergency.

As opposed to routine procedures, obstetric emergencies are infrequent but fatal when they do occur. Without regular skill drills, any amount of theoretical knowledge on the subject will be lost and handling the situation becomes chaotic. Skill drills remove the anxiety and uncertainty associated with the condition and avoid unnecessary confusion or mismanagement. This ensures better quality of care at the time of obstetric emergencies.

Simulation helps the team to be comfortable in handling unpredictable obstetric emergencies. It provides confidence to the team and helps to analyze team dynamics. It is a mode of training that is very effective. It also allows us to assess team readiness and analyze hospital protocols.

Obstetric skill drills are recommended by the Joint Commission to reduce maternal deaths in hospitals and "to train staff in the protocols, to refine local protocols, and to identify and fix systems problems that would prevent optimal care."[1]

■ METHODOLOGY

To conduct any skill drill, it is important to first define the emergency, describe the procedure, and identify the tools needed to address the situation. It is preferable to conduct drills in small groups for better understanding. When starting the drill, senior clinician should debrief the group regarding the standard protocol based on evidence-based guidelines. There should be another person enacting the role of patient encountering the emergency. The team participating in the drill should include all cadres such as doctors, nurses, and midwives.

The skill drill can be done as part of training using mannequins to demonstrate important maneuvers. Workshops organized with senior clinicians demonstrating the management protocol and allowing the juniors and other members of team to mimic maneuvers such as assisted breech delivery and instrumental delivery can help in passing on these vital procedures.

While performing any drill, the necessary equipment, protocol, preparation, and drill actions need to be formulated. The team involved should be intimated and there should be a senior monitoring the responses and correcting it as required. A checklist can be formed to help the team understand the protocol and further drills with other groups to help identify various deficiencies. A thorough analysis of the drill should be done, and corrective measures implemented with follow-up drills should ensure better understanding among the team.

The most important part of any drill is communicating the results to the team and pointing out the errors. This allows them to correct the mistake and have better memory of the situation rather than teaching them the theoretical aspect alone. At times, the drills can be recorded, and team can be allowed to review their video, identify their own mistakes, and allowed a post-training survey. This allows self-learning and better comprehension of the corrective measures needed.

Every member should know that drill is not to test individual skills, rather it tests the entire process, identifies gaps, and improves teamwork and communication.

■ FREQUENCY

The frequency of drills should be decided based on need. It can be as frequent as weekly or twice in a year depending on the problem addressed. In the first drill, the problems need to be identified and plans for improvement should be made. The following drills are to assess the efficacy of the corrective measures and ongoing assessment. It is important to continue the drills even after thorough understanding of the situation to ensure familiarity.

It is not necessary to perform skill drills only in hospital setting. These drills at primary healthcare (PHC) and other centers involving village health nurse (VHN) can help to identify a situation before it escalates into emergency and activate prompt referral services. For example, a drill of imminent eclampsia can help the midwife identify the warning signs, stress the importance of recording blood pressure (BP), and start the patient on oral nifedipine tablets and refer her to a higher center before she can develop into eclampsia, which results in maternal and neonatal mortality and morbidity. Using pictorial charts as in **Figures 1 and 2** and **Flowcharts 1 and 2** as ready reckoners pasted in the room can further stress the signs to look out for. Valarezo et al. found that training required four phases: (1) Exploration—form groups to address scenarios, (2) Planning—with reflective sessions and using flowcharts, (3) Action—training and forming protocols, and (4) Evaluation—assessing the improvement status. With this assessment, they found that skill drills brought about 90% improvement in levels of care.[2]

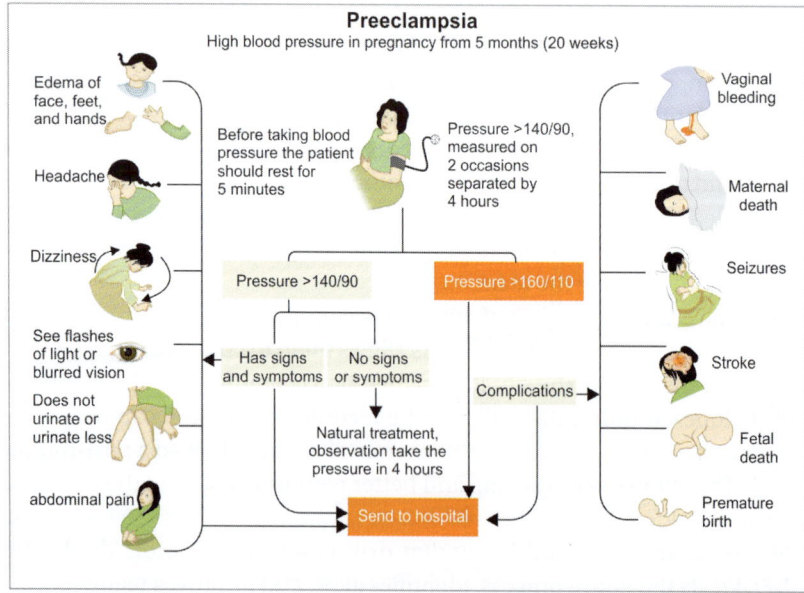

Fig. 1: Preeclampsia monitoring.

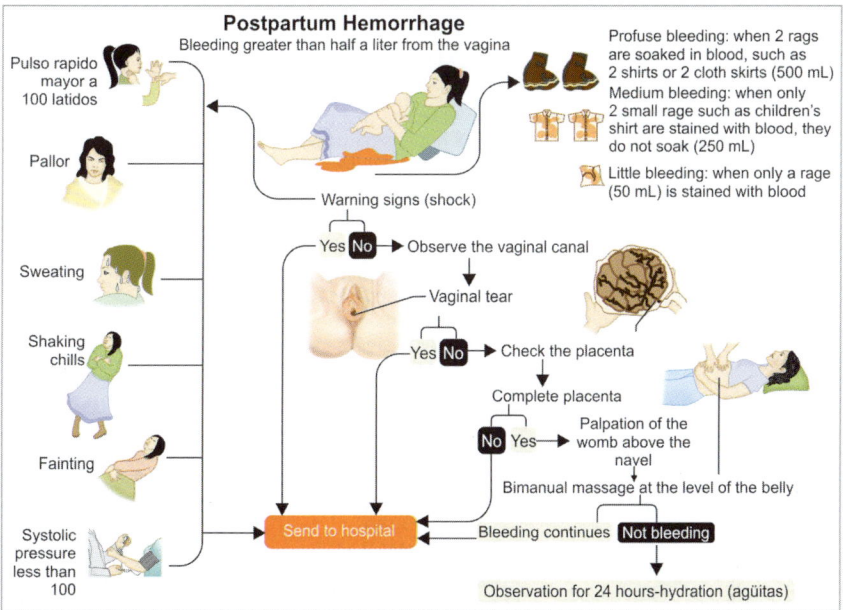

Fig. 2: Postpartum hemorrhage (PPH) management.

■ ADVANTAGES

There are many advantages in conducting regular skill drills, which are given as follows:
- The World Health Organization (WHO) and other studies have identified drills to be highly cost-effective.[4,5] Rather than setting up a specialized skill laboratory with multiple mannequins and costly equipment, skill drills are inexpensive and can be conducted at any place and simulate handling of real-time emergencies.
- It helps to identify areas of improvement and enables better quality of care.
- The team is well oriented and coordinated. They function as a unit rather than individually.
- Better preparedness for handling emergencies
- Handling the mock scenario—creates better memory and better organization of the team
- Improves teamwork
- Allows the team to practice and learn without any risk to patients
- Helps to improve infrastructure of facility to handle emergencies
- Can involve anybody ranging from final year undergraduate to super specialist and train their roles easily
- Can be a mode of teaching for undergraduate students
- Significantly reduces cost from medical liability

Flowchart 1: Eclampsia management algorithm.[3]

```
                          Eclampsia
                             ↓
```

New, otherwise unexplained, seizures in a pregnant lady
- Typically 3rd trimester up to 48 hours after delivery
- Consider other causes, e.g., blood sugar levels
- Confirmed if hypertensive and heavy proteinuria (catheterize and check)

Eclampsia Box in Resus Cupboard

ED management
Call obstetrics, Pediatrics and Anesthetics
(baby will need delivered)
Turn on to left side to avoid aortocaval compression
Support airway and deliver high flow oxygen
IV access + bloods (FBC, U&E, LFTs, COAG)
Catheterize

MAGNESIUM

Loading
4g IV bolus over 5 minutes
8 mL of 50% Mg^{2+} (4 g) mixed with 12 mL of saline (total 20 mL), then

Infusion
1 g per hour IV
20 mL of 50% Mg^{2+} (10 g) mixed with 30 mL of saline (total 50 mL)
Infuse at 5 mL/h

Recurrent Seizures on Infusion
2 g IV bolus over 5 minutes
4 mL of 50% Mg^{2+} (2 g) mixed with 6 mL of saline (total 10 mL)

BP control
Sys >150,
Dia >110, MAP >125

Loading
Labetalol 50 mg
IV over 5 min
(Can be repeated ×1), then

Infusion
Labetalol
50 mg/hr
Draw 40 mL of Labetalol (200 mg) undiluted and infuse in syringe driver (10 mL/h)
Can increase every 15 min (max 200 mg/hr) until BP controlled

Second line
Hydralazine 5 mg IV bolus
Hydralazine infusion (10 mg/hr)

Fluids
High risk for pulmonary edema

Fluid restrict
1 mL/kg/hr (max 85 mL/hr) inclusive of infusions

Urine output
Aim for around 25 mL/hr

3rd stage
AVOID Ergometrine/Syntometrine

Can give Syntocinon 10 IU IM/IV

Paralyse and ventilate if fits are prolonged or recurrent

(BP: blood pressure; ED: emergency department; FBC: full blood count; IV: intravenous; LFT: liver function test; U&E: urea and electrolyte)

- Decrease in maternal mortality and morbidity as well as neonatal mortality and morbidity

■ PLANNING

It is important to plan a skill drill involving all allied departments such as nursing, anesthesiology, neonatology, blood bank, and junior doctors. The department head proposes the skill drill after elaborating on pros and

Flowchart 2: Postpartum hemorrhage (PPH) algorithm.[3]

Postpartum hemorrhage
1° Postpartum hemorrhage >500 mL of blood in first 24 hours postdelivery *Tone (very common):* Uterine atony +/− distended bladder *Tissue (common):* Retained placenta or clots *Trauma (sometimes):* Lacerations of uterus, cervix or vagina *Thrombin (rate):* Pre-exisiting or acquired coagulopathy
ED management Call for help ABC resusctation Large bore IV access ×2 Blood + group and cross-match Low threshold for major hemorrhage protocol Fluid/blood product resuscitation Examine placenta for missing parts
Abdominal massage To stimulate contraction
Medications **Oxytocin** (Syntocinon) 10 IU slow IV Onset by 2 minutes and peak effect by 5 minutes Feel for uterine change when massaging and/or reduced PV blooding There is less duration of action if retained placental part and/or **Ergometrine** 0.5 mg IM (both uterotonics kept in fridge in resus) **Tranexamic acid** 1–2 g/hourly IV if above failed or thought due to trauma
Ensure bladder is empty Catheterize
Temporizing measures if drugs fail or not avaliable **Internal bimanual compression** Insert gloved fist into vagina and push up against uterus Press other hand on uterine fundus and compress between hands Maintain for at least 8–10 minutes **External aortic compression** Push hard with fist onto abdominal aorta (upper ado + left of midline) Successful compression is when femoral pulses no longer palpable

(ED: emergency department; IV: intravenous; PV: per vaginum)

cons and stressing that drills ensure patient safety. The need for planning is because skill drills are far better than slide teaching and allows learning in a no-consequence environment—the actions of team do not implicate any negative outcome for the hospital or patient.

Proper briefing is necessary to engage the team and a drill without team involvement is never complete. There should be a proper explanation on why the drill is needed, how it is going to be done, and what is going to be the evaluation.

The team should comprise a lead clinician, senior nurse, nursing team in charge, pharmacy, laboratory personnel, and other associated specialties. It can be done on the set date to allow the team to prepare themselves. Planned drills work better as there is no anxiety and team itself can review its actions. The drill can be repeated depending on the number of participants and follow-up frequency should also be determined. In case of large numbers, the teams can alternate performing the drill and debriefing. Every member of the team should be aware of his/her roles and responsibilities. Swapping the participants at the next quarterly drill allows training large numbers.

When debriefing, state learning objectives, review assumptions, understand how the drill went, and identify and stress takeaways while noting points for change. They should forward the main changes to administration. Also, the lead clinician should end the drill on a positive note by recognizing the correct protocol followed and build rapport among the team. The person debriefing should not be performing in the drill as he/she needs to evaluate the drill as a whole to identify mistakes.

Equipment should be available. If medicines are needed, they should be used without opening to avoid wastage. Drills are conducted to allow training, assess clinical performance, and perform research work. Some drills can be performed without long notice to ensure preparedness.

■ OBSTETRIC EMERGENCIES

Of the various obstetric emergencies, postpartum hemorrhage and eclampsia are the leading causes of maternal mortality. Skill drills can help the team to understand their role perfectly and perform appropriate actions. Birch et al. analyzed postpartum hemorrhage management among hospital staff and found that simulation-based training showed sustained improvement over long-term, better confidence, and communication skills over lecture-based teaching.[6] Lutgendorf et al., found that there was more comfort after skill drills rather than training alone. In handling hypertensive emergencies, it was 4.14 after skill drill versus 3.88 before skill drill; shoulder dystocia 4.29 versus 3.66, postpartum hemorrhage 4.35 versus 3.86 with less time needed to arrange required medicines and blood products after skill drills.[7]

■ OTHERS

Skill laboratories can be performed to teach various necessary but infrequently performed obstetric procedures such as instrumental delivery, assisted breech delivery, normal vaginal delivery, and neonatal resuscitation as in **Flowchart 3** and **Figures 3 and 4**. Performing drills gives the confidence

Importance of Obstetric Skill Drills

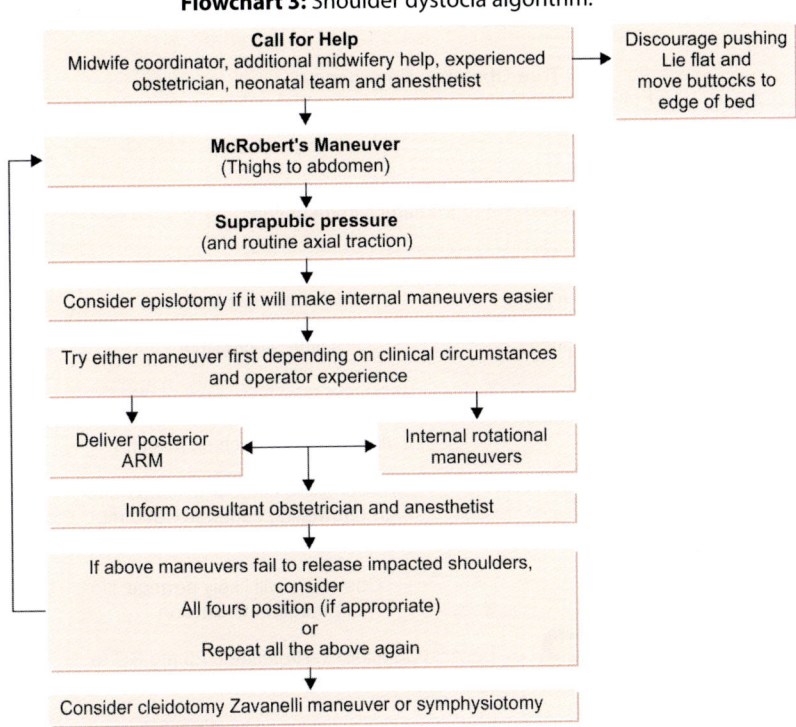

Flowchart 3: Shoulder dystocia algorithm.[9]

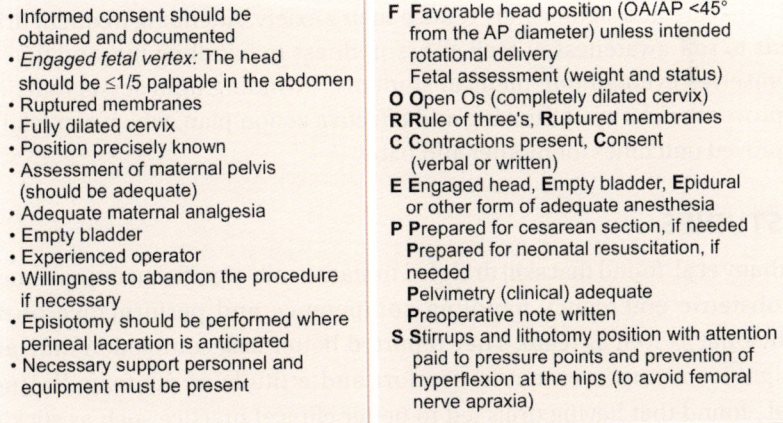

Fig. 3: Instrumental delivery algorithm.[10] (AP: anteroposterior; OA: occipital anterior)

to the attending clinician to proceed with the intervention when required. It allows reflective learning that improves confidence and decreases stress. The competence gained from repeated drills allows personnel to provide

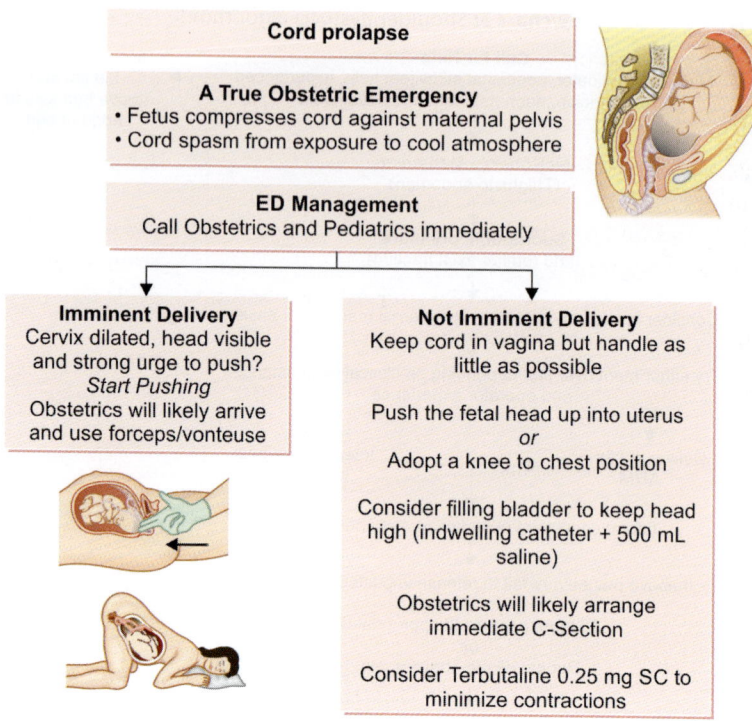

Fig. 4: Cord prolapse algorithm.[3] (C-section: cesarean section; ED: emergency department; SC: subcutaneous)

efficient care and significantly reduce their anxiety. Attending frequent drills leads to self-awareness as well as assuredness in handling the situation by themselves even among medical students.[8] Avoiding unnecessary anxiety improves the clarity of thinking and effective action plan, which can lead to improved outcomes for mother and baby.

■ STUDIES

Bethany et al. found that skill drills led to statistically significant improvement in obstetric emergency handling competence and performance of the individual as well as team. They reported better task completion time and insignificant improvement in comfort and attitude of the team.[11] Ameh et al., found that having drills led to better clinical practice such as sticking to protocols, proper resuscitation technique, better teamwork, and also improved outcomes such as less trauma for shoulder dystocia babies and lesser babies with hypothermia or hypoxia.[12] Cochrane review has shown that skill drills and simulation-based learning can improve team performance in terms of maternal and neonatal outcomes over no training such as reduced maternal and neonatal mortality and decreased birth trauma on analyzing with Kirkpatrick model for behavioral change and patient outcome.[13]

CONCLUSION

Obstetric emergencies are inevitable and the best way of risk management is training staff to handle the emergencies appropriately. Regular skill drills help to build better obstetricians who are well prepared to handle the emergency situation in a correct way. It builds better teams and improves communication and a chance of better performance. Skill drills are the best option to ensure safe practice in low-volume high-stake situations.

REFERENCES

1. The Joint Commission. (2010). Preventing maternal death. Sentinel Event Alert Issue 44. [online] Available from: https://jointcommission.org/assets/1/18/sea_44.pdf [Last accessed December, 2023].
2. Bautista-Valarezo E, Espinosa ME, Michels NRM, Hendrickx K, Verhoeven V. Culturally adapted flowcharts in obstetric emergencies: a participatory action study. BMC Pregnancy Childbirth. 2022;22(1);772.
3. St Mungo's. Skills & Drills. [online] Available from: https://stmungos-ed.com/skillsdrills [Last accessed December, 2023].
4. Ayres-de-Campos, D, Deering S, Siassakos D. Sustaining simulation training programmes—experience from maternity care. BJOG. 2011;118(Suppl 3):22-6.
5. WHO. Recommendations for Prevention and Treatment of PPH. Geneva: World Health Organization; 2012.
6. Birch L, Jones N, Doyle PM, Green P, McLaughlin A, Champney C, et al. Obstetric skill drills: evaluation of teaching methods. Nurse Educ Today. 2007;27(8):915-22.
7. Lutgendorf MA, Spalding C, Drake E, Spence D, Heaton JO, Morocco KV. Multidisciplinary in situ simulation-based training as a postpartum hemorrhage quality improvement project. Mil Med. 2017;182(3);1762-6.
8. Manella P, Antonelli R, Montt-Guevara MM, Caretto M, Palla G, Giannini A, et al. Simulation of childbirth improves clinical management capacity and self-confidence in medical students. BMJ Simul Tech Enhanc Learn. 2018;4(4);184-9.
9. RCOG. (2012). Shoulder dystocia (Green top guideline no. 42). [online] Available from: https://www.rcog.org.uk/guidance/browse-all-guidance/green-top-guidelines/shoulder-dystocia-green-top-guideline-no-42/# [Last accessed December, 2023].
10. Sinha P, Dutta A, Langford K. Instrumental delivery: how to meet the need for improvements in training. Obstet Gynaecol. 2010;12:265-71.
11. Robertson B, Schumacher L, Gosman G, Kanfer R, Kelley M, DeVita M. Simulation-based crisis team training for multidisciplinary obstetric providers. Simul Healthc. 2009 Summer;4(2):77-83.
12. Ameh CA, Mdegela M, White S, van den Broek N. The effectiveness of training in emergency obstetric care: a systematic literature review. Health Policy Plan. 2019;34(4):257-70.
13. Fransen FA, van de Ven J, Banga FR, Mol BWJ, Oei SG. Multi-professional simulation-based team training in obstetric emergencies for improving patient outcomes and trainees' performance. Cochrane Database Syst Rev. 2020;12(12):CD011545.

CHAPTER 8

Postpartum Collapse

Rajendra Saraogi, Rohan Palshetkar, Manisha Nandi

■ INTRODUCTION AND BACKGROUND

Maternal collapse is defined as an acute event that involves the cardiorespiratory or/and the central nervous system, resulting in an absent or reduced level of consciousness (and potentially leading to cardiac arrest and maternal death), at any of stage pregnancy till 6 weeks after birth. The sudden deterioration in maternal condition might occur in the postpartum period owing to a broad array of conditions, several of which are rare. Maternal survival solely depends on aggressive and rapid resuscitation protocols, precise diagnosis, and the commencement of disease-targeted therapy. Additionally, there might be further implications for future pregnancies.[1]

To note, the present-day prevalence of cardiac arrest in pregnancy is relatively rarer as compared to maternal collapse, around 1:36,000 maternities, and has a case fatality rate of 42%. The causes of maternal cardiac arrest differ and include hypovolemia, amniotic fluid embolism, and thromboembolism and, cardiac diseases with a significantly higher rate of mortality if it becomes apparent in the community setup. Around 25% of maternal collapses primarily occur due to obstetric anesthesia, after successful resuscitation. A modified warning score chart should be used with precise clinical skills for early identification of the patient who might become critical. One crucial subject on the same is that the obstetrics team should be skilled for initiation of effectual resuscitation methods and should be able to diagnose and investigate the primary cause of maternal collapse for individual patients so as to concede on an appropriately administered ongoing clinical management.[2]

■ CAUSES

General Causes

Maternal collapse might be due to many causes which might not be always related to pregnancy. A proper systematic approach helps in the assessment of the primary cause of collapse. If the cause of collapse is found to be reversible, the survival rate tend to be higher and for cases with existing specific treatment protocols available, must be rapidly considered for better management.

A systematic ABCDE approach should be implemented to allow the clinical team to identify the common causes of maternal collapse. Considering the 4 "H's" and 4 "T's" which include eclampsia and intracranial hemorrhage.

Hemorrhage

The major causes of hemorrhage include postpartum hemorrhage (PPH), antepartum hemorrhage (APH) from abruption, placenta previa, uterine rupture, and ectopic gestations. Concealed hemorrhage should never be ignored including ruptured ectopic pregnancies and following cesarean section. In cases of maternal collapse due to APH, the fetus and the placenta must be delivered on time to manage and control hemorrhage. In cases of massive placental abruption, the mode of delivery should be cesarean section even with a dead fetus to aid in the process of early control of the hemorrhage. IV administration of tranexamic acid has been effective in significantly reducing maternal mortality due to PPH.

Thromboembolism

Thromboembolic diseases account to be one of the leading causes of direct maternal death during or till 6 weeks after the termination of pregnancy. Identification of the risk factors and treatment should be initiated to avoid complications of thromboembolism.

Cardiac Diseases

Cardiac diseases are still one of the most common causes of indirect maternal death and pertains to be the most common cause of maternal death overall. The incidence of rheumatic and congenital heart diseases in pregnancy is still on the rise, secondary to a higher rate of survival owing to improved management skills. Additionally, patients with prosthetic heart valves are particularly at higher risk of complications during pregnancy. The other cardiac causes are—infective endocarditis, cardiomyopathy; acute left ventricular failure, dissection of the coronary artery, and pulmonary edema. After successful resuscitation, cardiac cases should be ideally managed by a skilled team of cardiologists.

Sepsis

Sepsis is one of the significant causes of maternal mortality. Bacteremia may be identified without pyrexia or a raised white blood cell count, and can rapidly progress toward septic shock inducing sudden collapse. Septic shock management should be ideally in accordance with the clinical guidelines.

Amniotic Fluid Embolism

It presents with maternal collapse during the period of labor or immediately after birth, or within 30 minutes of birth as respiratory distress, acute hypoxia, and hypotension. Seizures and cardiac arrest might also transpire. Subsequently acute coagulopathy develops in those patients who survive the inceptive event. The incidence is higher in patients with polyhydramnios, placenta previa, multiple pregnancy, induction of labor, and abruption. The management of amniotic fluid embolism (AFE) is provision of support rather than specific treatment. Coagulopathy needs early treatment, which includes the use of FFP. Recombinant factor VII to be administered only if coagulopathy failed to be corrected by blood component replacement therapy.

Eclampsia

Fits after 20 weeks of gestation mostly attributes to eclampsia, precisely if there is no prior history of epilepsy. To note, epilepsy must be always taken into consideration in cases of sudden collapse when associated with seizure. Intracranial hemorrhage (ICH) is one of the severe complications of uncontrolled hypertension, however also be a result arteriovenous malformations and ruptured aneurysms. The commencing presentation can be sudden collapse but, in most patients, severe headache precedes. Neurosurgeons and neuroradiologists should be part of the support and management of patients with ICH at the earliest hour.

Drug Overdose

Drug overdose and toxicity must be considered for all cases of sudden collapse. Substance abuse should be taken into account as one of the primary causes of maternal collapse especially outside of hospital premises. Therapeutic drug overdose and toxicity is a possibility with the commonly administered medications in obstetrics such as $MgSO_4$ in patients with renal impairment and the application of certain local anesthetic agents. The antidote to respiratory depression and cardiac arrhythmia caused by magnesium toxicity is the provision of 10 mL 10% calcium gluconate or 10% of calcium chloride by slow IV injection.

If toxicity due to administration of local anesthetic agents is suspected, one should immediately stop injecting. Lipid rescue should be commenced in patients of sudden collapse secondary to toxicity to local anesthetic agents.

Anaphylaxis

Anaphylaxis is a life-threatening systemic hypersensitivity reaction, leading to respiratory, circulatory, cutaneous changes, and collapse. A massive volume redistribution takes place, which decreases the cardiac output.

TABLE 1: Causes of postpartum collapse.

Reversible cause	Cause in pregnancy
4 H's	
Hypovolemia	Bleeding (obstetric/other; may be concealed) or relative hypovolemia due to dense spinal block, septic or neurogenic shock and anaphylaxis
Hypoxia	• Pregnant women can become hypoxic more quickly • Cardiac events—peripartum cardiomyopathy, myocardial infarction, aortic dissection, and large vessel aneurysms
Hypo/hyperkalemia	No more likely; severe hyperemesis
Hypo/hypernatremia	• May be caused by oxytocin use • Iatrogenic administration of fluids in labor/women's desire to "drink plenty of fluid" in labor
Hypothermia	No more likely
4 T's	
Thromboembolism	Amniotic fluid embolism, pulmonary embolus, air embolus, and myocardial infarction
Toxicity	Local anesthetic, magnesium, other
Tension pneumothorax	Following trauma/suicide attempts
Tamponade	Following trauma/suicide attempts
Eclampsia and preeclampsia	
Intracranial hemorrhage	

Acute ventricular function failure and myocardial ischemia might occur. Obstruction of airway owing to angioedema and bronchospasm contributes to hypoxia. In patients presenting with anaphylaxis, all the potential agents that might have contributed to anaphylaxis must be omitted, and the ABCDE (airway, breathing, circulation, disability, exposure) approach to assess and resuscitate should be followed.

The treatment for anaphylaxis is 1:1,000 adrenaline 500 μg (0.5 mL) intramuscularly. This dose is for intramuscular use only **(Tables 1 and 2 and Box 1)**.[2]

■ APPROACHES IN THE EVENT OF MATERNAL COLLAPSE

- One should ensure the safety to approach
- Assessment and stimulation of response

If patient responds:
- Call for help.
- Patient should be placed in her left lateral position or, one should manually displace the uterus gently by the placement of a hand just below

TABLE 2: Causes of sudden postpartum cardiorespiratory collapse.[3]

Cause	Incidence	Predisposing	Symptoms/signs
Massive postpartum hemorrhage	1:1,000	Abnormal placentation, placental abruption, severe preeclampsia, personal/family history, intrauterine fetal demise, high parity, and bleeding diathesis	
Pulmonary embolism	1:1,600	Multiple	Pleuritic chest pain, hemoptysis, dyspnea, signs deep vein thrombosis, signs pulmonary hypertension
Mitral stenosis	Variable	Rheumatic fever	Abrupt onset pulmonary edema, atrial fibrillation
Peripartum cardiomyopathy	1:3,000	African ethnicity, preeclampsia, multiple gestation, cocaine use	Dyspnea, cough, orthopnea, hemoptysis, edema, and signs heart failure
Aortic dissection	1:5,000	Marfan, Ehlers–Danlos, Loeys–Dietz and Turner's syndromes; bicuspid aortic valve, vasculitis	Chest/back pain, cardiac murmur, neurologic deficits
Uterine rupture	1:8,000	Loeys–Dietz and Ehlers–Danlos syndromes, abnormal placentation, older age, and multiple gestation	Fetal bradycardia, uterine pain and tenderness, vaginal bleeding
Uterine inversion	1:10,000	Macrosomia, rapid delivery, retained placenta, and severe preeclampsia	Vaginal bleeding, inability to palpate fundus, mass protruding from cervix
Septic shock	1:10,000	Premature rupture of membranes, chorioamnionitis, pyelonephritis, pneumonia, and puerperal sepsis	Peripherally shutdown, fever or hypothermia, altered mental status, abdominal pain
Myocardial infarction Coronary artery dissection	1:16,000	Connective tissue disease, vasculitis	Chest pain, dyspnea, presyncope
Atheromatous		Diabetes, smoking, hypertension, lipids	
Coronary artery spasm		Asian, migraine, Raynaud's	

Contd...

Contd...

Cause	Incidence	Predisposing	Symptoms/signs
Illicit drug use		Cocaine	
Amniotic fluid embolism	1:30,000	Preeclampsia, placental abnormalities	Sudden collapse in labor/within 30 minutes delivery, DIC, seizures
Anaphylaxis	1:40,000	Oxytocin, latex, misoprostol, antibiotics, anesthetic agents, and NSAIDs, breastfeeding	Angioedema, rash
Splenic aneurysm rupture	Rare	Portal hypertension	Left upper quadrant pain
Hepatic rupture	Rare	Preeclampsia, tumors, and acute fatty liver pregnancy	Right upper quadrant pain, abdominal distension
Pulmonary hypertension	Rare	Connective tissue disorders	Sudden collapse/death peripartum, signs right heart failure
Magnesium toxicity	Rare	Neuromuscular disorders	Respiratory failure
Cortisol deficiency	Rare	Prior glucocorticoid therapy, Sheehan's syndrome, hypophysitis, antiphospholid syndrome	Hyponatremia, hypoglycemia
Pheochromocytoma	Rare	Neurofibromatosis, MEN2, Von Hippel–Lindau syndromes	Cardiomyopathy, pulmonary edema
Tension pneumothorax	Rare	Marfan syndrome, lymphangioleiomyomatosis	Hypoxia, tracheal deviation, and absent breath sounds
Local anesthetic-induced sympathetic block/toxicity	Rare	Renal/liver/cardiac disease	Slurred speech, tinnitus, agitation, confusion, respiratory depression, seizures, hypotension, arrhythmias

(DIC: disseminated intravascular coagulation; MEN2: multiple endocrine neoplasia type 2; NSAIDs: non-steroidal anti-inflammatory drugs)
All may be associated with hypotension, tachycardia, or hypoxia.

> **BOX 1:** Physiological and anatomical changes in pregnancy that affect resuscitation.
>
> It is essential that anyone involved in the resuscitation of pregnant women is aware of the physiological differences. Aortocaval compression significantly reduces cardiac output from 20 weeks of gestation onwards and the efficacy of chest compressions during resuscitation. Changes in lung function, diaphragmatic splinting and increased oxygen consumption make pregnant women become hypoxic more readily and make ventilation more difficult. Difficult intubation is more likely in pregnancy. Weight gain in pregnancy, large breasts inhibiting the working space and laryngeal edema can all contribute to making intubation more difficult. Pregnant women are also at an increased risk of aspiration.
>
> *Management of the collapsed woman:* Maternal collapse resuscitation should follow the Resuscitation Council (UK) 2021 guidelines using the standard ABCDE approach, with some modifications for maternal physiology, in particular relief of aortocaval compression.

the uterus on the patient's right and push the uterus upward and to the left to aid in relieving aortocaval compression.
- High-flow oxygen should be provided so as to achieve an oxygen saturation of 94%.
- Commencement of MEOWS (modified early obstetric warning score) chart if not used already and escalation of the same whenever appropriate.
- Assessment of fetal wellbeing
- Blood glucose level monitoring
- Insertion of 16G intravenous cannula
- Collection of blood for:
    - Full blood count
    - Crossmatching
    - Blood urea
    - Serum electrolytes
    - Coagulation studies
    - ABG/VBG including lactate
    - Blood cultures

All samples must be processed as urgent by the pathology laboratory.

In case of NO response:
- Call for help alerting cardiac arrest
- One should ensure manual displacement of the uterus in patients above 20 weeks gestation or if the uterus is palpable at/above the level of umbilicus.

Airway

Open the airway of the patient:
- One should check for obstruction
- Approach should be—head tilt and chin lift

Assessment of breathing for 10 seconds:
- One should look for chest movement
- Assess breath sounds

When normally breathing:
- Turn the woman to recovery position
- Assessment of breathing, pulse rate, blood pressure, and fetal heart rate.

Not breathing:
Initiate cardiopulmonary resuscitation (CPR)

Resuscitation Council Guidelines (UK), 2021:
The airway management should be by a skilled anesthetist.
- Persons not involved directly with the resuscitation process should make sure that:
  - The security doors are open for emergency access
  - Cardiac arrest trolley ready for mobilization
  - Someone should be present to act as the "RUNNER"
  - The patient's records should be made available.
- Supplementation of O_2 at a flow rate of 10–15 L/minute. Bag and mask ventilation must be done till intubation.
- When the defibrillator is available, self-adhesive defibrillation pads should be used to access the rhythm. These should be applied along with chest compressions.

During Cardiopulmonary Resuscitation (Table 3)

- Establish IO/ IV access—ideally two wide bore cannulas should be inserted as soon as possible. If peripheral venous access is not possible early consideration of intraosseous access (IO), central venous access or venous cutdown should be considered.
- Give adrenaline as per advance life support algorithm.
- *Correct reversible cause:* 4 H's, 4T's

TABLE 3: Circulation.

Assess cardiac rhythm	
Shockable rhythm	**Non-shockable rhythm**
VF/pulseless VT	Asystole and PEA
Defibrillation with: • 200 J/300 J/360 J biphasic • 360 J monophasic	
CPR 30:2 for 2 minutes	Immediate CPR 30:2

Perimortem Cesarean Section

- Perimortem cesarean section (PMCS) should be seen as a resuscitative procedure to be performed primarily in the interests of maternal survival.
- Senior staff should be involved at an early stage.
- In women over 20 weeks of gestation, if there is no response to correctly performed CPR within 4 minutes of maternal collapse or if resuscitation is continued beyond this, then PMCS should be undertaken to assist maternal resuscitation. Ideally, this should be achieved within 5 minutes of the collapse.
- A scalpel and umbilical cord clamps should be available on the resuscitation trolley in all areas where maternal collapse may occur, including accident and emergency.
- Perimortem cesarean section should be performed where the resuscitation is taking place.
- The operator should use the incision which will facilitate the most rapid access. This may be a midline vertical incision or a suprapubic transverse incision.
- Where the outcome is not successful, the case should be discussed so as to determine whether a postmortem is required before any medical devices such as lines and endotracheal tubes are removed, as per the Royal College of Obstetricians and Gynecologists (RCOG) recommendations.[4]

What are the Outcomes for the Mother and the Baby?

Outcomes for mothers and babies depend on the cause of collapse, gestational age, and access to emergency care, with survival rates being poorer if the collapse occurs out of hospital. In maternal cardiac arrest maternal survival rates of over 50% have been reported.

Post-resuscitation Care

- Ongoing management depends on the underlying cause of the collapse.
- It is essential the woman and baby are transferred to an appropriate environment such as high dependency or critical care area.
- Accurate documentation is essential in all cases of maternal collapse and a critical incident form (RL) should be submitted whether or not resuscitation is successful.
- All cases of maternal death must be reported.
- All maternity staff should have annual formal multidisciplinary training in generic life support and the management of maternal collapse.
- Life support training improves resuscitation skills.
- Small group multidisciplinary interactive practical training is recommended to improve the management of maternal collapse.

- Debriefing is recommended for the woman, the family, and the staff involved in the event.

■ CONCLUSION

Postpartum collapse demands swift recognition and immediate intervention. Heightened awareness among healthcare providers and effective communication are crucial in addressing this medical emergency. Community education plays a vital role in empowering both professionals and new mothers to recognize warning signs and seek timely assistance. Continuous research is essential for refining protocols and improving maternal healthcare. By prioritizing, the well-being of mothers during the postpartum period, we contribute to creating a safer and more supportive environment for both women and their newborns. A collaborative effort from healthcare providers, communities, and policymakers is essential to enhance outcomes and save lives in cases of postpartum collapse.

KEY POINTS

Maternal collapse is a rare but life-threatening event, with a wide-ranging etiology. The outcome primarily for the mother, but also for the fetus, depends on prompt and effective resuscitation:
- An obstetric modified early warning score chart along with clinical judgments should be used for all women undergoing observation to allow for early recognition of the woman who is becoming critically ill.
- Consider four H's and four T's for the cause of maternal cardiac arrest, in the pregnant woman add eclampsia and intracranial hemorrhage.
- Maternal collapse resuscitation should follow the resuscitation guidelines using the standard ABCDE approach, with some modifications for maternal physiology, in particular relief of aortocaval compression.
- If maternal cardiac arrest occurs in the community setting, basic life support should be administered and rapid transfer arranged.
- Senior staff with appropriate experience should be involved at an early stage.
- Perimortem cesarean section (PMCS) should be seen as a resuscitative procedure to be performed primarily in the interests of maternal survival.

■ REFERENCES

1. Nanda S, Penna LK. Postpartum collapse. Obstet Gynaecol Reprod Med. 2009;19(8):221-8.
2. Liu B, Bhide A. Sudden postpartum maternal collapse. In: Chandraharan E, Arulkumaran SS (Eds). Obstetric and Intrapartum Emergencies: A Practical Guide to Management [Internet]. 2nd edition. Cambridge: Cambridge University Press; 2021. pp. 139-46.
3. Morton A. Postpartum collapse. Obstet Med. 2021;14(1):46-9.
4. Sharma C, Mistry K. Chapter-26 Postpartum collapse. In: Sharma A (Ed). A Practical Guide to Third Trimester of Pregnancy and Puerperium. New Delhi: Jaypee Brothers Medical Publishers; 2016. pp. 225-34.

9 Hydrops Fetalis

Vandana Bansal, Rupal Parekh

■ INTRODUCTION

Hydrops fetalis is a Greek word for water. It is a condition characterized by abnormal accumulation of serous fluid in two or more body cavities (pericardial effusion, pleural effusion, and ascites) and skin edema.[1] Hydrops is frequently associated with anemia, placentomegaly, polyhydramnios, and hepatosplenomegaly. Diagnosis is made prenatally by ultrasound and postnatal clinical evaluation of the fetus.

It is not a disease but rather a symptom of an underlying disorder that affects the fetus. The underlying pathophysiology of fetal hydrops is increased fluid transudation from intravascular to extravascular compartment due to increased interstitial fluid production or high capillary permeability or impaired lymphatic circulation. This may result from a wide range of conditions with varying pathophysiological mechanism, each with the potential of severely affecting the fetus.

Hydrops fetalis is classically divided into two broad categories:
1. Immune hydrops fetalis is caused by presence of maternal circulating antibodies against red blood cells and is responsible for 10% of cases of hydrops.
2. Nonimmune hydrops fetalis (NIHF) is caused by etiologies other than immune with absence of hemolytic antibodies and is responsible for 76–87%% of cases.[2]

■ EPIDEMIOLOGY

Prevalence of hydrops fetalis is about one in 2,000 births. With the widespread use of anti-D immunoglobulin postnatally to all Rhesus (Rh)-negative mother with Rh-positive neonates, the prevalence of RhD-alloimmunization and associated immune hydrops has drastically declined.[3]

■ ETIOPATHOGENESIS

Immune Hydrops

It occurs due to maternal antibodies coated on fetal red blood cells causing hemolysis and fetal anemia.

- Rh-isoimmunization—due to Rh-incapability (Rh-negative mother with Rh-positive fetus)
- ABO incompatible—due to ABO mismatch between mother and fetus. The RBC are lysed rapidly in this case and not enough timeframe for immune system to form antibodies.
- Atypical antibodies—Kell, Duffy antibodies, anti c, C, e, E antibodies

The latter two are to be suspected when immune hydrops occur in Rh-positive pregnant women.

Nonimmune Hydrops Fetalis

It may occur at various gestational age and is due to wide array of conditions as presented in **Table 1** along with their etiopathogenesis. It is important to note that 1/3rd of NIHF have a genetic etiology and hence high chances

TABLE 1: Etiopathogenesis of nonimmune hydrops fetalis.

Cardiac causes	17–35% of all NIHF. They are most common cause of NIHF
	
	Mechanism:
	• Increased central venous pressure resulting from increased right heart pressure or volume overload
	• Inadequate diastolic ventricular filling in rhythm disturbances or in cardiomyopathies
		Most common congenital cardiac defect associated with NIHF are right-sided heart defects:
		• Cardiac tumors
		• Subendocardial fibroelastosis
		• *Arrhythmia* is an important cause.
		  – Tachyarrhythmia; Supraventricular tachycardia (most common); Atrial flutter
		  – Bradyarrhythmia commonly due to congenital heart block in maternal autoimmune condition like Sjögren's syndrome and anti-Ro, anti-La antibodies. Heart block may also occur due to structural defect affecting the cardiac conduction fibers as in heterotaxy

		Once hydrops develops in case of third-degree heart block, prognosis is poor
		The prognosis of NIHF due to cardiac structural abnormalities is also poor due to the severity of the heart defects that cause in utero congestive heart failure

Contd...

Contd...

Chromosomal	7–16% of NIHF *Mechanism:* Impaired lymphatic microcirculation	• Mainly aneuploidy Turner syndrome (45, XO) and trisomy 21, 13, 18 　– Turner syndrome is associated with cystic hygroma and impaired lymphatic circulation 　– Trisomy 21 may be associated with abnormal myelopoiesis leading to leukemia/anemia and hydrops • Other genetic syndromes: Tuberous sclerosis, Noonan syndrome, arthrogryposis
Fetal anemia/ hematologic (nonimmune causes)	4–12% of NIHF *Mechanism:* Any condition (not immune mediated) which has underlying defect in hemoglobin/RBC production or hemolysis will cause fetal anemia and cardiac failure leading to hydrops	• *Inherited conditions* 　– Hemoglobinopathy (particularly alpha-thalassemia is very common in Southern Asian countries) 　– Disorders of RBC membranes, for example, hereditary spherocytosis 　– Defects of RBC production, for example, Diamond–Blackfan anemia, Fanconi anemia 　– G6PD deficiency 　– Leukemias • *Acquired conditions:* 　– Parvovirus infection (transient anemia due to bone marrow suppression) 　– Fetomaternal hemorrhage leading to anemia. It can be isolated acute event or a chronic ongoing hemorrhage
Infections	5–7% of NIHF *Mechanism:* Increased capillary permeability, bone marrow suppression causing anemia and myocarditis	• Most common infectious cause of NIHF is Parvovirus B19 • It causes transient bone marrow suppression • Poor outcome expected if infection occurs <20 weeks gestation. Late in gestation it is a transient and resolves • Others include CMV infection, syphilis and toxoplasmosis

Contd...

Contd...

Structural anomalies	6–10 % of NIHF
	
	Mechanism:
	• Intrathoracic mass effect leads to venocaval obstruction
	• Increased intra-abdominal pressure due to any abdominal lesion decreases venous return
	• Reduced colloid oncotic pressure
		• *Thorax lesions:*
		  – Mass lesions like congenital pulmonary airway malformation (CPAM)
		  – Hydrothorax/chylothorax
		• *GIT lesions:*
		  – Congenital diaphragmatic hernia, volvulus, GI obstruction, meconium peritonitis, liver and hemangioma
		• Skeletal dysplasia
		• *Neuromuscular disorder:*
		  – Akinesia deformities
		• *Fetal tumors:*
		  – Neuroblastoma, sacrococcygeal teratoma, hemangioma, rhabdomyoma in tuberous sclerosis Leading to high output cardiac failure and NIHF
		• *Congenital nephrosis* with hypoproteinemia

Placental or cord lesions	2–3% of NIHF *Mechanism:* High output cardiac failure	Large lesions like chorioangioma >5 cm function like a large arteriovenous shunt and lead to high output cardiac failure causing NIHF
Inborn error of metabolism	1–2 % NIHF Rare causes of NIHF but better to be alert especially for idiopathic hydrops. Prone for recurrence *Mechanism:* Visceromegaly and obstruction of venous return, decreased erythropoiesis and anemia, and/or hypoproteinemia from liver failure	• Lysosomal storage disorders • Mucopolysaccharidosis, Gaucher's and Niemann–Pick disease • Gangliosidosis To examine for enlarged liver, spleen, bone marrow, and placental findings in cases of hydrops after birth or in case of neonatal death
Twins	3–10 % of NIHF *Mechanism:* High cardiac output and hypervolemia in the recipient twin	In cases of monochorionic twins, one or both twin can develop hydrops: • Twin-to-twin transfusion syndrome • Twin reversed arterial perfusion sequence

of recurrence. A thorough evaluation of etiology is imperative in NIHF to determine recurrence risk and plan prenatal diagnosis in subsequent pregnancy. Common causes have been broadly enumerated while frequently it may remain unclear in 15–25% of cases. The success of identifying the cause would depend on thoroughness of efforts to establish the diagnosis.
- Chromosomal aneuploidy
- Hematological abnormalities
- Cardiovascular abnormalities
- Skeletal dysplasia
- Inborn error of metabolism
- Infections

■ SONOGRAPHIC FINDINGS IN HYDROPS FETALIS

The most common findings detected during early pregnancy are ascites and skin edema in the fetal head, back of the neck, thorax, and abdomen **(Fig. 1)**. Polyhydramnios and placental edema are most commonly seen before 20 weeks, whereas pleural effusion and pericardial effusion in the fetus is rarely seen before 15 weeks of gestation.[4] Hydrops due to chromosomal abnormalities is usually detected during early pregnancy, whereas cardiac causes are detected in the second or third trimester.

Skin edema is defined as the subcutaneous tissue thickness on the scalp **(Fig. 2)** or prenasal edema >5 mm **(Fig. 3)**. Placentomegaly is defined as placental thickness >4 cm **(Fig. 4)**.[5] Polyhydramnios is an increased quantity of liquor amnii measured vertically as single deepest pocket of >8 cm or an amniotic fluid index of >24 cm.[6]

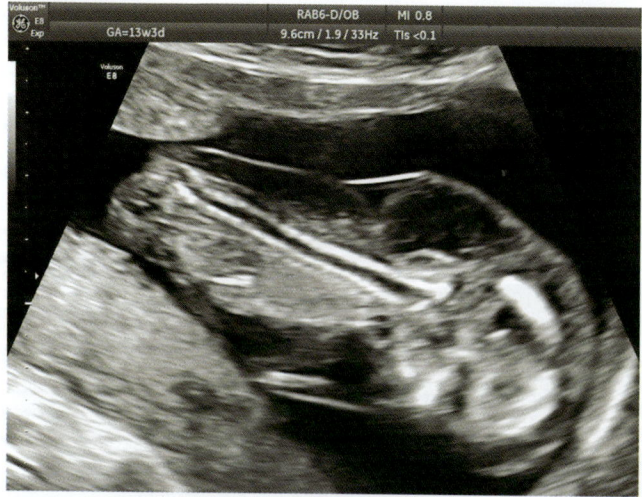

Fig. 1: Generalized edema at early gestation.

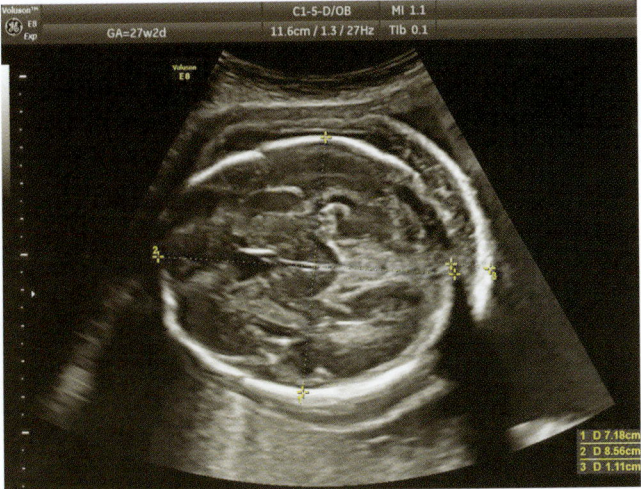

Fig. 2: Scalp edema.

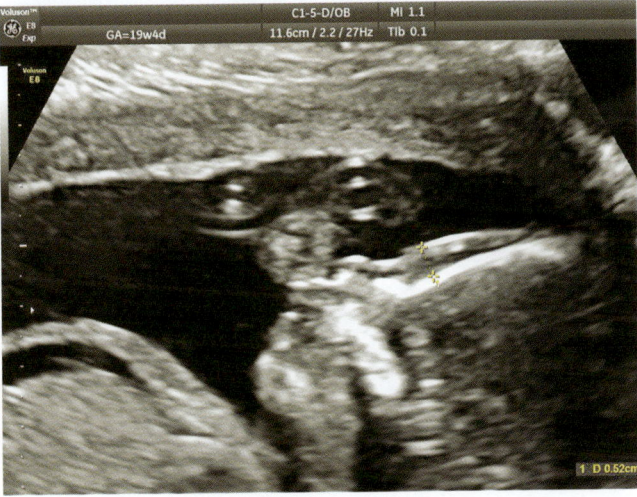

Fig. 3: Prenasal edema.

Ascites can be an early manifestation of hydrops fetalis and is seen as early as 20 weeks of gestation **(Fig. 5)**. Isolated fetal ascites is seen in many other systemic diseases. Hence it is essential to differentiate hydrops fetalis from other causes of ascites.

Pleural effusion can be unilateral **(Fig. 6)** or bilateral. Mild effusions can cause respiratory distress at birth and severe effusions result in lung hypoplasia and respiratory/circulatory disorders associated with poor prognosis after birth.[7] Pericardial effusion is commonly seen in the hydropic fetus of Rh-sensitized mother.[8]

Hydrops Fetalis

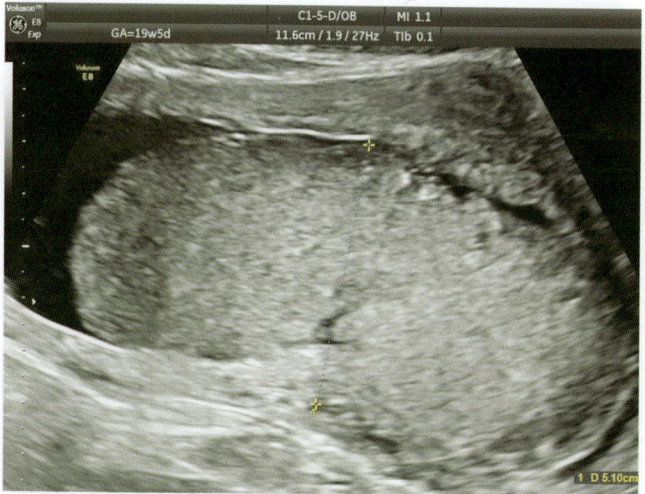

Fig. 4: Placentomegaly.

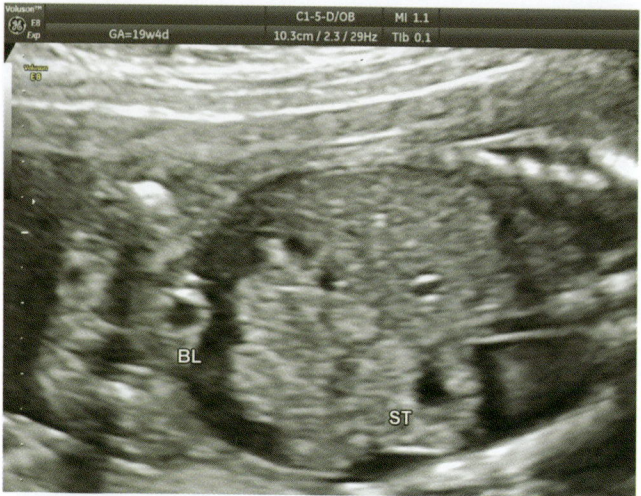

Fig. 5: Ascites secondary to fetal infection with liver calcification.

■ MATERNAL EFFECTS OF FETAL HYDROPS

- Mirror syndrome is considered a form of preeclampsia where mother's body mimics (mirrors) the hydropic fetus. Maternal edema is pronounced in 90% of cases. Hypertension and proteinuria is mostly (but not always) present. The definitive treatment of mirror syndrome is delivery but in cases where hydrops is due to correctable cause then antenatal treatment of hydrops also leads to resolution of the mirror syndrome.
- Polyhydramnios and preterm labor are commonly associated with fetal hydrops.

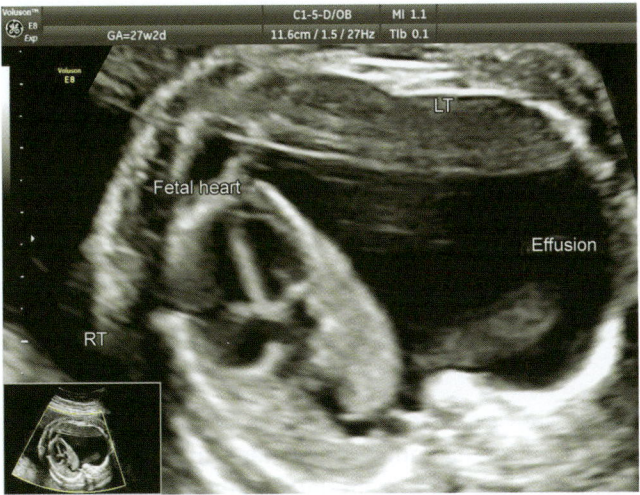

Fig. 6: Unilateral massive pleural effusion.

INVESTIGATIONS IN FETAL HYDROPS: ROLE OF INDIVIDUAL TESTS AND ALGORITHM FOR HYDROPS FETALIS WORKUP

- *Meticulous sonographic examination:* The foremost step is to look for sonographic clues to the underlying etiology as it has a direct influence on prognosis and management.
- Rule out any structural defect (e.g., thoracic mass, tumors)
- Detailed cardiac evaluation by fetal echocardiography and identify any arrhythmia
- Placental or cord lesions
- Color Doppler examination of middle cerebral artery peak systolic velocity (MCA-PSV) for noninvasive assessment of fetal anemia.[9] If fetal anemia has occurred due to any cause (immune or nonimmune) it reflects as high velocity in MCA-PSV which is quantified using multiple of median (MoM values). When fetal MCA-PSV is >1.5 MoM, it indicates severe fetal anemia and is indication for fetal intrauterine blood transfusion.[10,11]
- *Maternal blood tests:*
  - Tests indicating *immune hydrop:* Maternal blood group, indirect Coombs test **(Table 2)** and Rh-titers.
  - If any acute/chronic event for *fetomaternal hemorrhage (FMH) is suspected,* then Kleihauer–Betke (KB) test or flow cytometry to detect fetal hemoglobin in maternal circulation is done. The KB test is based on principle of differential resistance of fetal and adult RBC to acid elution. The adult RBCs become ghost cells and the amount of fetal RBC are used to quantify the hemorrhage. The KB test is sensitive but drawback is lack of reproducibility and inter observer variation.

TABLE 2: Understanding direct and indirect Coombs test.

Indirect Coombs test	Direct Coombs test
• Done on maternal serum • Aim to identify circulating antibody in maternal serum • When the isoimmunized maternal serum is added to RBC with known antigens, it will show coagulation • Positive ICT indicates Rh-sensitized mother	• Done on fetal RBC (fetal or neonatal blood sample) • Aim to identify the fetal RBC coated with maternal antibody • When the "antibody coated RBCs" are added to Coombs reagent (anti-human globulin), it shows coagulation • Positive DCT indicates fetal RBCs are antibody coated, i.e. affected fetus

If KB test shows equivocal result or large FMH, then flow cytometry is used to confirm the finding. The latter is more accurate and based on principle of dual fluorescent detection of two intracellular antigens, hemoglobin F (HbF) and carbonic anhydrase (CA) present in adult Hb. Also note that maternal serum alpha-fetoprotein value is high if fetomaternal hemorrhage has occurred.

- *Role of maternal serology for TORCH [toxoplasmosis, others (syphilis, hepatitis B), rubella, cytomegalovirus, herpes simplex] and Parvovirus:* IgM positive indicates recent infection and IgG indicates past infection. However these antibodies remain positive for many months or IgG can be positive for many years, and hence it gives a poor estimation of possible infection during antenatal period. IgG avidity testing should always be done when IgG antibodies are seen. High avidity report suggests infection >3 months old and low avidity suggests recent infection within 3 months. However, one must be alert for the limitation of avidity in late gestation because a 3-month timeframe could still not rule out a first trimester infection. The most definitive test for TORCH and Parvovirus infection is via PCR on a fetal sample (see below).
- *Anti SS-A/SS-B* antibodies are done in fetal hydrops secondary to complete heart block in mothers with Sjögren's syndrome.
- *Invasive testing (amniocentesis/fetal cord blood sampling):*
  - The fetal sample (cord blood or liquor amnii) is to be analyzed for genetic disorders using FISH, microarray and whole exome testing. NIHF is a shared, severe presentation of many genetic disorders. An important step in the evaluation of NIHF is to exclude a genetic abnormality. Genetically transmitted disorders account for about one-thirds of cases of NIHF, and include chromosomal abnormalities, hemoglobinopathies, skeletal dysplasias, metabolic storage disorders, and erythrocyte enzymopathies. A complete family history is thus imperative to rule out a known inherited disorder in the family and to assess for consanguinity, which will increase the likelihood of a recessive disorder.

Standard genetic testing with karyotyping or chromosomal microarray analysis identifies the cause of only 25% of NIHF cases and does not detect single-gene disorders. The contribution of single-gene disorders to NIHF is unknown but is potentially substantial. An accurate diagnosis enables focused prenatal management and early neonatal care to improve outcomes for this severe condition and helps in determining recurrence risk in next pregnancy. Fetal DNA can be saved to analyze single gene disorders, metabolic disorders if required.
- TORCH, parvovirus PCR on the amniotic fluid sample if infection is suspected. Sonographic clues to TORCH infections can be looked for such as ventriculomegaly, intracranial calcifications, hepatic calcifications, and hepatosplenomegaly, echogenic bowel, etc.
- Fetal hemoglobin, blood group, direct Coombs test **(Table 2)** can be performed direct from the cord blood sample.

■ TREATMENT/FETAL THERAPY

The diagnosis and management of hydrops fetalis have improved in recent years with advances in prenatal diagnostic and therapeutic interventions together with the advances in neonatal intensive care. However, it is still associated with a high mortality rate. Overall survival rate in nonimmune hydrops is about 21.8%.

The cornerstone of management for this condition is a thorough evaluation for the underlying etiology of the hydrops. Pregnancy management decisions will depend on the etiology, in particular whether there is a treatable cause and the gestational age that NIHF develops or is first identified.

Cases generally fall into three categories—those amenable to fetal therapy which often require urgent treatment or referral to a specialized center; those with a lethal prognosis, for whom pregnancy termination is the only options; and cases in which the etiology is idiopathic, and the prognosis is likely poor but uncertain. It is important to counsel that the potential for maternal complications with expectant management be anticipated, including mirror syndrome. Serial evaluation of maternal blood pressure is therefore recommended. Ultrasound follow-up is needed every 2–3 weeks to monitor the evolution of hydrops with an aim to achieve gestational maturity as much as possible.

Counseling for pregnancies with NIHF amenable to fetal therapy should include a discussion of potential risks, benefits, and alternatives that takes into consideration the severity of the underlying condition and the anticipated response to the intervention.

Structural cardiac abnormalities and aneuploidy cannot be intervened with, and prognosis is poor. Hence they need to be excluded. Treatment as per the etiology has been shown in **Flowchart 1 and Table 3**.

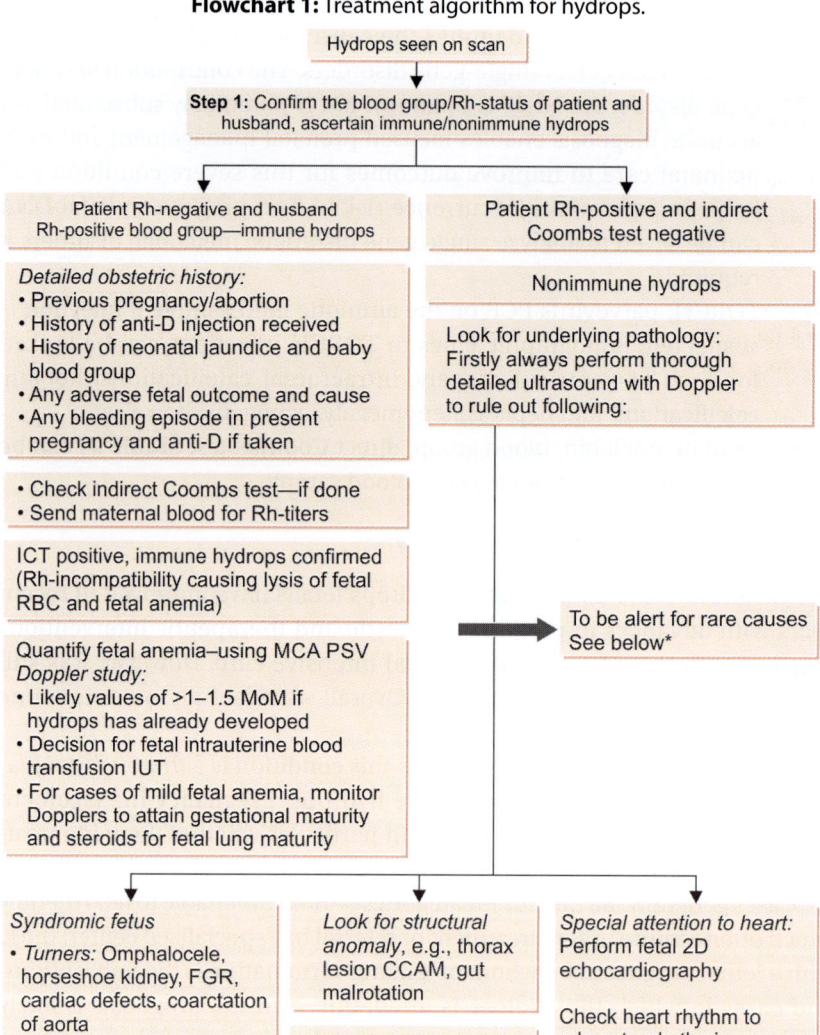

Flowchart 1: Treatment algorithm for hydrops.

TABLE 3: Treatment as per the etiology of hydrops.

Cardiac tachyarrhythmia, supraventricular tachycardia, atrial flutter, or atrial fibrillation	Maternal transplacental administration of antiarrhythmic medication(s)	Treatment with antiarrhythmic medication unless near term gestation where delivery is an option
Fetal anemia due to Rh-isoimmunization or secondary to parvovirus infection or fetomaternal hemorrhage	Fetal blood sampling followed by intrauterine transfusion	• Confirm fetal Hb, blood group, DCT, and intrauterine blood transfusion • IUT in these cases is life-saving and hydrops resolves if transient causes of fetal anemia-like parvovirus • If immune hydrops, then each IUT buys time of few weeks to gain fetal maturity
Fetal hydrothorax, chylothorax, or large pleural effusion associated with bronchopulmonary sequestration **(Fig. 7)**	If large effusion/hydrothorax/chylothorax is causing mediastinal shift and impaired venous return so as to cause NIHF, then drainage is indicated	• Fetal needle drainage of pleural effusion or placement of thoracoamniotic shunt • Send aspirated fluid sample for cytology. Lack of infection with >80% lymphocytes suggests chylothorax • Good prognosis if hydrops resolves after aspiration
Fetal CPAM	• Most cases of CPAM can be conservatively managed by only monitoring • Only few cases lead to NIHF in which case decision of invasive therapy can be taken in macrocystic type	• *Macrocystic type:* Fetal needle drainage of effusion or placement of thoracoamniotic shunt; • *Microcystic type:* Maternal administration of corticosteroids, betamethasone 12 mg—2 doses, 24 hours apart
TTTS or TRAP	• Laser ablation or radiofrequency ablation • Balance risk of procedure with risk of prematurity (monitoring only and preterm delivery)	• If *both fetus are salvageable*, then fetoscopic laser ablation of anastomotic vessels • If *only one fetus is salvageable*, then selective fetal reduction using radiofrequency ablation of the twin with poor prognosis

Postnatal management includes initial resuscitation, identification, and treatment of the underlying cause. Most of the infants with hydrops fetalis will require endotracheal intubation because of respiratory depression. Thoracentesis, paracentesis, and sometimes cardiocentesis are performed if

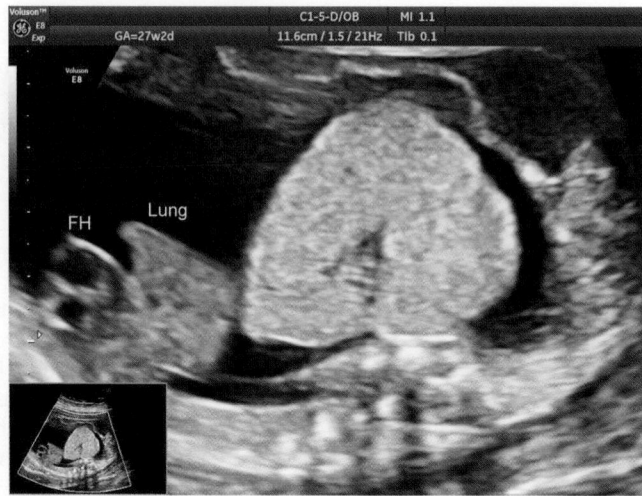

Fig. 7: Hydrops due to extrapulmonary sequestration, a correctable disorder.

the neonate presents with pleural effusion, ascites, and pericardial effusion. In cases of severe anemia, a blood transfusion or exchange transfusion is required. Further, close monitoring is needed if tachyarrhythmias are transient or intermittent. If severe, they are corrected with cardioversion, antiarrhythmic drugs, and pacing. Despite aggressive treatment, the survival rate is as low as 10% with neurodevelopmental and cognitive defects in surviving infants.

■ PROGNOSIS AND RECURRENCE

The prognosis of hydrops fetalis is dependent mainly on the underlying cause whether immune or nonimmune, treatable or not, gestational age at the time of the diagnosis, time of delivery, amount of fetal edema, intrauterine interventions, Apgar scores, extent of resuscitation in the delivery room, and whether the newborn requires transport.[12]

Neonates who present with thoracic causes and bronchopulmonary malformations have a good prognosis, while those with chromosomal abnormalities, structural abnormalities, and other genetic metabolic disorders are associated with poor prognosis.

Hydrops fetalis is not a consequence of heart failure but rather due to hypervolemia and the high vascular permeability of the fetus. In contrast, heart failure is a very late consequence of a long-standing overworked heart in hydrops. Presence of cardiac dysfunction in hydrops confers a poor prognosis.[13] The fetal cardiovascular profile score can be used in the surveillance of hydropic fetuses for prediction of the presence of congestive heart failure and as an aid for predicting fetal outcome **(Table 4)**.[14]

TABLE 4: Cardiovascular profile score.

CVPS Parameters	Principle	Normal score = +2	Minus 1	Minus 2
Hydrops	Measure of intravascular hydrostatic pressure/capillary permeability	No	In one compartment	Subcutaneous tissue
Venous Doppler umbilical vein (UV) and ductus venosus (DV)	• Measure of central venous pressure? • RV diastolic function	UV and DV normal	UV normal, DV reversal	UV pulsation
Heart size	Measure of heart remodeling in response to overload	0.25–0.35	0.35–0.5	>0.5
Heart function	TR and ventricular shortening are measures of afterload monophasic filling suggests severe diastolic filling abnormality	• Normal TV, MV • SF LV ≥0.28 • Biphasic diastolic filling	Holosystolic TR or SF LV ≤0.28	• Holosystolic MR/TR or dP/dT <400 or • Monophasic filling
Arterial Doppler: Umbilical artery (UA)	Measure of placental resistance	UA normal	UA = AEDF	UA = REDF

(AEDF: absent end diastolic flow; dP/dT: change in pressure over time of TR jet; LV: left ventricle; MR: mitral regurgitation; MV: mitral valve; REDF: reversal of end diastolic flow; SF LV: ventricular shortening fraction; TR: tricuspid regurgitation; TV: tricuspid valve)

Two points for each parameter. Normal score is 10 i.e. If there are no abnormal signs. Each abnormal finding reflects minus 1 or 2 points as above.

■ CASES OF HYDROPS WITH POTENTIAL OF RECURRENCE[15]

- Aneuploidy/genetic disorders—low-to-moderate recurrence depending on the type of defect and inheritance
- Red blood cell isoimmunization—high
- Metabolic disorders—25%
- Structural fetal defects, fetal infection have no increased risk of recurrence.

Overall hydrops fetalis has guarded prognosis (depending on cause) and often results in intrauterine fetal demise or neonatal death. Fetal autopsies, including histopathologic evaluation, placental examination, molecular and genetic studies, must be performed to determine the cause and recurrence.

Dealing with a bad prognosis for a fetus is challenging for the couple and often they are not keen on detailed workup. Option of invasive testing and DNA save must always be given in such cases. DNA can be analyzed at a later stage, before planning next pregnancy. The importance of precious sample of the index case (affected fetus) must be explained.

■ IMMUNE HYDROPS

This is a special category of hydrops with good results on intrauterine transfusion. Erythroblastosis fetalis, as it is also called, is due to maternal alloantibodies directed against paternal antigen on fetal cells resulting in hemolysis of fetal RBC causing anemia. A total of 97% of all cases of immune hydrops are caused by maternal antibodies against RhD antigen on fetal red blood cells. The C and E antigen usually cause alloimmunization via blood transfusions and usually not following fetomaternal bleed. Other rare atypical antigens systems that have potential to cause hemolytic disease are Kell, Duffy, Kidd, and MNS.

Pathophysiology of Immune Hydrops

When a fetomaternal bleed occurs in an Rh-negative mother with an Rh-positive fetus, maternal immune system is stimulated and B-lymphocytes clones that recognize the RhD antigen are established. The initial primary immune response produces anti-rhesus IgM antibodies which are short lived and have a molecular weight too large to cross the placental barrier. This primary immune response is followed by synthesis of IgG antibodies which can cross the placenta and destroy fetal erythrocytes and cause fetal anemia. Fortunately this alloimmune response takes few weeks to months (6 weeks–12 months) to occur and ensures that the first pregnancy is not at risk (primary sensitized pregnancy). However the mother will remain sensitized and anti-D antibodies remain in maternal circulation throughout her life and in every subsequent pregnancy.

Once a sensitized mother has a second Rh-positive fetus, Rh-positive fetal D antigen will trigger an amnestic secondary immune response from a previously primed maternal immune system and produces IgG antibodies rapidly (usually measured in days). These IgG immunoglobulins cross the placenta and enter fetal circulation and attack fetal blood cells. In the event of an appropriate fetal antigen being present in the fetal blood, the maternal IgG antibodies bind to these antigens and cause an antigen antibody reaction leading to hemolysis of the fetal RBCs in the fetal reticuloendothelial system leading to fetal anemia. Depending upon the severity of hemolysis the clinical presentation may be congestive cardiac failure with hydrops fetalis, hepatosplenomegaly, and placentomegaly, death in utero to hyperbilirubinemia/kernicterus (icterus gravis neonatorum) or just mild congenital anemia of the newborn.

Anemia if severe leads to structural, functional and hemodynamic changes in the liver, spleen, and portal system along with hyperdynamic systemic circulation. Fetal hemolysis leads to compensatory extramedullary hematopoiesis causing hepatosplenomegaly. Normal hepatic protein synthesis is deranged which along with the increased portal vein pressure leads to hypoproteinemia, fetal ascites, pleural effusion, and generalized edema. There is an alteration in the fluid distribution across the various compartments leading to fetal hydrops. Cardiomegaly ensues due to hyperdynamic circulation with increased cardiac output. Congestive cardiac failure develops subsequent to high output failure. Increased umbilical vein pressure develops along with placentomegaly and polyhydramnios. Placentomegaly leads to preeclampsia like syndrome in the mother called as "mirror syndrome".

■ SEROLOGY TO DETECT ISOIMMUNIZATION

The presence of anti-D antibodies in the maternal serum by indirect Coombs test is diagnostic of maternal alloimmunization. If indirect Coombs test is positive, Rh-antibody titers are quantified by double dilution of test serum that is able to produce agglutination with RBCs. The reciprocal of the highest dilution that causes agglutination is taken as the titer. Critical titer is the titer at or below which no fetal death or severe alloimmunization occurs. Its value varies with different laboratories and the same laboratory should be used for subsequent titer analysis. For most laboratories the critical titer is ≥1:16 (range >1:8–1:32).

Tests for Determining Amount of Fetomaternal Bleed (Kleihauer–Betke Acid Elution Test)

Kleihauer–Betke test is based on the fact that an acid solution elutes adult hemoglobin but not fetal hemoglobin from the red blood cells. A monolayer of blood film or smear of red cells are fixed using alcohol. An acid buffer is used to elute (remove) HbA as it is more soluble than HbF which is the predominant Hb in fetal red cells. This slide is then counterstained with eosin. Cells containing HbF stain darkly whereas HbA cells appear as ghost cells (pale and unstained). This test can detect as little as 0.2 mL of fetal blood cells in 5 mL of maternal blood.

The KB test is required only when massive fetomaternal hemorrhage is suspected (0.1% of deliveries) as in abruption placenta, abdominal trauma, unexplained fetal demise, placenta previa, multifetal gestation, manual removal of placenta, etc. The dosage of anti-D immunoglobulin would, then need to be increased as per the amount of fetomaternal bleed.

Noninvasive Diagnosis of Fetal Anemia by Ultrasound Doppler

Use of middle cerebral artery peak systolic velocity as a noninvasive method for fetal anemia has been a practice changing discovery in the field of Rh-isoimmunization. The landmark study by Mari et al., in 1995 showed that increased velocity in the middle cerebral artery above 1.5 MoM is extremely accurate method for diagnosing moderate to severe fetal anemia with a sensitivity of almost 100% and a false positive rate of 12%.[8] This noninvasive monitoring has resulted in reduction of invasive procedures by 70% and is now the standard of care for diagnosis and management of fetal anemia.

Technique for Middle Cerebral Artery Peak Systolic Velocity Measurement

The middle cerebral artery was selected for use because of its ease of sampling while maintaining almost 0° angle for accurate and reproducible measurement of velocity of blood flow. Anemia causes a reduction in the viscosity of blood leading to increased velocity blood flow. It can be reliably measured between 18 and 35 weeks of gestation.

Middle cerebral artery on ultrasound can be seen in an axial plane of the brain at the level of the sphenoid bone, thalami, and cavum septum pellucidum **(Fig. 8)**. MCA of the cerebral hemisphere closer to the ultrasound beam is sampled at proximal portion as it originates from the circle of Willis taking care that the angle of insonation is as close to 0°. The highest point on the peak is measured using electronic calipers and are plotted on Mari et al., chart. The threshold for diagnosis of severe fetal anemia is 1.5 MoM for that gestational age. The measurements can be falsely increased if measurements are taken during fetal movement, uterine contraction or late in gestation after 35 weeks.

Rh-negative isoimmunized mother with previously affected fetus or those with Rh-antibodies titers above critical levels are monitored noninvasively by Doppler of MCA-PSV to identify moderate-to-severe anemia prior to development of hydrops. MCA-PSV correlates well with the degree of fetal anemia. A cut-off value of MCA-PSV of 1.5 MoM for the period of gestation

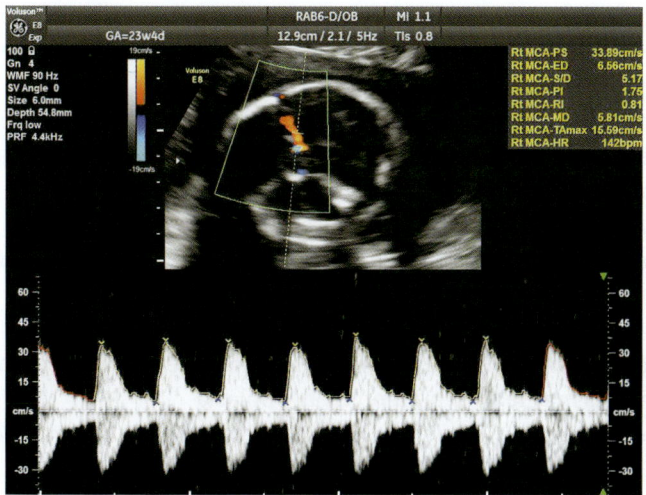

Fig. 8: Middle cerebral artery peak systolic flow for noninvasive monitoring of fetal anemia.

or evidence of hydrops on ultrasound indicates severe anemia (hematocrit <30%) requiring intrauterine transfusion.

This noninvasive method has superseded the traditional technique of serial amniocentesis for the spectral analysis of amniotic fluid at 450 nm (delta OD450) first described by Liley in 1961. Liley's technique was used to measure bilirubin in amniotic fluid, an indirect measure of fetal hemolysis to determine time for intrauterine transfusion. These invasive techniques for determining fetal hemolysis have now been completely abandoned.

If untreated, the anemic fetus would develop hepatosplenomegaly, cardiomegaly, placentomegaly, polyhydramnios and end-stage hydropic fetus which may die in utero or postnatally of cardiac failure or develop kernicterus with its sequela.

Other B Mode Ultrasound Assessment for Fetal Anemia in Immune Hydrops

- Hepatomegaly occurs due to compensatory extramedullary hematopoiesis. Increase in the measurement of the abdominal circumference maybe seen (since liver occupies about two-thirds of the fetal abdomen). Nomograms to compare fetal liver length with degrees of fetal anemia are available.
- *Splenomegaly:* An increase in 3–4 times the original size, due to extramedullary hematopoiesis may be noted.
- Increased blood flow through the umbilical vein due to hyperdynamic circulation leading to increase in the diameter of the umbilical vein and intrahepatic portal vein.

- Presence of fluid collection in the various serous cavities. Pericardial space is the first site in immune hydrops. Abnormal if the pericardial thickness of fluid is >2 mm.
- *Ascites:* First feature is clear delineation of the intestinal loops due to presence of free fluid in between. Several mechanisms have been proposed for the development of fetal ascites:
  - Increased portal venous pressure
  - Decreased hepatic protein synthesis, due to disruption of hepatic architecture due to extramedullary hematopoiesis
  - Increased transudation into the peritoneal cavity
- Pleural effusion and diaphragmatic elevation due to hepatosplenomegaly and ascites may lead to pulmonary hypoplasia
- Skin edema—skin thickness >5 mm. Ideal site is the forehead while imaging the facial profile
- *Changes in the fetal heart:*
  - The right atrium is the first chamber to dilate due to increased venous return due to increased flow in the umbilical and portal veins. Subsequently this leads to right ventricular dilatation and subsequent tricuspid regurgitation. Finally, the left heart also dilates leading to generalized cardiomegaly.
  - Cardiomegaly is diagnosed when the cardiac circumference (CC)—thoracic circumference (TC) is >50% (normal CC: TC 33–50%)
- Placentomegaly—thickness >4 cm
- Polyhydramnios
- Hydrops presents as end-stage sign of fetal anemia and is observed once the hemoglobin deficit is 7g/dL below the mean for the gestational age. Usually below a hemoglobin of 4–6 gm%.

Fetal Blood Sampling

It is a direct access to the umbilical cord vessels by ultrasound-guided needle puncture and is done once the MCA-PSV increases to a range requiring intrauterine transfusion so as to document the exact hematocrit. Due to the extreme accuracy of MCA PSV in predicting fetal anemia, most centers perform cordocentesis simultaneous with intrauterine transfusion. Sample prior to transfusion is collected for hemoglobin/hematocrit and blood group.

■ TREATMENT OF IMMUNE HYDROPS AND FETAL ANEMIA

Intrauterine transfusion is the treatment of choice for fetal anemia. It is indicated if the MCA-PSV reaches above 1.5 MoM suggesting severe fetal anemia or development of immune hydrops or a fetal hematocrit of <30% at cordocentesis and the fetus is not mature enough to be delivered (<35 weeks). This intervention is more effective if started prior to development of hydrops.

Intraperitoneal Transfusion

Initially when high-resolution ultrasound was not available clinicians used the peritoneal cavity for transfusions. In non-hydropic fetus, the rate of absorption is estimated to be 10–15% per 24 hours. Absorption is slower if hydrops is evident. Because of the erratic absorption, especially in hydropic fetuses intravascular fetal transfusion has largely replaced the intraperitoneal technique.

However intraperitoneal transfusion is still indicated if the need for transfusion is early in gestation <18 weeks or if the direct access to cord is not feasible.

The volume calculated for transfusion: (Weeks of gestation–20) × 10.

Intravascular Transfusion

Two sites used for direct vascular access are intrahepatic portion of umbilical vein or the umbilical vein at the cord insertion site into the placenta **(Fig. 9)**. The procedure is done after detailed counseling of the couple regarding the technique, advantages, and risk. Pre-procedure tocolysis and antibiotic may be given. Operation theater may be kept standby in case of need for emergency LSCS, if bradycardia ensues. A paralyzing agent such as vecuronium/pancuronium may be given intramuscular in the fetal deltoid or intravascular to minimize fetal movements during transfusion.

Under ultrasound guidance intrauterine transfusion is done of double packed (hematocrit of 75–80%) fresh within 72 hours, O-negative blood, leukodepleted, CMV negative, gamma-irradiated, cross-matched with mothers blood into the intravascular (cord insertion site or hepatic portal vein), or intraperitoneal compartment. Volume of blood to be transfused is

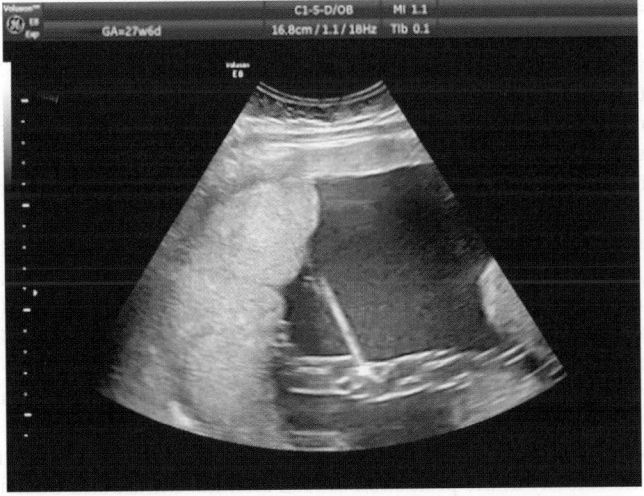

Fig. 9: Intrauterine intravascular transfusion.

calculated depending on the initial fetal hematocrit, donor hematocrit, and fetoplacental blood volume. A target hematocrit to be achieved at the end of procedure is 40–50%.

In experienced hands, intrauterine transfusion is considered relatively safe with survival rates of about 90% for red cell alloimmunization.[16] However, the procedure related loss rate is 1–3% and includes preterm labor, premature rupture of membranes, cord hematoma, fetal bradycardia, cardiac overload, infection, fetomaternal bleed, and fetal demise.[17] Post-transfusion follow-up is done using MCA-PSV. Repeat transfusion is usually required in 1–2 weeks and is calculated by a 1% drop of hematocrit per day from the final post-transfusion hematocrit or when MCA-PSV reaches 1.5 MoM again.

Intrauterine transfusion to the fetus is a top-up transfusion done for temporary correction of anemia so as to prevent or reverse the sequel of anemia in-utero. In short, it helps to buy time till the baby is mature to be delivered. Intrauterine transfusion of blood to these anemic fetuses is one of the best fetal therapies available with extremely good results.

■ CONCLUSION

Hydrops fetalis is challenging to evaluate and manage, however if approached meticulously one can achieve best outcome for treatable causes and/or determine cause/recurrence for the ones with poor prognosis.

■ REFERENCES

1. The Fetal Medicine Foundation. Hydrops Fetalis. [online] Available from https://fetalmedicine.org/education/fetal-abnormalities/hydrops-fetalis-1/overview [Last accessed December, 2023].
2. Bellini C, Hennekam RC, Fulcheri E, Rutigliani M, Morcaldi G, Boccardo F, et al. Etiology of nonimmune hydrops fetalis: a systematic review. Am J Med Genet Part A. 2009;149(5):844-51.
3. Vanaparthy R, Mahdy H. Hydrops fetalis. In: StatPearls. 2022. StatPearls Publishing.
4. Jauniaux E. Diagnosis and management of early non-immune hydrops fetalis. Prenat Diagn. 1997;17(13):1261-8.
5. Radiopaedia. (2021). Placental Thickness [online]. Available from radiopaedia.org/articles/placental-thickness [Last accessed December, 2023].
6. Society for Maternal-Fetal Medicine (SMFM). Electronic address: pubs@smfm.org, Dashe JS, Pressman EK, Hibbard JU. SMFM Consult Series #46: Evaluation and management of polyhydramnios. Am J Obstet Gynecol. 2018;219(4):B2-8.
7. Nakayama A, Oshiro M, Yamada Y, Hattori T, Wakano Y, Hayashi S, et al. Prognostic factors of hydrops fetalis with pleural effusion. Pediatr Int. 2017;59(10):1053-7.
8. Shenker L, Reed KL, Anderson CF, Kern W. Fetal pericardial effusion. Am J Obstet Gynecol. 1989;160(6):1505-7; discussion 1507-8.
9. Teixeira JM, Duncan K, Letsky E, Fisk NM. Middle cerebral artery peak systolic velocity in the prediction of fetal anemia. Ultrasound Obstet Gynecol. 2000;15(3):205-8.

10. Abdelshafi S, Okasha A, Elsirgany S, Khalil A, El-Dessouky S, AbdelHakim N, et al. Peak systolic velocity of fetal middle cerebral artery to predict anemia in Red Cell Alloimmunization in un-transfused and transfused fetuses. Eur J Obstet Gynecol Reprod Biol. 2021;258:437-42.
11. Hernandez-Andrade E, Scheier M, Dezerega V, Carmo A, Nicolaides KH. Fetal middle cerebral artery peak systolic velocity in the investigation of non-immune hydrops. Ultrasound Obstet Gynecol. 2004;23(5):442-5.
12. An X, Wang J, Zhuang X, Dai J, Lu C, Li X, et al. Clinical features of neonates with hydrops fetalis. Am J Perinatol. 2015;32(13):1231-9.
13. Thammavong K, Luewan S, Wanapirak C, Tongsong T. Ultrasound features of fetal anemia lessons from hemoglobin Bart disease. J Ultrasound Med. 2021;40(4):659-74.
14. Hofstaetter C, Hansmann M, Eik-Nes SH, Huhta JC, Luther SL. A cardiovascular profile score in the surveillance of fetal hydrops. J Matern Fetal Neonatal Med. 2006;19(7):407-13.
15. Society for Maternal-Fetal Medicine (SMFM), Norton ME, Chauhan SP, Dashe JS. Society for maternal-fetal medicine (SMFM) clinical guideline #7: nonimmune hydrops fetalis. Am J Obstet Gynecol. 2015;212(2):127-39.
16. Alkhaibary A, Ali M, Tulbah M, Al-Nemer M, Khan RM, Al Mugbel M, et al. Complications of intravascular intrauterine transfusion for Rh-alloimmunization. Ann Saudi Med. 2021;41(6):313-7.
17. Van Kamp IL, Klumper FJ, Oepkes D, Meerman RH, Scherjon SA, Vandenbussche FP, et al. Complications of intrauterine intravascular transfusion for fetal anemia due to maternal red-cell alloimmunization. Am J Obstet Gynecol. 2005;192(1):171-7.

CHAPTER 10

Social Egg Freezing

Nandita Palshetkar

■ INTRODUCTION

The range of assisted reproductive technology (ART) has significantly expanded since the birth of Louise Brown in 1978. Embryo and sperm cryopreservation are established treatments, however oocyte cryopreservation has only recently become available as an extra fertility preservation option for women.[1]

Female fertility experiences a gradual but considerable drop beyond the age of 32 years, with the decline accelerating after the age of 35 years. The primary reason for the drop in fertility associated with age is the reduction in the number of follicles and the decline in the quality of oocytes, which increases the likelihood of fetal chromosomal disorders and subsequent fetal loss.[2]

For several unmarried ladies who are advancing in age, the biological clock symbolizes a significant menace that endangers the potential of conceiving a biological offspring. Typically, the prospect of "running out of time" causes significant pressure for individuals, typically accompanied by additional social pressure and criticism from their surroundings. Cryopreserving oocytes presents a promising possibility to relieve this burden, contingent upon the emergence of a suitable partner. Oocyte cryopreservation is becoming increasingly popular since it enhances a woman's confidence in her capacity to conceive biological children of her own.[3]

Elective egg freezing does not ensure the ability to conceive, but it empowers women to have greater control over their reproductive potential.[4]

■ TERMINOLOGY

Oocyte cryopreservation, often known as "social egg freezing", is a widely used method for women to delay pregnancy and safeguard their fertility.

Currently, there is a lack of consensus over the terminology.

The phrase "social egg freezing" refers to the socioeconomic limitations that prompt women to undergo oocyte cryopreservation, although "elective egg freezing" is generally deemed acceptable by the majority of women. Some authors opt to utilize the term "fertility preservation" due to its proven usage in the realm of gamete cryopreservation for medical purposes. As a result, the practice of "nonmedical egg freezing" or "egg freezing for nonmedical purposes" emerged. Some argued against the use of "nonmedical freezing" as it was not deemed suitable. They claimed that the decision to cryopreserve oocytes for the purpose of safeguarding women against age-related fertility decrease should be regarded as a form of preventative medical treatment. The authors proposed the term "AGE banking" (oocyte banking for anticipated gamete exhaustion) as a more accurate description of the method to predict gamete exhaustion. Other terms commonly used to refer to social egg freezing include "planned oocyte cryopreservation", "oocyte cryopreservation for age-related fertility loss", and "elective egg freezing".[5]

■ SOCIAL VERSUS MEDICAL EGG FREEZING

Medical egg freezing refers to the use of egg freezing techniques for medical purposes, such as oncofertility. In many countries, the acceptance of certain behaviors is influenced by the perception that they are related to a condition and medically essential. This perception grants individuals a morally valid justification to seek and utilize these services.[5]

Social egg freezing refers to the practice of freezing eggs for nonmedical purposes. A primary incentive for healthy women opting for social egg freezing is their absence of a stable relationship or other significant milestones they deem necessary prior to starting a family. Some individuals view social egg freezing as contentious due to its artificial nature, potential concerns for women's health, and the medicalization of a societal issue. Social egg freezing is widely recognized as a rapidly expanding assisted reproductive technology in Europe, the UK, and other global regions, notwithstanding the debates surrounding it.[5]

■ PROCEDURE

Egg freezing is a procedure that entails the use of hormones to stimulate the ovaries, followed by the retrieval of a woman's eggs through the vagina. These eggs are then frozen and stored for future use. Vitrification, a flash-freezing technique, is the preferred method for egg freezing since it has shown higher rates of oocyte survival after thawing and greater chances of conception. This approach is approved by professional medical societies. Vitrification is a process that utilizes cryoprotectants and extremely fast cooling to harden cells, preventing the creation of ice crystals.[6]

Controlled Ovarian Stimulation Protocol and Oocyte Retrieval

The ovarian stimulation protocols consist of the gonadotropin-releasing hormone (GnRH) antagonist protocol, progestin-primed ovarian stimulation (PPOS) protocol, short GnRH agonist protocol, and long GnRH agonist protocol. Serum levels of follicular stimulating hormone, luteinizing hormone, and estradiol are assessed on either day 2 or day 3 of the menstrual cycle. The levels of hormones and the diameters of follicles are monitored on either day 5 or day 6 of stimulation, as well as on the following days. Oocyte final maturation is initiated when the size of two follicles reaches 18 mm and the estradiol level reaches around 150 pg/mL per follicle. The oocyte retrieval procedure is scheduled to take place 34–36 hours after triggering.[7]

Oocyte Denudation and Oocyte Freezing

Following retrieval, the oocytes are stripped of their surrounding cells, a process known as denudation, and subsequently examined to determine their maturity status. The oocytes are cryopreserved 2 hours after they are retrieved. Both metaphase II (MII) and metaphase I (MI) oocytes have been cryopreserved. Following a consultation with the patient, the remaining immature oocytes are cryopreserved. There are two methods for freezing oocytes—gradual freezing and vitrification. The cryopreserved oocytes are stored in cryogenic tanks filled with liquid nitrogen until the patients' subsequent visits.[7]

Oocyte Thawing

The Kitazato thawing kit (manufactured by Kitazato Supply Corporation) is utilized for vitrified oocytes. The Cryotop vitrification device, manufactured by Kitazato Supply Corporation, is put directly into the thawing solution and remains stationary for a duration of 1 minute. Following detachment from the Cryotop, the oocytes undergo a 3-minute treatment with the diluent solution, followed by a 5-minute treatment with the washing solution. Subsequently, they were transferred to the fundamental solution at a temperature of 20ºC during a time frame of 1 minute. The oocytes are placed in the human tubal fluid culture medium and kept at a temperature of 37ºC till insemination.[7]

Insemination, Embryo Culture, and Transfer

Fertilization is achieved by utilizing the matured oocytes that have endured a 3-hour incubation period. The chosen fertilization technique is intracytoplasmic sperm injection (ICSI). The initial examination of the embryos is performed 16–18 hours after ICSI. A normally fertilized embryo is characterized by the presence of two pronuclei (2PN) and a second polar body. An embryo culture is conducted using a sequential culture medium. The patients are engaged in discussions regarding the quantity and timing of embryo transfer, which are determined by the quality of the embryos. If blastocyst formation is detected, the remaining embryos are cultivated and then preserved through vitrification.[7]

■ OPTIMAL TIMING OF OOCYTE CRYOPRESERVATION

Strategies to improve the clinical and ethical aspects of social freezing involve three distinct steps—raising public awareness, providing personalized, age-specific information and counseling, and offering predictive tests such as anti-Müllerian hormone measurements or antral follicle count. The primary goal of these efforts is to persuade women who are most likely to gain advantages from social freezing to seek medical attention before reaching the age of 35 years. Additionally, these measures aim to deter fertility clinics from explicitly focusing on women who have already exceeded the age at which favorable outcomes can be anticipated.[8]

Effective counseling should inform women that freezing their oocytes does not guarantee protection against age-related infertility, but rather provides an additional chance at conception.[2]

■ OPTIMAL NUMBER OF EGGS TO FREEZE

An additional significant concern pertains to the quantity of eggs to be preserved in order to ensure the possibility of conceiving at least one offspring. Determining the optimal number of oocytes is a complex task due to various aspects such as maternal age, maternal health, ovarian reserve, reproductive objectives, and paternal health. There is no amount of oocytes that can provide a guarantee. Most clinics advise the preservation of approximately 20 eggs, necessitating multiple procedures for the majority of women. According to two American prediction models that focus on in vitro fertilization (IVF)/ICSI treatments, it is estimated that around 20 oocytes are required to have a 75% chance of successfully having at least one kid, as long as the mother is under the age of 38 years. The models also demonstrate that the likelihood of success is strongly influenced by age and validate that the endeavor of preserving fertility in women beyond the age of 40 years is improbable to be successful.[4]

For women under the age of 35 years, freezing 8 or 10 oocytes resulted in a 40.8% or 60.5% chance of a successful live delivery per warmed oocyte, respectively. In order to have a reasonable possibility of achieving a pregnancy, it is necessary to have a minimum of 8–10 cryopreserved oocytes.[2]

■ CHANCE OF HAVING A CHILD

An appropriate inquiry pertains to the probability of conceiving a child. Prior research has demonstrated that frozen eggs are comparable in quality to fresh ones. However, there is a lack of conclusive evidence about the success rates of nonmedical elective egg freezing in achieving pregnancy. Primarily, we have heavily depended on results obtained from traditional IVF procedures. However, there is now emerging data regarding the utilization of egg freezing techniques.[4]

Cobo et al., reported on a cohort of 137 women out of a total of 1,468 who underwent autologous IVF and subsequently returned for follow-up. A total of 9% of the women who froze eggs did so for elective purposes, encompassing both medical and nonmedical motivations. The overall pregnancy success rate, measured as the cumulative ongoing pregnancy rate/live birth rate (OPR/LBR) per patient, was about 60%.[4]

■ BENEFITS

The process of social egg freezing offers two significant advantages to women who plan on conceiving at a later stage in life—it grants them the opportunity to become a biological parent by utilizing their frozen and thawed eggs, and it diminishes the likelihood of having offspring with chromosomal abnormalities linked to ovarian aneuploidy.

The potential advantages of oocyte vitrification include increased fertility preservation at younger ages for several reasons:
- Enhanced success rates;
- Reduced number of unsuccessful IVF cycles caused by advanced maternal age, thereby minimizing emotional and financial distress; and
- Decreased reliance on donor oocytes if women freeze and store their own eggs.[3]

■ RISKS

Medical Risks of Social Egg Freezing and In Vitro Fertilization

The primary medical hazards linked with egg freezing are primarily attributed to ovarian stimulation, notably ovarian hyperstimulation syndrome. Mild-to-moderate ovarian hyperstimulation syndrome is characterized by symptoms such as fatigue, nausea, headaches, abdominal pain, breast tenderness, and irritability. However, these negative consequences may typically be effectively managed. Nevertheless, a small percentage of people, ranging from 0.1 to 2%, may encounter a severe condition known as ovarian hyperstimulation syndrome. This condition can lead to the formation of blood clots, difficulty breathing, abdominal pain, dehydration, and vomiting, which require hospitalization.

Women who undergo the process of using their frozen-thawed eggs to produce pregnancy will be exposed to the potential hazards associated with IVF. The hazards encompass the occurrence of numerous pregnancies, pregnancy-induced hypertension, preterm birth, cesarean delivery, and infants with low birth weight.[6]

Medical Risks of Pregnancy at an Advanced Age

Women who inquire about social egg freezing should be informed about the medical hazards to themselves and their potential kids that are linked to pregnancy at an advanced age, namely when the projected birth occurs after the age of 35 years.[6]

Women who conceive at a later stage in life face a higher likelihood of developing gestational diabetes, preeclampsia, requiring a cesarean delivery, and delivering a baby prematurely with low birth weight. Nevertheless, the extent of these dangers differs significantly, contingent upon the woman's health condition, and escalates with the advancing age of the mother at the time of childbirth.[6]

It is important to note that elective oocyte cryopreservation for nonmedical purposes does not mitigate the risk of maternal morbidity in women who conceive at an advanced age. Indeed, advanced maternal age is correlated with an increased likelihood of ectopic pregnancy and various problems such as preeclampsia, gestational diabetes, premature delivery, and low birth weight. Hence, it is imperative to enforce obligatory counseling for women who choose to cryopreserve oocytes, in order to inform them about the potential hazards associated with pregnancy at a later stage of life. The absence of significant obstetric and perinatal hazards in pregnancies resulting from the use of frozen oocytes is a reassuring indication that oocyte cryopreservation is not associated with any negative effects. Furthermore, the extended freezing of oocytes in liquid nitrogen does not have any impact on the success rates of IVF or the rate of having a normal number of chromosomes (euploidy).[2]

Risks to Offspring

Aside from the negative consequences related to premature birth and low birth weight, there is evidence indicating a slight rise in the likelihood of congenital structural abnormalities in children born through IVF. Furthermore, certain studies suggest that these children may have a small yet elevated risk of developing cancer and structural cardiac anomalies. Additional investigation is required to validate the hazards posed to offspring born through IVF and ascertain whether there are any special concerns linked with births resulting from cryopreserved eggs. The number is six.

Due to the new development of the vitrification technology, there is currently a lack of data regarding the long-term monitoring of children who have had this procedure. It is important to mention that variations in the levels of potentially harmful cryoprotectants lead to a theoretically distinct risk assessment following vitrification, in comparison to the traditional slow-freezing method.[9]

■ USE OF STORED OOCYTES

There is limited data available regarding the proportion of women who utilize their cryopreserved oocytes. The metric in question is referred to as the "usage rate", and it serves as a crucial concern for the practice of egg freezing for nonmedical purposes. Four survey-based studies have examined follow-up data on individuals working in the banking industry. One study revealed that just 50.8% of women who froze their eggs believed they would utilize them in the future. After 3 years, 29.2% of the women found it less probable to use cryopreserved oocytes compared to when they were frozen. This was related to their age range of 33–41 years at the time of vitrification and having recovered 6–20 oocytes. Out of these, only three women achieved successful conception of a child. According to a separate poll of 23 women, it was found that just two women had utilized their cryopreserved eggs at the time of the interview, and one of them successfully gave birth to a live baby. Noteworthy findings from these studies encompass the inclination to provide surplus oocytes for research purposes or to assist other women in infertility treatment. It is crucial to acknowledge that the afore-mentioned stance was taken at the time of their oocyte cryopreservation, but attitudes about donation may evolve with time.[2]

■ SOCIAL AND ETHICAL IMPLICATIONS

As previously mentioned, the term "social" is used to characterize the component of the medical strategy that is related to social interactions. Egg freezing serves as a means to counteract decreasing fertility rates and provide optimism for future families, representing the realization of an innate reproductive instinct.[2]

Oocyte cryopreservation can provide the possibility of having a biological child in the future, alleviating feelings of uncertainty, such as anxiety and tension. It also offers women the flexibility to make choices and ensures that any decision they make will be appropriate. Many women view oocyte cryopreservation as a potential solution for a future need, if they have established a stable family with a dependable and trustworthy spouse. In contrast, critics contend that this type of regulation incentivizes women to prioritize their careers at the expense of their families. Both of these stances demonstrate distinct perspectives on autonomy, with one advocating for social egg freezing as a suitable response to the broader social environment, while the other suggesting a potential diminishment of decision-making authority. Put simply, the conversation pertains to the concept of relational autonomy as it applies to decision-making. Human beings are inherently social creatures, and as such, they are never completely autonomous. Critics argue that this lack of complete independence results in a diminished ability to make individual decisions. The social backdrop, encompassing political and cultural factors, has the ability to influence decisions in one direction or another.

Psychological Impact

It is crucial to provide women with accurate information regarding the current uncertainty regarding the effectiveness and safety of using their oocytes for reproductive purposes in the future. It is important for them to understand that the approach does not provide a guarantee of success, regardless of the quantity of preserved oocytes.[9,10]

■ CONCLUSION

Additional knowledge regarding fertility challenges and potential solutions for age-related infertility is valuable not only for delaying parenthood, but also for achieving a more definite and deliberate reproductive independence. This is desirable regardless of career demands and limited support services, in order to promote responsible parenting. Nevertheless, this information processing must also consider other equally significant considerations involving the potential creation of elevated and potentially inaccurate expectations, as well as the introduction of medical procedures to women of reproductive age.[11,12]

■ REFERENCES

1. Argyle CE, Harper JC, Davies MC. Oocyte cryopreservation: where are we now? Hum Reprod Update. 2016;22(4):440-9.
2. Alteri A, Pisaturo V, Nogueira D, D'Angelo A. Elective egg freezing without medical indications. Acta Obstet Gynecol Scand. 2019;98(5):647-52.
3. Cobo A, García-Velasco JA, Coello A, Domingo J, Pellicer A, Remohí J. Oocyte vitrification as an efficient option for elective fertility preservation. Fertil Steril. 2016;105(3):755-64.
4. Wennberg AL. Social freezing of oocytes: a means to take control of your fertility. Ups J Med Sci. 2020;125(2):95-8.
5. De Proost M, Paton A. Medical versus social egg freezing: The importance of future choice for women's decision-making. Monash Bioeth Rev. 2022;40(2):145-56.
6. Petropanagos A, Cattapan A, Baylis F, Leader A. Social egg freezing: risk, benefits and other considerations. CMAJ. 2015;187(9):666-9.
7. Yang IJ, Wu MY, Chao KH, Wei SY, Tsai YY, Huang TC, et al. Usage and cost-effectiveness of elective oocyte freezing: a retrospective observational study. Reprod Biol Endocrinol. 2022;20(1):123.
8. Mertes H, Pennings G. Social egg freezing: for better, not for worse. Reprod Biomed Online. 2011;23(7):824-9.
9. Soop D. Social oocyte freezing. Facts Views Vis Obgyn. 2010;2(1):31-4.
10. Wennberg AL, Schildauer K, Brännström M. Elective oocyte freezing for nonmedical reasons: a 6-year report on utilization and in vitro fertilization results from a Swedish center. Acta Obstet Gynecol Scand. 2019;98(11):1429-34.
11. Tozzo P, Fassina A, Nespeca P, Spigarolo G, Caenazzo L. Understanding social oocyte freezing in Italy: a scoping survey on university female students' awareness and attitudes. Life Sci Soc Policy. 2019;15(1):3.
12. Inhorn MC. The egg freezing revolution? Gender, technology, and fertility preservation in the twenty-first century. In: Emerging Trends in the Social and Behavioral Sciences. Hoboken, NJ: John Wiley and Sons; 2017. pp. 1-4.

Ovarian Tissue Cryopreservation

CHAPTER

Rohan Palshetkar, Nandita Palshetkar, Manisha Nandi

■ INTRODUCTION

Ovarian tissue cryopreservation (OTC) can be offered as an alternative to preserve fertility in young patients at risk of premature ovarian insufficiency (POI). The clinical application was supported by large animal experimentations in the 1990's demonstrating the efficacy of the procedure to restore ovarian function and fertility. OTC is still considered as experimental in many countries, and legislations and regulations vary. However, recently the American Society for Reproductive Medicine (ASRM) suggested to consider it as an established option for selected patients [Practice Committee of the American Society for Reproductive Medicine (2019)].

The OTC technique has the advantages of being feasible within a short timeframe in both post- and pre-pubertal patients and does not require any preceding drug treatment. The success of the procedure was demonstrated several years after first storage, and its use as an alternative to oocyte/embryo cryopreservation (or in combination) has developed rapidly over the last two decades.[1]

■ PATIENT SELECTION

Patient selection criteria and indications vary by center offering OTC. Formalized recommendations regarding the indications for OTC, i.e., the Edinburgh criteria included:
- Patients younger than 35 years old with >50% of risk of chemotherapy-induced ovarian failure

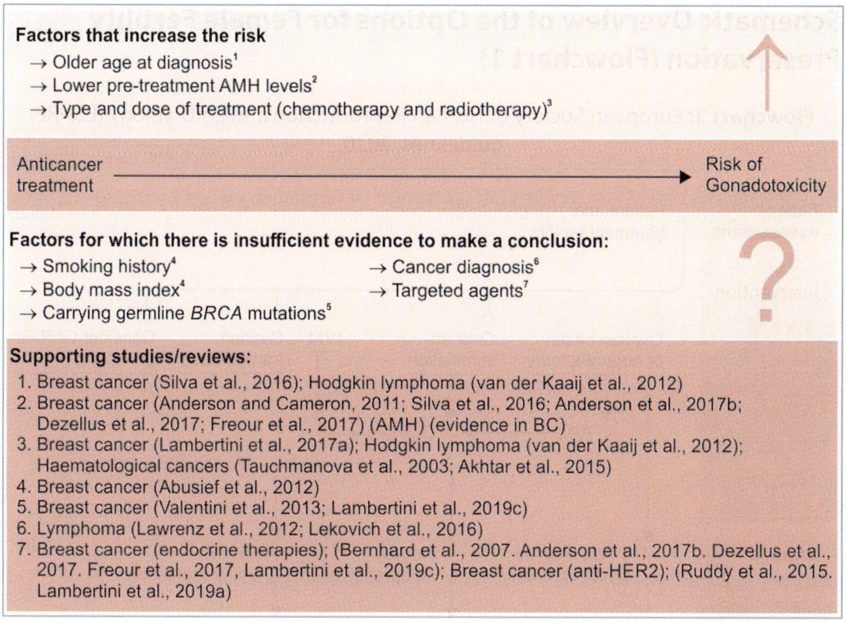

Factors that increase the risk
- → Older age at diagnosis[1]
- → Lower pre-treatment AMH levels[2]
- → Type and dose of treatment (chemotherapy and radiotherapy)[3]

Anticancer treatment ⟶ Risk of Gonadotoxicity

Factors for which there is insufficient evidence to make a conclusion:
- → Smoking history[4]
- → Body mass index[4]
- → Carrying germline *BRCA* mutations[5]
- → Cancer diagnosis[6]
- → Targeted agents[7]

Supporting studies/reviews:
1. Breast cancer (Silva et al., 2016); Hodgkin lymphoma (van der Kaaij et al., 2012)
2. Breast cancer (Anderson and Cameron, 2011; Silva et al., 2016; Anderson et al., 2017b; Dezellus et al., 2017; Freour et al., 2017) (AMH) (evidence in BC)
3. Breast cancer (Lambertini et al., 2017a); Hodgkin lymphoma (van der Kaaij et al., 2012); Haematological cancers (Tauchmanova et al., 2003; Akhtar et al., 2015)
4. Breast cancer (Abusief et al., 2012)
5. Breast cancer (Valentini et al., 2013; Lambertini et al., 2019c)
6. Lymphoma (Lawrenz et al., 2012; Lekovich et al., 2016)
7. Breast cancer (endocrine therapies); (Bernhard et al., 2007. Anderson et al., 2017b. Dezellus et al., 2017. Freour et al., 2017, Lambertini et al., 2019c); Breast cancer (anti-HER2); (Ruddy et al., 2015. Lambertini et al., 2019a)

Fig. 1: Factors to be considered when estimating the risk of gonadotoxicity.[2]

- No previous gonadotoxic treatment
- No surgical contraindication and a realistic chance of survival

The Oncofertility Consortium Consensus Statement (US) recommends:
- The procedure for patients aged up to 42 years who could or did not want to cryopreserve oocytes or embryos.

Practice Committee of the American Society for Reproductive Medicine

- Ovarian tissue cryopreservation is no longer considered to be experimental and can be used in prepubertal patients when there is no time for ovarian stimulation.
- Ovarian transposition may be offered to patients undergoing pelvic radiation **(Fig. 1)**.

Schematic Overview of the Options for Female Fertility Preservation (Flowchart 1)

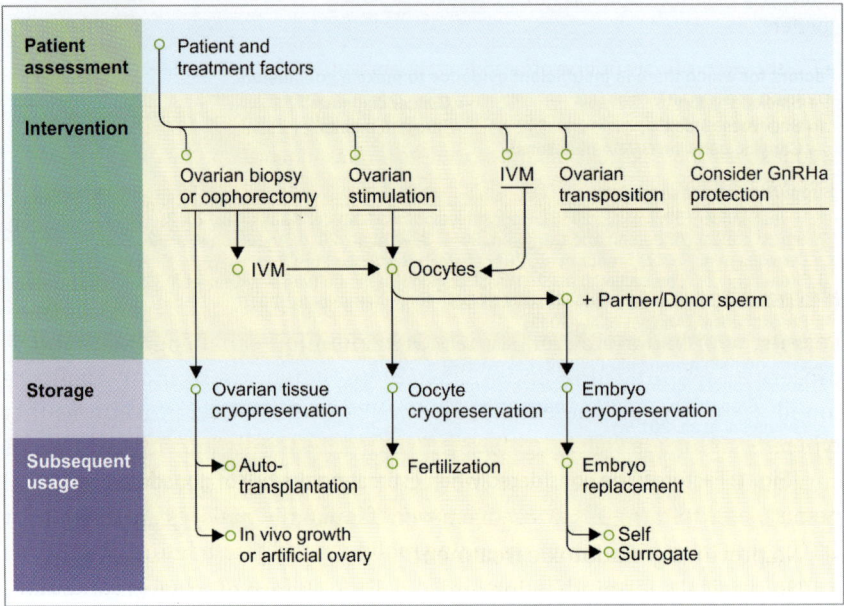

Flowchart 1: European Society of Human Reproduction and Embryology (ESHRE) guidelines, 2020.

SPECIAL CLINICAL CONSIDERATIONS FOR OVARIAN TISSUE CRYOPRESERVATION (TABLE 1)

Breast Cancer

While standard ovarian stimulation (employing injectable gonadotropins) is a reasonable choice, providers may wish to offer treatment incorporating coadministration of aromatase inhibitors to decrease circulating estrogen levels or tamoxifen as an estrogen-receptor blocker. Breast cancer patients who are not comfortable with the potential impact of COS on their disease or who lack sufficient time to undergo oocyte retrieval may be candidates for IVM or ovarian tissue-preservation protocols.

Gynecological Malignancies

Early-stage disease should be eligible for procedures that preserve reproductive potential by way of fertility sparing surgery, oophoropexy, and/or egg/embryo cryopreservation. The success depends on the diagnosis and treatment (97–100). If a hysterectomy is performed, these patients should be counseled regarding surrogacy.

TABLE 1: Recommendations: European Society of Human Reproduction and Embryology (ESHRE), 2020.

It is recommended to offer OTC in patients undergoing moderate/high-risk gonadotoxic treatment where oocyte/embryo cryopreservation is not feasible, or at patient preference	STRONG	⊕OOO
OTC should probably not be offered to patients with low ovarian reserve (AMH <0.5 ng/mL and AFC <5) or advanced age considering the unfavorable risk/benefit. Current evidence suggest that the efficiency of OTC procedure is questionable >36 years of age	WEAK	⊕OOO

Hematological Malignancies

Patients with hematologic disorders present unique challenges to fertility-preservation counseling and management. Often, these individuals are too ill at diagnosis to be eligible for fertility-preservation procedures that typically require a delay in therapy of days to weeks and involve minor surgical procedures that pose increased risks in patients with abnormal hematologic parameters. Moreover, even if leukemic patients are eligible for OTC, there is concern about reseeding malignant cells with future autologous transplantation of tissue. While patients with lymphoma are better candidates for fertility-preservation techniques, initial therapies do not have a substantial risk of gonadotoxicity.

Children and Adolescents

Ovarian tissue cryopreservation is currently the only way to cryopreserve gametes in prepubertal girls. Working with these individuals and their parents requires an approach that is sensitive to various levels of physical and psychological development. Given that this is a particularly vulnerable population, careful counseling and informed consent are especially required.[3]

KEY TECHNICAL ASPECTS OF OVARIAN TISSUE CRYOPRESERVATION

- It is necessary to have appropriate equipment, quality control and training for the healthcare team before performing OTC.
- Local legal aspects should also be taken into account, including the need for ethical approval.
- Laparoscopy caries a low-risk (in healthy women) and is considered as the standard surgical procedure to collect ovarian tissue. However, patients referred for OTC may have an increased risk of surgical complications.

- It is possible to perform the laparoscopy in the referring center and transport the tissue under strict conditions for up to 20 hours before processing.
- Both unilateral oophorectomy and biopsy are acceptable for collecting ovarian tissue.
- The choice will depend on the patient's characteristics, their scheduled treatments, and available expertise in the center.
- In the majority of patients, the removal of two-thirds of the ovarian cortex surface from one ovary is sufficient to achieve pregnancy.[2]

■ OVARIAN TISSUE CRYOPRESERVATION PROCEDURE

Either an ovarian cortex biopsy (the location of the primordial follicle pool) or one whole ovary can be retrieved at any time during the menstrual cycle and the cortex is cryopreserved for future restoration of ovarian function. Several centers perform ovarian biopsy (1/3 to 2/3 of one ovary), while others routinely perform unilateral oophorectomy. Oophorectomy by single-incision laparoscopic surgery was shown not to be inferior to standard 2- or 3-port laparoscopy in terms of complication rate, duration of the procedure, hospital stay, and delay to start chemotherapy.

For ovarian biopsy, large fragments of cortex at a distance from the hilum and from any large visible follicles or corpus luteum should be harvested and careful hemostasis should be achieved after tissue removal. An advantage is to maintain two ovarian sites for future transplantation and to limit the invasiveness of the procedure, given the uncertainty over loss of ovarian function from the proposed chemotherapy in many cases **(Fig. 2)**.

Vitrification versus Slow-freezing

The protocol most widely used for ovarian cryopreservation is slow-freezing and rapid thawing of the ovarian tissue. Vitrification has been widely implemented in fertility laboratories as a standard method for the cryopreservation of embryos and oocytes and has been suggested as an alternative technique for OTC. Vitrification has several potential advantages, as it avoids cell damage induced by ice formation, it is less time-consuming, and it does not require an expensive controlled rate freezer **(Table 2)**.

■ REPLACING OVARIAN TISSUE: SAFETY ISSUES

- Surgical complications
- Risk of reintroducing malignancy
- Oncological outcomes in hormonal-sensitive diseases
- Risk for offspring.
- Long-term risk of ovarian tissue transplantation (OTT)

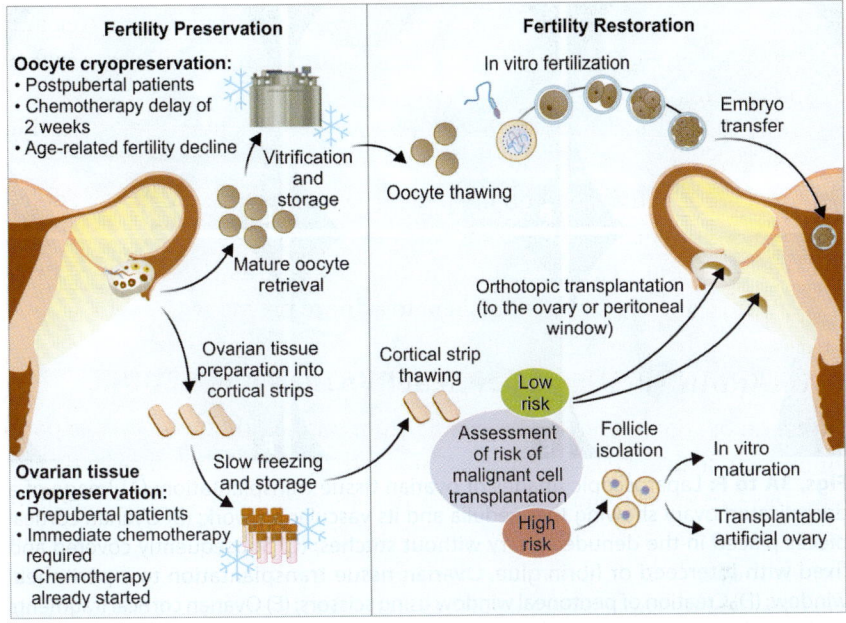

Fig. 2: Ovarian tissue freezing and transpostition.

TABLE 2: Current recommendations.		
The slow-freezing protocol should be used for OTC as it is well-established and considered as standard	STRONG	⊕OOO
Vitrification of ovarian tissue should only be offered within a research program	RESEARCH ONLY	
For ovarian tissue transplantation (OTT), a one-step laparoscopy procedure should be performed as it is considered safe without causing additional surgical risk	STRONG	⊕⊕OO
OTT at the orthotopic site is recommended to restore fertility	STRONG	⊕⊕OO

Surgical Technique

Ovarian tissue transplantation at the orthotopic site, either on the remaining ovaries or in the nearby peritoneal site, is usually performed by laparoscopy, and more rarely by mini-laparotomy, under general anesthesia. The transplantation procedure is usually performed in one-step laparoscopy using standard or robot-assisted techniques. A two-step laparoscopy (1-week interval) to prepare the transplantation site and induce neovascularization has been proposed, but is not widely used, and there is no evidence for the superiority of the two-step procedure in terms of ovarian function recovery and pregnancy rate **(Figs. 3A to F)**.[2]

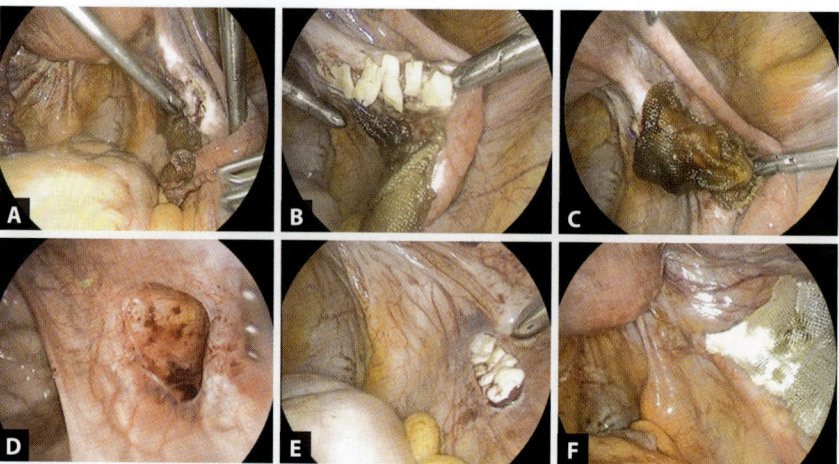

Figs. 3A to F: Laparoscopic images of ovarian tissue transplantation: (A) Image of a decorticated ovary showing the medulla and its vascular network; (B) Ovarian cortical pieces placed in the denuded ovary without stitches; (C) Subsequently covered and fixed with Interceed or fibrin glue. Ovarian tissue transplantation to a peritoneal window; (D) Creation of peritoneal window using scissors; (E) Ovarian cortical fragments positioned with the cortex surface facing the abdominal cavity; (F) Covered and fixed with Interceed of fibrin glue.[4]

Risk of Reintroducing Malignancy

Ovarian metastases have been reported in >20% of female autopsies from non-gynecological malignancies, both hematological, and solid tumors. In cancer patients, the risk of the presence of residual cancer cells in the cortex should always be carefully evaluated using the most sensitive techniques, according to the disease. These may include immunohistology, molecular markers and/or a xenograft model when available. Before OTT, the patient should be in good health and free of the disease for a sufficient period which will vary according to the type of cancer and the stage. Information regarding the oncological follow-up should be reported at least during 2 years after OTT in order to evaluate the involvement of grafted ovarian tissue in a possible relapse (Andersen, et al., 2018).

Ovarian and Adnexal Tumors (Tables 3 and 4)

Ovarian tissue transplantation is not recommended in patients treated for borderline ovarian tumor (BOT) or ovarian cancer. BOT is bilateral at diagnosis in 15–40% of the cases and if the disease is unilateral at diagnosis, the risk of recurrence in the contralateral ovary remains high.

TABLE 3: Summary of Guideline Development Group (GDG) recommendations for specific patient groups.

Disease	Considerations for OTC/OTT	Recommendation for OTT
Ovarian or adnexal tumor	Ovarian tissue cryopreservation (OTC) should only be carried out after careful consideration, when other options are not feasible, bearing in mind that replacement may not be available to the patient in the foreseeable future due to the high risk of recurrence and the risk of cryopreserved ovarian tissue involvement	Ovarian tissue transplantation (OTT) is *probably not recommended* considering the high risk of ovarian tissue involvement. The safety of OTT with removal after pregnancy needs to be further investigated
Leukemia	Ovarian tissue should ideally be collected at the time of complete bone marrow remission (after first chemotherapy regimen) and it should be tested using molecular detection techniques before OTT. If molecular markers are not available, xenograft experiments should be performed	OTT should be considered with *extreme caution* considering the high risk of ovarian involvement by leukemia cells. Additional data are needed regarding the safety of OTT
Tumors of the central nervous system (CNS)	• Data are limited regarding the risk of reintroducing the disease in patients treated for CNS tumors • Medulloblastoma and neuroblastoma are considered at higher risk	OTT should be considered with *extreme caution*. Additional data are needed regarding the safety of OTT
Non-Hodgkin lymphoma	OTC/OTT can be performed in patients with non-Hodgkin lymphoma with no evidence of distant metastasis or pelvic involvement at diagnosis	OTT appears to be *safe* if pelvic involvement is excluded at diagnosis. OTT can be considered after appropriate ovarian tissue testing using histology and molecular approaches when available
Hodgkin lymphoma	OTC/OTT appears to be safe in patients with Hodgkin lymphoma when pelvic involvement was excluded at diagnosis	OTT appears to be *safe* if ovarian involvement is excluded at diagnosis. OTT can be considered after appropriate ovarian tissue testing using histology

Contd...

Contd...

Disease	Considerations for OTC/OTT	Recommendation for OTT
Cervical tumors	Ovarian involvement is rare at diagnosis, and more frequent in adenocarcinoma than in squamous cell carcinoma	OTT appears to be *safe* in patients treated with fertility-spearing strategy although more data are requested regarding the risk of ovarian tissue involvement in patients after OTC
Other solid tumors	OTC/OTT appears to be safe in patients with solid tumor such as sarcoma, breast cancer, gastrointestinal, and colorectal malignancies when distant metastasis and pelvic involvement was excluded at diagnosis	OTT appears to be *safe* in nonmetastatic disease at OCT. OTT can be considered after appropriate ovarian tissue testing, using histology and molecular markers when available

TABLE 4: Recommendations: European Society of Human Reproduction and Embryology (ESHRE), 2020.

The decision to perform ovarian tissue transplantation (OTT) in oncological patients requires a multidisciplinary approach	GPP	
It is recommended to evaluate the presence of residual neoplastic cells in the ovarian cortex (and in the residual medulla when available) using appropriate techniques in all cancer survivors before OTT and patients should be informed about this risk	STRONG	⊕OOO
OTT is not recommended in cases where the ovary is involved in the malignancy	STRONG	⊕OOO
OTT and pregnancy can be considered in hormone-sensitive tumors such as endometrial cancer treated by fertility-sparing strategy or breast cancer, after complete remission of the disease	STRONG	⊕⊕OO

Transplantation at the peritoneal site of ovarian tissue collected from the contralateral ovary, free of any cancer cells after analysis, has been described. However, studies have concluded that the peritoneal site is not recommended as it is difficult to completely remove the graft after achieving pregnancy.

Risks for the Offspring

The rate of congenital abnormalities in the children was estimated to be 1.2%, which is comparable to the rate of major malformation occurring in the general population. In a recent study on the fertility outcomes after OTT in 22 patients who received first-line chemotherapy before OTC, the authors reported 13 pregnancies in seven patients, resulting in eight healthy children **(Table 5)**.

Long-term Risk of Ovarian Tissue Transplantation

Breast cancer gene (BRCA) mutation carriers have a high risk of ovarian cancer, justifying a prophylactic bilateral oophorectomy at the age of 40 years or before. Therefore, some oncologists do not recommend the transplantation of cryopreserved ovarian tissue in these cases or to choose a site where close monitoring is feasible. Another approach is to transplant the tissue only on the ovarian site and to perform bilateral oophorectomy as soon as patient has completed her family.

Animal studies have shown that ovarian tissue transplantation into a hormonal-sensitive organ such as liver can induce hepatocellular neoplasms. In the rat model, granulosa/theca cell tumors were observed during long-term follow-up after transplantation of cryopreserved or fresh ovarian tissue into the spleen. The authors suggested that the high level of gonadotropins stimulated the development of sex-cord tumors in this model. Despite the lack of clinical relevance of these transplantation sites, it raises the question of the long-term outcome of the heterotopic-transplanted tissue in humans **(Table 6)**.

Success Rate of Ovarian Tissue Cryopreservation

The success rate of OTC—defined as at least one child per transplanted patient—was estimated to be around 40%. In contrast to established MAR research practice, data are not generally presented per patient starting the intervention (i.e. from the time OTC is first discussed). Overall, the usage rate of cryopreserved ovarian tissue remains low (Diaz-Garcia, et al., 2018, Hoekman, et al., 2020) but may increase with time **(Box 1)**.

TABLE 5: Recommendation: European Society of Human Reproduction and Embryology (ESHRE), 2020.		
There appears to be no increased risk of congenital abnormalities for children born after OTT.	WEAK	⊕OOO

TABLE 6: Recommendations.		
Long-term risks in human are considered to be low but a long-term follow-up of patients after OTT is recommended	GPP	
OTT can be offered in BRCA patients, as an alternative when egg or embryo freezing is not feasible, but the ovarian tissue must be completely removed after subsequent pregnancy	WEAK	⊕OOO

> **BOX 1:** Research recommendations.
> - Evaluate the effectiveness of OTC in restoring fertility in larger cohorts of patients
> - Evaluate long-term safety of OTC and replacement for patients and their children (long-term follow-up)
> - Develop highly sensitive methods for detection of neoplastic cells within the ovarian cortex of high-risk patients

■ CONCLUSION

The feasibility of freezing and thawing ovarian tissue is nowadays widely documented. However, OTT is happening at a much slower pace, and clinical experience is somewhat limited. The focus is on surgical techniques and OTT outcomes, reproductive outcomes, the impact of chemotherapy before OTC, the risk of relapse, and endocrine resumption and longevity of transplanted tissue. The risk of relapse due to reimplantation of ovarian tissue appears to be very low according to current data. Recovery of endocrine function is seen in almost all women undergoing transplantation of ovarian tissue, and about one-in-four gives birth to a healthy child. The efficacy of in vitro fertilization in these patients is not very high, however, and needs to be substantially improved. Radiation to the pelvis, especially with relatively high doses, appears to considerably decrease the likelihood of a successful pregnancy and may be contraindicated. Chemotherapy before OTC does not impair the chances of success, depending, of course, on the total dose and type of chemotherapy administered. At this early stage of development of OTT for restoration of fertility, the results are encouraging and demonstrate clear potential. However, the method is far from being fully developed and requires continued research efforts to optimize our approach.

■ REFERENCES

1. Anderson RA, Wallace WHB, Telfer EE. Ovarian tissue cryopreservation for fertility preservation: clinical and research perspectives. Hum Reprod Open. 2017;2017(1):hox001.
2. ESHRE Guideline Group on Female Fertility Preservation, Anderson RA, Amant F, Braat D, D'Angelo A, Chuva de Sousa Lopes SM, et al. ESHRE guideline: female fertility preservation. Hum Reprod Open. 2020;2020(4):hoaa052.
3. ASRM.ORG. (2020). Micro-presentation: fertility preservation in patients undergoing gonadotoxic therapy or gonadectomy. [online] Available from https://www.asrm.org/resources/videos/learn-on-the-go---short-videos/committee-document-micro-presentations/videos/micro-presentation-fertility-preservation-in-patients-undergoing-gonadotoxic-therapy-or-gonadectomy/ [Last accessed December, 2023].
4. Dolmans MM, von Wolff M, Poirot C, Diaz-Garcia C, Cacciottola L, Boissel N, et al. Transplantation of cryopreserved ovarian tissue in a series of 285 women: a review of five leading European centers. Fertil Steril. 2021;115(5):1102-15.

CHAPTER 12
Relevance of Magnetic Resonance Imaging in Gynecology

Atul Ganatra, Freni Shah

■ INTRODUCTION

The imaging methodology of preference for female pelvis has forever been ultrasonography as it is generally accessible, extensively acknowledged by the patients as a known test and reasonable. High-definition imaging of transvaginal ultrasound gives high analytic precision to pelvic pathology. In any case, there are few limitations with this methodology, for example, restricted field of view, obscuration of pelvic organs by the presence of bowel gas, inherent limitation reliant upon patient size and its reliance on the expertise and experience of the administrator.[1]

Magnetic resonance imaging (MRI) has progressively been utilized to assess pelvic pathology on account of its characteristics, for example, high-contrast resolution, capacity to give great tissue characterization and its multiplanar abilities. There being tremendous distinction between the expense of X-ray and ultrasound, we precisely need to be aware to allude which patient for MRI for female pelvic pathology assessment.

Magnetic resonance imaging is a noninvasive imaging technology that produces three-dimensional detailed anatomical images. It is based on technology that excites and detects the change in the direction of the rotational axis of protons found in the water that makes up living tissue.

A solid magnetic field is delivered with the assistance of magnets that force the protons in the body to line up with that field. The protons are subsequently excited and spin out of equilibrium when a radiofrequency current is pulsed into the patient, pushing against the magnetic field's pull. The energy produced as the protons realign with the magnetic field can be detected by the MRI sensors when the radiofrequency field is switched off. The duration for proton realignment with the magnetic field, as well as the energy release, varies based on the surrounding conditions and the molecular composition. Physicians can distinguish between various types of tissues by analyzing their magnetic characteristics. Intravenous administration of contrast agents, typically containing gadolinium, can be employed before or during an MRI to expedite the realignment of protons with the magnetic field. The speed at which the protons realign directly correlates with the intensity of the image.

■ T1 AND T2 WEIGHTED SCANS

There are two fundamental categories of MRI scans: T1-weighted and T2-weighted images. The timing of radiofrequency pulse sequences employed for generating T1 pictures yields images that accentuate fatty tissue within the organism. The combination of radiofrequency pulse sequences employed for generating T2 pictures leads to the production of images that accentuate the concentrations of fat and water in the body.

T1 scans display prominent signals for fatty tissues.

The T2 scans exhibit high-signal intensity for both fat and water.

Adnexal mass: Hemorrhagic cyst, endometrioma, dermoid, or ovarian neoplasm may represent as complex echogenic adnexal lesion on ultrasound. A cystic adnexal mass >5 cm in a woman who has not yet reached menopause, or >3 cm in a woman who has already reached menopause, that maintains or grows in size on a subsequent ultrasound examination, should be subjected to additional evaluation using MRI. Accuracy of an MRI in diagnosing an adnexal mass as malignant or benign is almost 93–95%. Therefore, any solid or solid cystic tumor that exhibits internal color flow on Doppler ultrasonography should be reassessed using MRI. Therefore, the use of MRI is economically advantageous in such instances since it diminishes needless surgical interventions.

Hemorrhagic cysts typically possess thicker walls compared to normal cysts and may display wall enhancement on post-contrast pictures.

With an accuracy of almost 98%, MRI can easily detect *endometrioma* in cases suspected of adnexal mass, clinically. The stage and amount of blood products in an endometrioma decide its appearance on MRI.[2]

When the result of ultrasound with Doppler is equivocal in a case of *ovarian torsion*, MRI may be performed. Indications on MRI that indicate ovarian torsion include displacement of the uterus toward the affected side, dilation of blood vessels toward the affected side, and a little amount of fluid accumulation in the abdomen (ascites). Signs of a twisted adnexal tumor include the tumor protruding toward the affected side, presence of thick, straight blood vessels enveloping the tumor, and complete absence of enhancement.

Fallopian tubal abnormalities **(Fig. 1)** typically arise from salpingitis, endometriosis, or adhesions and appear as an adnexal mass. MRI is valuable for diagnosing extensive scarring and locating the nearby ovary. MRI enables easy identification of the tubular structure, distinguishing it from a possible cystic mass in the ovary. The administration of contrast reveals a strong augmentation in both the tubo-ovarian abscess and the inflammation in the surrounding tissue.

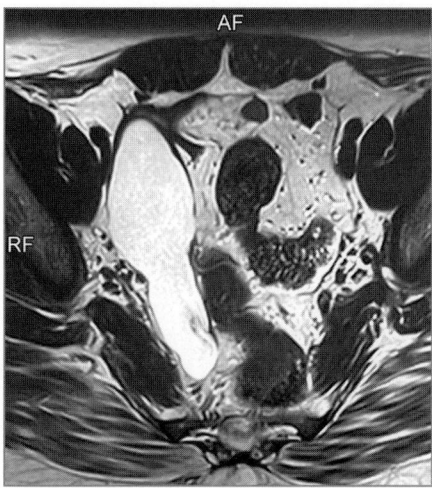

Fig. 1: Hydrosalpinx.

Dermoid cysts, also known as mature cystic teratomas, are typically discovered by chance in young women and make up 95% of all ovarian germ cell tumors. The conventional therapy is surgical removal due to the risk of ovarian torsion or cyst rupture. Additionally, there exists a low probability of malignant transformation into squamous cell carcinoma. The echogenic appearance can be attributed to either a hemorrhagic cyst or the nearby bowel.

Magnetic resonance imaging is highly sensitive in detecting the presence of fat inside the sebaceous component, a distinguishing feature of almost all these lesions. Chemical shift imaging, using in- and out-of-phase sequences, aids in distinguishing the uncommon lesion that contains little fat. The images in malignant patients exhibit the solid component extending along the whole wall and frequently invading nearby pelvic tissues.

Differentiating fibromas and fibrothecomas from other solid ovarian tumors and pedunculated fibroids on ultrasonography can be challenging. Larger lesions may exhibit small regions of cystic degeneration and edema, which often demonstrate little enhancement when gadolinium contrast is used **(Fig. 2)**. Follicles in the adjacent ovarian tissue aid in distinguishing uterine leiomyomas from solid tumors.

The preclinical phase for ovarian cancer is typically estimated to be <2 years. Consequently, the identification of ovarian cancer in its first phase is a challenge due to the absence of any screening method other than ultrasonography and CA-125, which lacks specificity for ovarian cancer.

Magnetic resonance imaging is a cost-effective option when the results of ultrasonography are inconclusive. MRI surpasses CT in detecting peritoneal implants and exhibits higher accuracy in identifying ovarian cancer when

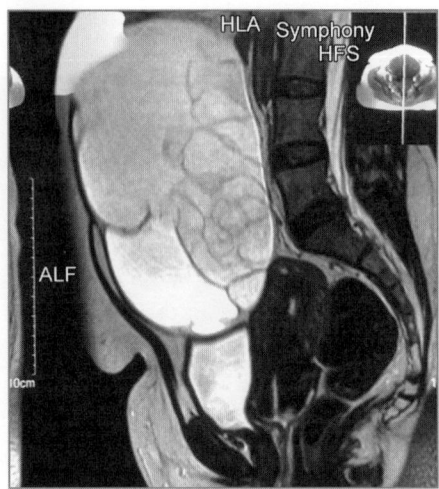

Fig. 2: Complex ovarian cyst.

compared to CT and Doppler sonography. The utilization of gadolinium-enhanced MRI results in a depiction rate of 93% for benign lesions and 95% for malignant lesions.[10-11]

An MRI examination can provide both characterization and staging of an ovarian mass, particularly when the mass has malignant characteristics. Ascites, peritoneal, or serosal metastases, as well as hydronephrosis, can be identified.

Magnetic resonance imaging is useful for precisely determining the location and source of a pelvic mass, allowing for an accurate differential diagnosis. It can help identify conditions such as peritoneal inclusion cysts, pedunculated fibroid cysts, para-ovarian cysts, paratubal cysts, or lymphadenopathy. MRI can accurately identify cystic midline lesions such as Gartner's duct cyst, Bartholin's cyst, and urethral diverticula.

When dealing with uterine leiomyoma, MRI is more effective than ultrasonography for identifying and locating individual myomas inside a big uterus or when there are numerous myomas present. On MRI, the uterus with leiomyomas will exhibit an increased size and display an atypical shape. Calcifications are commonly found in leiomyomas, particularly in elderly women. Calcified myomas can provide substantial interference on ultrasonography and can hide neighboring tissues. Due to varying levels of deterioration in larger myomas (>3–5 cm), the improvement in their condition tends to be uneven and lower than that of the surrounding muscular tissue (myometrium).

Magnetic resonance imaging is the modality of choice in evaluating leiomyomas before and after treatment with uterine artery embolization (UAE).[3,4] MRI is the most effective method for evaluating the location of leiomyoma and precisely assessing pedunculated lesions prior to embolization. It is also valuable for generating post-embolization comparative images to evaluate the presence of persistent augmenting fibroids and to compare the size before and after treatment.

Magnetic resonance imaging is superior to ultrasound for the diagnosis of *adenomyosis*.[5] A junctional zone measuring 8 mm or less effectively rules out the presence of the disease.

Magnetic resonance imaging is a crucial tool for determining the stage of diagnosed endometrial cancer.[6] MRI can distinguish between cancers that invade superficial and deep muscle layers by employing a mix of T2-weighted imaging and contrast-enhanced MRI. This can greatly modify the surgical approach. Endometrial carcinomas typically have lower enhancement levels compared to the myometrium.

Identifying transmyometrial involvement is facilitated by a disruption in the usual low signal intensity of the serosal surface. Similarly, alterations in signal intensity observed in the parametrial fat on T1-weighted images indicate the presence of parametrial involvement. Lymph node involvement is indicated by the presence of nodes with a diameter >1 cm in the short axis on T1W images. MRI is capable of identifying tumor expansion beyond the actual pelvis, as well as invasion of the bladder and rectum.[7]

Magnetic resonance imaging is employed to determine the extent of disease in women who have received a confirmed diagnosis by a Pap screen or biopsy. MRI is highly reliable in evaluating more advanced conditions, such as invasion of the pelvic sidewall and blockage of the distal ureter. MRI aids in establishing the appropriate course of treatment (radiotherapy or chemotherapy) by precisely identifying the location of the tumor and assessing the presence or absence of ureteral obstruction.

Magnetic resonance imaging has become the gold standard in identifying *M*üllerian duct anomalies, thus determining presence or absence of uterus, *cervix, or vagina*.[8-11] Distinguishing between bicornuate and septate uteri is crucial due to their prevalence as the most frequent types of Müllerian ductal abnormalities, as well as the distinct difficulties and therapies associated with each. An accurate assessment of the external fundal contour is crucial for distinguishing between bicornuate and septate uteri. The most accurate assessment can be made by examining a plane that intersects the longitudinal axis of the uterus. The external outline of the septated uterus is either convex or flat, with a concavity of <10 mm. The external shape of a bicornuate uterus or uterus didelphys should have a concavity of >10 mm between the right and left uterine horns.

Table 1 explaining how certain conditions can be identified on an MRI scan.[1]

TABLE 1: Diagnosis of Pathologies on MRI.

T1W image	T2W image
Hemorrhagic cyst **(Fig. 3)**: High signal intensity with fat suppression	*Hemorrhagic cyst* **(Fig. 3)**: Intermediate-to-high signal intensity, fluid-fluid level
Endometrioma: High signal	*Endometrioma:* Intermediate-to-low signal, referred as "T2-shading"
Endometriosis implants on serosal or peritoneal surfaces: Hyperintense T1 signal seen on non-enhanced fat-suppressed images	
	Pyosalpinx: Shading or hypointense area (from the protein content)
Dermoid: High signal intensity with fat suppression	
Fibromas/fibrothecoma: Low-to-intermediate signal	*Fibromas/fibrothecoma:* Low signal intensity
	Leiomyoma **(Figs. 4 and 5)**: Sharply marginated lesions of low signal intensity. Intramural or subserosal leiomyoma can be identified as having high signal intensity rim *Calcified leiomyoma:* Calcification appears as a signal void
Adenomyosis **(Figs. 6 and 7)**: A junctional zone >8 mm, poorly defined margins of the junctional zone and foci of high signal intensity (indicate the presence of endometrial cysts). The foci of high signal may represent ectopic endometrium, cystically dilated endometrial glands, or hemorrhage.[11] The external shape of a bicornuate uterus or uterus didelphys should have a concavity of >10 mm between the right and left uterine horns	*Adenomyosis* **(Figs. 6 and 7)**: Diffuse thickening (>12 mm) of the junctional zone (smooth muscle hyperplasia)
Endometrial polyp: Intermediate signal intensity	• *Endometrial polyp:* The signal strength is intermediate to high, surpassing that seen in endometrial cancer • The fibrous core is shown by the central point of low signal intensity
• *Endometrial carcinoma* **(Fig. 8)**: Isointense to the myometrium and endometrium • *Vaginal involvement:* Disruption of low intensity signal	• *Endometrial carcinoma* **(Fig. 8)**: Signal intensity is commonly hyperintense • *Myometrial invasion:* Appears as a disruption or an irregularity of the junctional zone by a mass of intermediate signal intensity

Contd...

Contd...

T1W image	T2W image
	• *Cervical cancer:* Mass of higher signal intensity than the adjacent fibrous cervical stroma, but of lower signal intensity than the endometrium
	• *Lower than Stage IIB:* The low signal intensity of the inner cervical stroma preserved

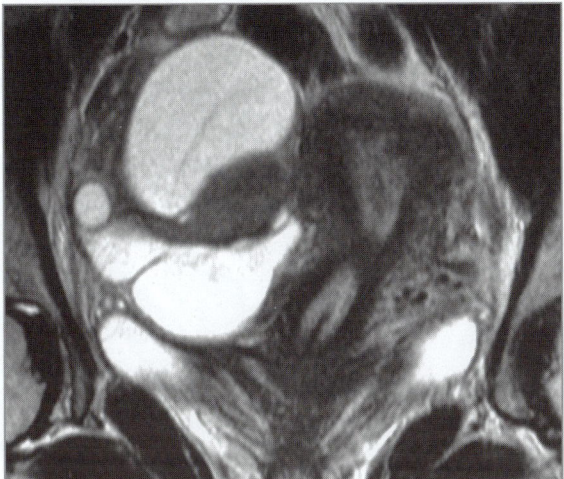

Fig. 3: Hemorrhagic cyst.

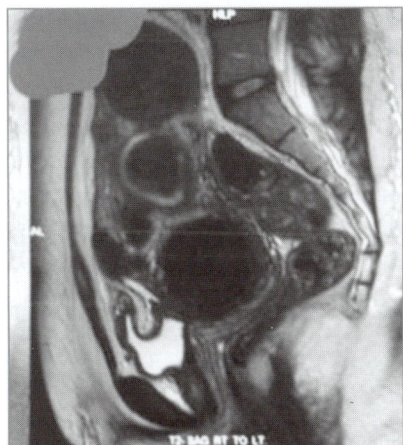

Fig. 4: Multiple leiomyomas.

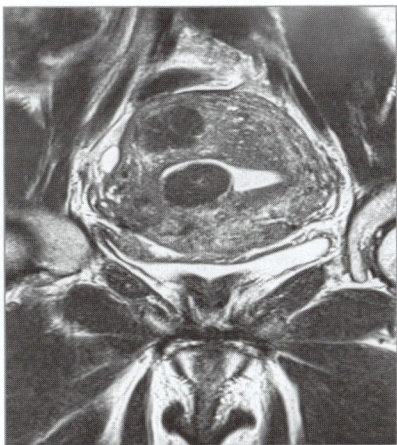

Fig. 5: Submucous leiomyomas.

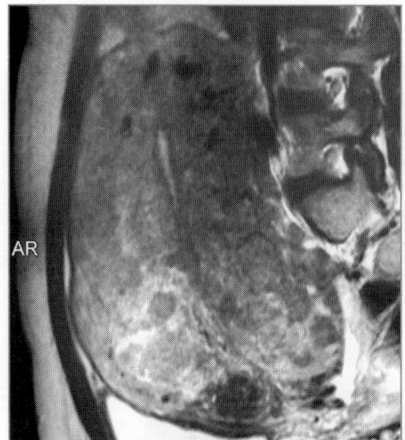

Fig. 6: Adenomyosis.

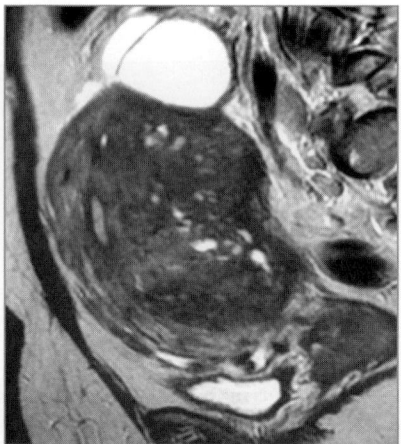

Fig. 7: Focal posterior-wall adenomyosis.

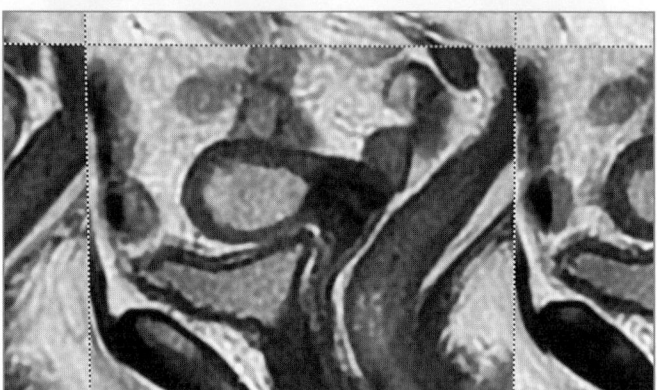

Fig. 8: CA endometrium.

■ CONCLUSION

In conclusion, MRI has become indispensable in gynecology, offering non-invasive and high-resolution imaging for precise diagnosis of a wide array of reproductive and pelvic health issues. Its ability to capture dynamic changes in real-time enhances our understanding of reproductive processes, contributing to personalized treatment plans. As technology evolves, the expanding role of MRI in gynecology promises improved early detection and tailored management, marking a significant advancement in women's reproductive healthcare.

■ REFERENCES

1. (Oct 11, 2011). Imaging the female pelvis: When should MRI be considered? Appl Radiol. 2012;1(1):1.

2. Togashi K, Nishimura K, Kimura I, Tsuda Y, Yamashita K, Shibata T, et al. Endometrial cysts: diagnosis with MR imaging. Radiology.1991;180(1):73-8.
3. Burn PR, McCall JM, Chinn RJ, Vashisht A, Smith JR, Healy JC. Uterine fibroleiomyoma: MR imaging appearances before and after embolization of uterine arteries. Radiology. 2000;214(3):729-34.
4. Ascher SM, Arnold LL, Patt RH, Schruefer JJ, Bagley AS, Semelka RC, et al. Adenomyosis: Prospective comparison of MR imaging and transvaginal sonography. Radiology. 1994;190(3):803-6.
5. Harman M, Zeteroglu S, Arslan H, Sengül M, Etlik O. Predictive value of magnetic resonance imaging signal and contrast-enhancement characteristics on post-embolization volume reduction of uterine fibroids. Acta Radiol. 2006;47(4):427-35.
6. Yamashita Y, Mizutani H, Torashima M, Takahashi M, Miyazaki K, Okamura H, et al. Assessment of myometrial invasion by endometrial carcinoma: transvaginal sonography vs contrast-enhanced MR imaging. Am J Roentgenol.1993;161(3):595-9.
7. Hricak H, Finck S, Honda G, Göranson H. MR imaging in the evaluation of benign uterine masses: value of gadopentetate dimeglumine-enhanced T1-weighted images. Am J Roentgenol. 1992;158:1043-50.
8. Siewert B, Hochman M, Levine D. Problems and pitfalls in MR evaluation of uterine anomalies. J Womens Imaging. 2002;4:100-07.
9. Troiano RN. Magnetic resonance imaging of Müllerian duct anomalies of the uterus. Top Magn Reson Imaging. 2003;14(4):269-79.
10. Pellerito JS, McCarthy SM, Doyle MB, Glickman MG, DeCherney AH. Diagnosis of uterine anomalies: relative accuracy of MR imaging, endovaginal sonography, and hysterosalpingography. Radiology. 1992;183(3):795-800.
11. Carrington BM, Hricak H, Nuruddin RN, Secaf E, Laros RK Jr, Hill EC. Müllerian duct anomalies: MR imaging evaluation. Radiology. 1990;176(3):715-20.

CHAPTER 13

Modern Management of Endometrial Cancer

Niranjan Chavan, Zeba Pathan

■ INTRODUCTION

In 2023, the American Cancer Society estimates about 66,200 new cases of endometrial cancer and about 13,030 deaths are estimated in year 2023.[1] It is the most common gynecologic malignancy in the United States (US) and the only gynecologic cancer with increasing incidence and mortality.[2] Tran and Gehrig[3] outlined the genetic bases of endometrial cancer, novel surgical treatment, molecular targeted therapeutics, and current clinical trial. There have been several important advances in understanding and therapy, including surgical staging and the utility of sentinel lymph node (SLN) mapping, adjuvant treatment for high-risk disease and human epidermal growth factor receptor 2 (HER2)/neu-positive serous tumor, combination therapy for recurrent disease, molecular biology, and immunotherapy. We focus on these recent advances **(Fig. 1)**.

Treatment of endometrial cancer depends mostly on the stage at which it is detected. But other factors given further can also affect your treatment options **(Flowchart 1)**.

- The type of cancer
- Age and overall health
- Whether the female wants to get pregnant.

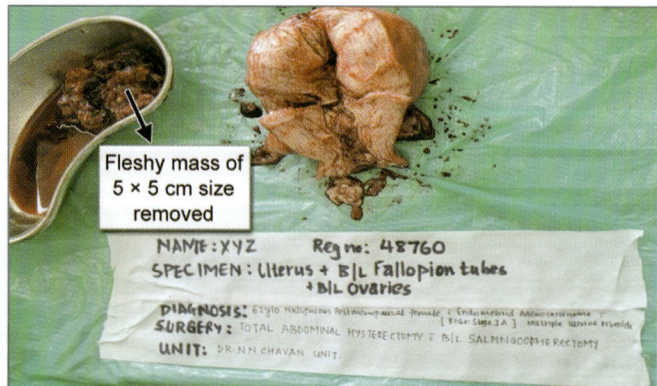

Fig. 1: Gross specimen of endometrial carcinoma.

Flowchart 1: Overview of treatment of endometrial cancer.

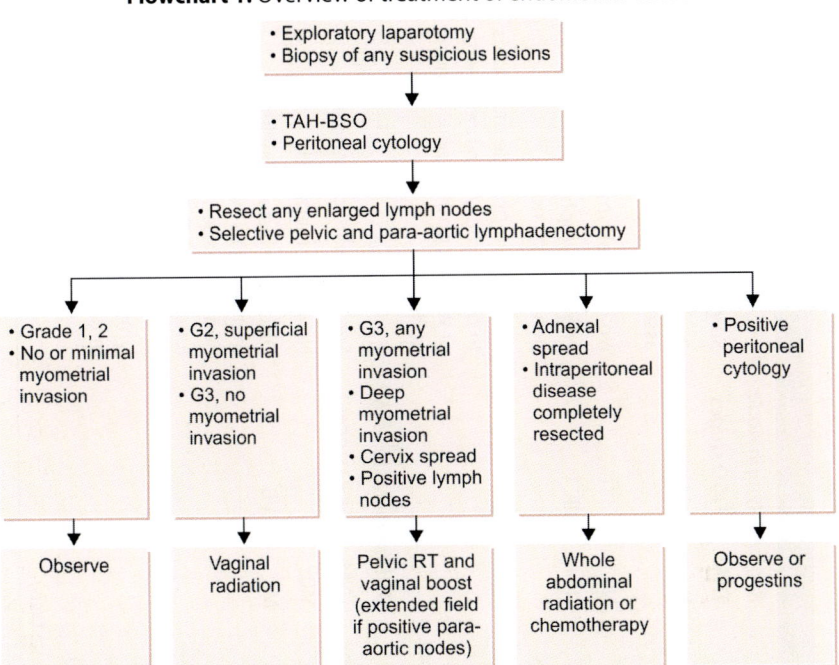

(RT: radiotherapy; TAH-BSO: total abdominal hysterectomy with bilateral salpingo-oophorectomy)

For nearly all endometrial cancer patients, surgery is the initial line of treatment. The uterus, fallopian tubes, and ovaries are all removed during the procedure. Thus, total abdominal hysterectomy with bilateral salpingo-oophorectomy (TAH/BSO), or complete hysterectomy bilateral salpingo-oophorectomy. In order to check for malignant spread, lymph nodes from the pelvis and the area around the aorta may also be removed [a pelvic and para-aortic lymph node dissection (LND) or sampling]. Pelvic washings are also possible. To determine the extent of cancer's spread, the tissues removed after surgery are examined (the stage). Other therapies, such as radiation and/or chemotherapy, may be advised depending on the stage of cancer.

Surgery may be postponed for a while and alternative treatments may be tried in place of it for some women who still want to be able to become pregnant **(Table 1 and Figs. 2A to D)**.

■ STAGE I CANCERS

Stage I is only in the uterus. It has not spread to lymph nodes or distant sites.

TABLE 1: TNM and FIGO staging of endometrial carcinoma.

Primary tumor (T)

TNM	FIGO stages	Surgical–pathologic findings
TX		Primary tumors cannot be assessed
T0		No evidence of primary tumor
Tis		Carcinoma in situ (preinvasive carcinoma)
T1	I	Tumor confined to corpus uteri
T1a	IA	Tumor limited to endometrium or invades less than one half of the myometrium
T1b	IB	Tumor invades one half or more of the myometrium
T2	II	Tumor invades stromal connective tissue of the cervix but does not extend beyond uterus
T3a	IIIA	Tumor involves serosa and/or adnexa (direct extension or metastasis)
T3b	IIIB	Vaginal involvement (direct extension or metastasis) or parametrial involvement
	IIIC	Metastases to pelvic and/or para-aortic lymph nodes
T4	IV	Tumor invades bladder mucosa and/or bowel mucosa, and/or distant metastases
T4	IVA	Tumor invades bladder mucosa and/or bowel mucosa (bullous edema is not sufficient to classify a tumor as T4)

Regional lymph nodes (N)

TNM	FIGO stages	Surgical–pathologic findings
NX		Regional lymph nodes cannot be assessed
N0		No regional lymph node metastasis
N1	IIIC1	Regional lymph node metastasis to pelvic lymph nodes
N2	IIIC2	Regional lymph node metastasis to para-aortic lymph nodes, with or without positive pelvic lymph nodes

Distant metastasis (M)

TNM	FIGO stages	Surgical–pathologic findings
M0		No distant metastasis
M1	IVB	Distant metastasis (includes metastasis to inguinal lymph nodes, intraperitoneal disease, or lung, liver, or bone metastases; it excludes metastasis to para-aortic lymph nodes, vagina, pelvic serosa, or adnexa)

(FIGO: International Federation of Gynecology and Obstetrics; TNM: tumor-node-metastasis)

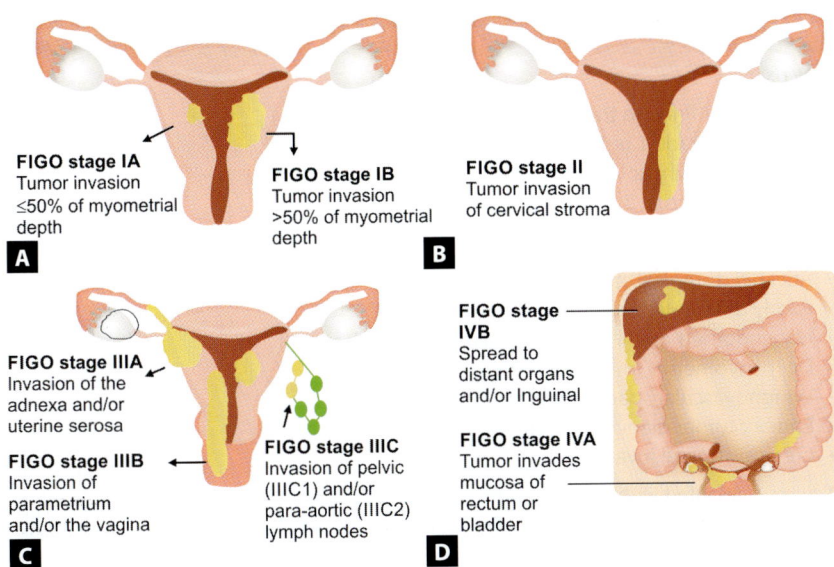

Figs. 2A to D: Diagrammatic representation of FIGO staging. (International Federation of Gynecology and Obstetrics)

Stage I Endometrioid Cancers

Surgery to stage and remove the cancer is a component of standard care. In some cases, this is the only therapy required. The patient is then constantly monitored for recurrent symptoms.

Radiation will probably be suggested as a postoperative treatment for women with higher grade malignancies. Radiation to the pelvis, vaginal brachytherapy (VB), or both are options.

The uterus may be removed without the ovaries in some younger women with early endometrial cancer. By doing this, menopause and the problems that can accompany it are avoided. The likelihood of the cancer returning is also increased by this, but the likelihood that you will pass away from the disease is unaffected.

Radiation therapy is frequently the only kind of treatment for women who cannot have surgery owing to additional health issues or who are frail due to age.

Management for Stage IA Grade 1 Endometrioid Tumors that Spare Fertility

Surgery may be delayed for young women who still desire to become mothers, while the malignancy is treated with progestin medication. A woman may be able to conceive after receiving progestin treatment if cancer shrinks or temporarily disappears. This is still experimental and if the patient is not constantly monitored, it might be dangerous. Every 3–6 months, a dilation

> **BOX 1:** Low-risk versus high-risk endometrial cancers.
>
> *Low risk:*
> - Disease confined to the uterus
> - Histologic grade 1 or 2
> - Endometrioid histologic subtype
> - <50% myometrial invasion
>
> *High risk:*
> - Advanced surgical stage
> - Poorly differentiated histologic grade
> - Nonendometrioid histologic subtype (serous, clear cell)
> - Deep myometrial invasion (>50%)
> - Lymphovascular space invasion
> - Primary tumor diameter >2 cm
> - Cervical stromal invasion
>
> *Source:* 1. Adapted with permission from Pecorelli S, Ngan HYS, Hacker NF (Eds). Staging Classifications and Clinical Practice Guidelines for Gynaecological Cancers. London, UK: FIGO; 2006. pp. 63-83.
> 2. H. Lee Moffitt Cancer Center and Research Institute, Inc. Cancer Control©. 2009.

and curettage (D&C) or endometrial biopsy should be performed. After 6 months, if there is still no sign of malignancy, the woman can try for a baby. Every 6 months, she will continue to have cancer screenings. Doctors advise TAH/BSO when childbearing is finished because the malignancy frequently returns.

Other Types of Stage I Endometrial Cancers

When cancers such as papillary serous carcinoma, clear cell carcinoma, or carcinosarcoma are discovered, they are more likely to have spread outside the uterus. Women with these tumors do not fare as well as those with cancers of a lower grade. The procedure could be more involved in the biopsy performed before surgery reveals a high-grade malignancy. In addition to a total hysterectomy and removal of the ovaries, fallopian tubes, and para-aortic lymph nodes, the omentum is frequently removed as well.

Following surgery, chemotherapy may be administered with or without radiation therapy to help prevent cancer from returning. Drugs other than carboplatin and paclitaxel may also be utilized throughout the chemotherapy **(Box 1)**.

■ STAGE II CANCERS

When endometrial cancer reaches stage II, it has penetrated the cervix's connective tissue, but it has not yet developed outside of the uterus.

Radiation therapy after surgery is one possible course of treatment. The procedure is a radical hysterectomy, in which the entire uterus, the tissues surrounding it, and the upper portion of the vagina are removed. It also involves the removal of the fallopian tubes and ovaries (BSO) as well as the pelvic and para-aortic lymph nodes (LND) or sampling. After the patient has fully recovered from surgery, radiation therapy, which frequently includes both external pelvic radiation and VB, may be administered. An alternative strategy is to administer radiation therapy first, followed by a straightforward hysterectomy, BSO, and potentially an LND or lymph node sampling.

In addition to a total hysterectomy, removal of the fallopian tubes and ovaries, pelvic and para-aortic LND, and pelvic washings, surgery for women with high-grade cancers, such as papillary serous carcinoma or clear cell carcinoma, may also involve an omentectomy and peritoneal biopsy. Radiation therapy, chemotherapy, or both may be administered following surgery to help prevent cancer from returning. Carboplatin and paclitaxel, or perhaps cisplatin and doxorubicin, are two of the common medications used during chemotherapy.

The same kind of surgery used for a high-grade tumor is frequently performed on a patient with stage II uterine carcinosarcoma. Following surgery, radiation, chemotherapy, or combined treatments may be employed. Although paclitaxel and carboplatin are frequently used in chemotherapy, ifosfamide may also be used.

∎ STAGE III CANCERS

Stage III endometrial cancers have spread outside of the uterus.

The ovaries and fallopian tubes are removed during a hysterectomy if the surgeon believes that all visible cancer can be removed. Sometimes, a radical hysterectomy is necessary for women with stage III cancer. Possible procedures include pelvic and para-aortic LND. There will be pelvic cleanings and the omentum might be taken out.

In rare instances, radiation therapy may be administered prior to any surgery if tests performed before surgery reveal that cancer has spread too far to be completely eliminated. It might reduce the tumor to the point where surgery is feasible. The immunotherapy medicine pembrolizumab may be used to treat advanced endometrial malignancies that cannot be treated surgically or with radiotherapy.

Stage IIIA

The serosa, the tissue that covers the uterus, as well as other tissues in the pelvis, such as the ovaries or fallopian tubes, have been affected by the cancer (the adnexa). Following surgery, these cancers may be treated with chemotherapy, radiation, or a combination of the two. The pelvis may receive radiation, as well as the abdomen (belly). Additionally, VB is frequently employed.

Stage IIIB

The cancer has reached the vagina at this point. Stage IIIB cancer may be treated with chemotherapy and/or radiation after surgery.

Stage IIIC

Stage IIIC comprises malignancies that have progressed to the lymph nodes surrounding the aorta and the lymph nodes in the pelvis (stage IIIC1) (stage IIIC2). Surgery is first, followed by chemotherapy and/or radiation therapy.

Following surgery, radiation, chemotherapy, or combined treatments may be employed. Chemotherapy frequently uses the drugs paclitaxel and carboplatin, although it is also possible to employ ifosfamide in addition to paclitaxel or cisplatin. For certain women, targeted and/or immunotherapy may also be alternatives.

■ STAGE IV CANCERS

Stage IVA

When endometrial cancer spreads into bowel or bladder, it is called stage IVA.

Stage IVB

The lymph nodes outside the pelvic or para-aortic region have been affected by these endometrial malignancies. Cancers that have progressed to the liver, lungs, omentum, or other organs are also included in this stage.

Most stage IV endometrial cancer cases cannot be fully treated surgically because cancer has gone too far. It is still possible to do a hysterectomy and remove the ovaries as well as the fallopian tubes in order to stop heavy bleeding. Another option for this is radiation therapy. Hormone therapy may be utilized if cancer has progressed to other bodily parts. However, hormone therapy is unlikely to be effective in treating high-grade malignancies or those with cancer cells that do not express progesterone or estrogen receptors. Some women may experience temporary relief from chemotherapy medication combinations. Paclitaxel, doxorubicin, and either carboplatin or cisplatin are the medications that are most frequently utilized. Combining these medicines is a common practice. The same chemotherapy regimen is frequently used to treat stage IV carcinosarcoma. It is also possible to mix paclitaxel, ifosfamide, and cisplatin.

■ RECURRENT ENDOMETRIAL CANCER

When cancer returns after therapy, it is referred to as recurrent cancer. Recurrence might occur locally (near where it first occurred) or far (spread to organs such as the lungs or bone). The type of treatment utilized the first time, as well as the amount and location of cancer, all affect the course of treatment.

Surgery is performed for local recurrences, such as those in the pelvis, occasionally with radiation therapy afterward. Radiation therapy alone or in conjunction with hormone therapy is frequently utilized for women whose other medical issues prevent them from undergoing surgery.

When the cancer is limited in a few, small areas, surgery and/or focused radiation therapy may be performed to treat the distant recurrence (like in the lungs or bones). Women with more widespread cancer recurrences are treated similarly to those with stage IV endometrial cancer.

There have been some significant developments in endometrial cancer research and treatment during the past several years. We emphasize surgical staging clinical trials, SLN mapping, and adjuvant therapy for high risk.

Surgical Staging: Sentinel Lymph Node Evaluation

In endometrial cancer, lymph node involvement is a crucial determinant in determining prognosis and adjuvant therapy. Adjuvant chemotherapy has been shown to improve survival in patients with stage III endometrial cancer, as will be covered in more detail further; however, those with locally progressed illnesses may not have a similar benefit.[4-6]

The National Comprehensive Cancer Network (NCCN) and the Society of Gynecologic Oncology (SGO) both encourage SLN evaluation due to its reduced morbidity, high sensitivity, and high negative predictive value; nevertheless, some surgeons may decide to restrict its usage to intermediate-risk groups until further data are gathered **(Figs. 3A to C and Table 2)**.[13-17]

The majority of endometrial malignancies are curable with just surgery. However, many malignancies in the advanced stages and some in the early stages will return. The risk of postsurgical recurrence has been defined in numerous studies and efforts have been made to develop adjuvant therapy to lower it. Tumor stage, tumor size, cell type, myometrial invasion depth, lymphovascular space invasion (LVSI), and stage[7-9] are high-risk characteristics.

Chemotherapy has improved overall survival (OS) in patients with advanced cancer but not in those with high-risk, early-stage disease. Although local control can be achieved with radiation therapy relatively successfully, OS has not improved.[6,8,10,11] The outcomes of three significant trials that assessed the effectiveness of combining radiation and chemotherapy to lower risks of both local and distant recurrence were recently presented **(Figs. 4 and 5)**.

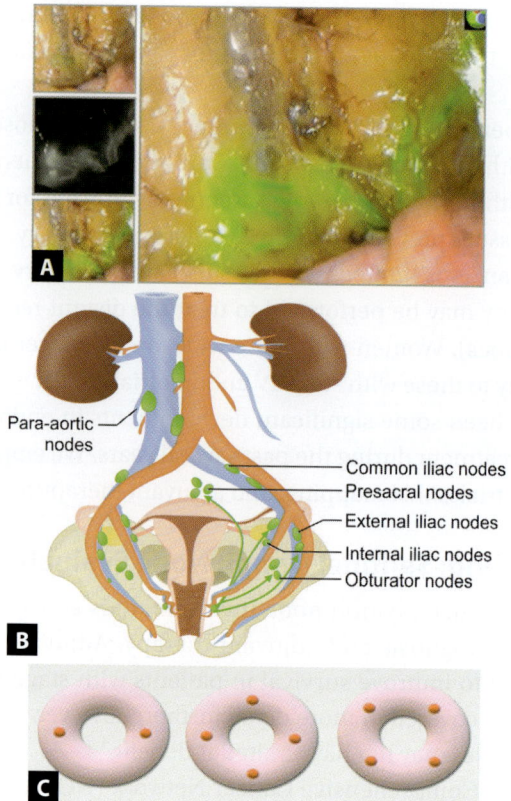

Figs. 3A to C: Sentinel lymph nodes for endometrial carcinoma.

TABLE 2: Histological classification of the endometrial cancer.				
	A	B	C	D
Histological type	Endometrioid	Endometrioid	Serous	Clear cell
Histological grade	Low	High	High	High
Metastasis	Uncommon	• Lymph nodes • Distant organs	• Lymph nodes • Peritoneal • Distant organs	• Lymph nodes • Peritoneal –/+
Prognosis	Favorable	Poor	Poor	Poor
Molecular markers[18-21]				
ER/PR expression	+	±	±	–
PTEN expression	±	±	+	+
DNA MMR loss	±	±	–	±
Aberrant P53	–	±	+	±
Ki-67/MIB-I	Low	High	High	Low or high

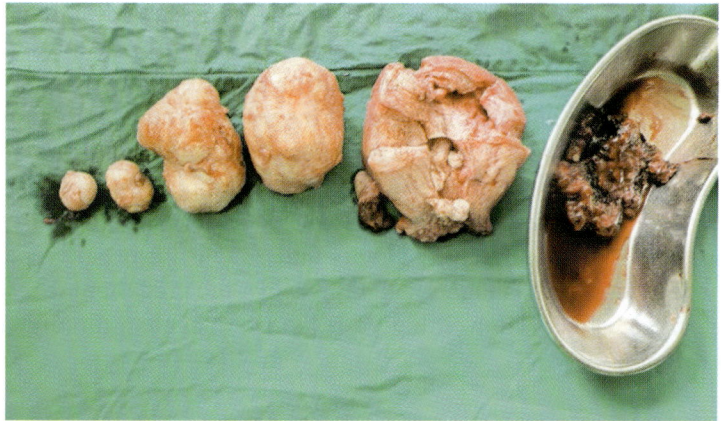

Fig. 4: Gross specimen of endometrial carcinoma along with multiple fibroids.

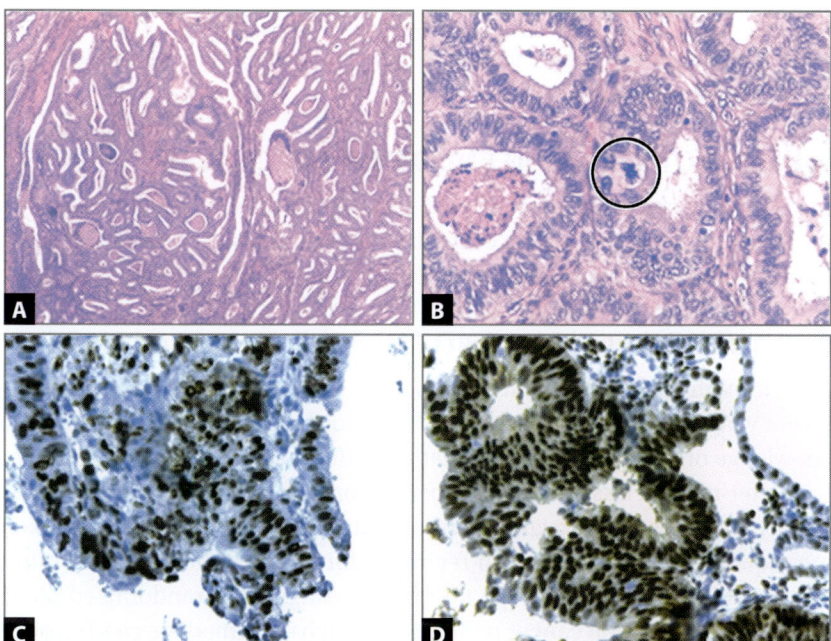

Figs. 5A to D: Immunology of endometrial carcinoma. (A) Back-to-back endometrial-type glands with little to no intervening stroma; (B) Endometrial-type glands with several mitotic figures (magnification lens); (C) Moderate expression of Ki-67 proliferation index; (D) Highly positive (>90%) estrogen receptor (ER) status.

Treatment of Recurrent Endometrial Cancers

Endometrial cancer that has spread throughout the body is typically regarded as incurable and has a dismal prognosis. In recurrent endometrial cancer, a number of Gynecologic Oncology Group (GOG) trials have examined single medicines (etoposide, paclitaxel, dactinomycin, liposomal doxorubicin, pyrazoloacridine, topotecan, oxaliplatin, irofulven, flavopiridol, and bevacizumab) and alternating cycles of megestrol acetate and tamoxifen. Given that many endometrial malignancies are hormonally driven and the relatively low level of toxicity associated with hormonal therapy, hormone therapy is a desirable choice in cases of recurrent endometrial cancer. Although 33% of ER-negative patients and 25% of PR-negative patients experienced responses, patients with ER-positive and progesterone receptor- (PR)-positive cancers showed higher response rates than tumors lacking either receptor.

UNDERSTANDING THE MOLECULAR BIOLOGY OF ENDOMETRIAL CANCER

With improvements in molecular profiling, we may be able to better stratify risk and recommend therapy for endometrial cancer. Systemic therapy in the context of recurring disease is increasingly being guided by biomarkers and molecular changes **(Table 3)**.

IMMUNOTHERAPY IN ENDOMETRIAL CANCER

More investigation is being done to determine a combinatorial strategy with radiation, systemic therapy, or other immunotherapies to boost the effects of immunotherapy in endometrial cancer.

FUTURE DIRECTIONS AND CURRENT CLINICAL TRIALS

Even though endometrial cancer research has made significant strides in recent years, there is still more work to be done as we strive to improve our knowledge of and approaches to treating endometrial cancer.

Better tumor classification will be a priority in order to more effectively enroll patients in clinical trials according to their profile. Improved biomarkers are required and combinatorial regimens for targeted therapies, hormone treatment, and immunotherapy must be investigated. A randomized phase III trial in endometrial cancer patients with high–intermediate risk factors is one of the trials that is currently enrolling participants.

- Investigate the role of an integrated clinicopathological and molecular risk profile to guide adjuvant therapy [PORTEC-4a (postoperative radiation therapy in endometrial carcinoma 4a)]
- A phase II trial of paclitaxel, carboplatin, and pembrolizumab in measurable advanced or recurrent endometrial cancer
- A phase II trial of vaginal cuff brachytherapy followed by adjuvant chemotherapy with carboplatin and dose-dense paclitaxel in patients with high-risk endometrial cancer

TABLE 3: Expression of biomarkers in type 1 and type 2 endometrial cancer.

Target	Function	Change	Type 1 (%)	Type 2 (%)	Outcome	Potential targeted therapy
HER2/neu	Oncogene	Enhanced expression	Rare	18–80	Poor prognosis, aggressive tumor[27]	HER2 inhibitors (afatinib,[28] trastuzumab, and lapatinib[29])
ER and PR	Transcription factor	Enhanced expression	70–73	19–24	Improved overall survival[30]	Tamoxifen, megestrol acetate[12], medroxyprogesterone acetate[31], letrozole[23,24]
p53	Tumor suppressor	Mutation	5–10	80–90	Poor prognosis[32]	Anti-VEGF (bevacizumab)[33-37]
PIK3CA	Oncogene	Mutation	26–90[53]	26–36	No association with survival, except exon 9 charge-changing mutations associated with worse survival[67]	mTOR inhibitor[38,39] (everolimus and temsirolimus[40]) ± letrozole[23]
PTEN	Tumor suppressor	Mutation, deletion, methylation	35–55	0–11	Poor prognosis[41-43]	mTOR inhibitor[38,39] (everolimus and temsirolimus), evaluating combination with olaparib
EZH2	Transcription factor	Enhanced expression	16	36	Poor prognosis, aggressive tumor[44]	EZH2 inhibitor
MLH1	DNA repair	Methylation	20–35	0–10	No association with survival[22]	Checkpoint inhibitor: Pembrolizumab[25,49]

Contd...

Contd...

Target	Function	Change	Type 1 (%)	Type 2 (%)	Outcome	Potential targeted therapy
PD-L1	Ligand for PD-1, immune checkpoint receptor on tumor-infiltrating lymphocytes	Expression on tumor cells	14–48[48,50]	33[51,52]	Trend toward improved survival[53]	Checkpoint inhibitor: Pembrolizumab[54]
MSI	Downstream evidence of deficient DNA mismatch repair system	Mutation	13–26	0–10	Poor prognosis[45]	MEK inhibitor[46,47] (trametinib, cobimetinib, and selumetinib), GOG-2290 evaluating trametinib ± Akt inhibitor

(DNA: deoxyribonucleic acid; ER: estrogen receptor; EZH2: enhancer of zeste homolog 2; HER2: human epidermal growth factor receptor 2; MLH1: MutL homolog 1; MSI: microsatellite instability; PD-L1: programmed death-ligand 1; PR: progesterone receptor; PTEN: phosphatase and tensin homolog; VEGF: vascular endothelial growth factor; mTOR: mammalian target of rapamycin)

- A phase I study of the Wee1 kinase inhibitor AZD1775 in combination with radiotherapy and cisplatin in cervical, upper vaginal, and uterine cancers
- A randomized phase II studies comparing single-agent olaparib, single-agent cediranib, or combination cediranib/olaparib in women with recurrent, persistent, or metastatic endometrial

CONCLUSION

In summary, modern management of endometrial cancer emphasizes individualized treatment plans based on tumor characteristics. Minimally invasive surgeries, such as laparoscopy, are standard, and the role of lymphadenectomy is evolving. Adjuvant therapies, including targeted treatments and immunotherapy, are increasingly relevant. Patient-centered care, shared decision-making, and survivorship considerations play crucial roles in optimizing outcomes. Ongoing research is shaping the landscape, promising continued advancements in endometrial cancer management.

REFERENCES

1. American Cancer Society. Cancer Facts & Figures 2023. Atlanta, Ga: American Cancer Society; 2023.
2. Evans T, Sany O, Pearmain P, Ganesan R, Blann A, Sundar S. Differential trends in the rising incidence of endometrial cancer by type: data from a UK population-based registry from 1994 to 2006. Br J Cancer. 2011;104(9):1505-10.
3. Tran AQ, Gehrig P. Recent Advances in Endometrial Cancer. F1000Res. 2017;6:81.
4. Hogberg T. Adjuvant Chemotherapy in Endometrial Cancer. Int J Gynecol Cancer. 2010;20(Suppl 2):S57-9.
5. Rossi EC, Kowalski LD, Scalici J, Cantrell L, Schuler K, Hanna RK, et al. A comparison of sentinel lymph node biopsy to lymphadenectomy for endometrial cancer staging (FIRES trial): a multicentre, prospective, cohort study. Lancet Oncol. 2017;18(3):384-92.
6. Randall ME, Filiaci VL, Muss H, Spirtos NM, Mannel RS, Fowler J, et al. Randomized phase III trial of whole-abdominal irradiation versus doxorubicin and cisplatin chemotherapy in advanced endometrial carcinoma: a Gynecologic Oncology Group Study. J Clin Oncol. 2006;24(1):36-44.
7. Creasman WT, Morrow CP, Bundy BN, Homesley HD, Graham JE, Heller PB. Surgical pathologic spread patterns of endometrial cancer. A Gynecologic Oncology Group Study. Cancer. 1987;60(8 Suppl):2035-41.
8. Keys HM, Roberts JA, Brunetto VL, Zaino RJ, Spirtos NM, Bloss JD, et al. A phase III trial of surgery with or without adjunctive external pelvic radiation therapy in intermediate risk endometrial adenocarcinoma: A Gynecologic Oncology Group study. Gynecol Oncol. 2004;92(3):744-51.
9. Mariani A, Dowdy SC, Cliby WA, Gostout BS, Jones MB, Wilson TO, et al. Prospective assessment of lymphatic dissemination in endometrial cancer: a paradigm shift in surgical staging. Gynecol Oncol. 2008;109:11-8.

10. Creutzberg CL, van Putten WL, Koper PC, Lybeert ML, Jobsen JJ, Wárlám-Rodenhuis CC, et al. Surgery and postoperative radiotherapy versus surgery alone for patients with stage-1 endometrial carcinoma: Multicentre randomised trial. PORTEC Study Group. Post Operative Radiation Therapy in Endometrial Carcinoma. Lancet. 2000;355(9213):1404-11.
11. Creutzberg CL, Nout RA, Lybeert MLM, Wárlám-Rodenhuis CC, Jobsen JJ, Mens JW, et al. Fifteen-year radiotherapy outcomes of the randomized PORTEC-1 trial for endometrial carcinoma. Int J Radiat Oncol Biol Phys. 2011;81(4):e631-8.
12. Fiorica JV, Brunetto VL, Hanjani P, Lentz SS, Mannel R, Andersen W. Gynecologic Oncology Group study. Phase II trial of alternating courses of megestrol acetate and tamoxifen in advanced endometrial carcinoma: a Gynecologic Oncology Group study. Gynecol Oncol. 2004;92(1):10-4.
13. Slayton RE, Blessing JA, Delgado G. Phase II trial of etoposide in the management of advanced or recurrent endometrial carcinoma: a Gynecologic Oncology Group Study. Cancer Treat Rep. 1982;66(8):1669-71.
14. Lincoln S, Blessing JA, Lee RB, Rocereto TF. Activity of paclitaxel as second-line chemotherapy in endometrial carcinoma: a Gynecologic Oncology Group study. Gynecol Oncol. 2003;88(3):277-81.
15. Moore DH, Blessing JA, Dunton C, et al. Dactinomycin in the treatment of recurrent or persistent endometrial carcinoma: a Phase II study of the Gynecologic Oncology Group. Gynecol Oncol. 1999;75(3):473-5.
16. Homesley HD, Blessing JA, Sorosky J, Reid G, Look KY. Phase II trial of liposomal doxorubicin at 40 mg/m(2) every 4 weeks in endometrial carcinoma: a Gynecologic Oncology Group Study. Gynecol Oncol. 2005;98(2):294-8.
17. Plaxe SC, Blessing JA, Husseinzadeh N, Webster KD, Rader JS, Dunton CJ. Phase II trial of pyrazoloacridine in patients with persistent or recurrent endometrial carcinoma: a Gynecologic Oncology Group Study. Gynecol Oncol. 2002;84(2):241-4.
18. Miller DS, Blessing JA, Lentz SS, Waggoner SE. A phase II trial of topotecan in patients with advanced, persistent, or recurrent endometrial carcinoma: a gynecologic oncology group study. Gynecol Oncol. 2002;87(3):247-51.
19. Fracasso PM, Blessing JA, Molpus KL, Adler LM, Sorosky JI, Rose PG. Phase II study of oxaliplatin as second-line chemotherapy in endometrial carcinoma: a Gynecologic Oncology Group study. Gynecol Oncol. 2006;103(2):523-6.
20. Schilder RJ, Blessing JA, Pearl ML, Rose PG. Evaluation of irofulven (MGI-114) in the treatment of recurrent or persistent endometrial carcinoma: A phase II study of the Gynecologic Oncology Group. Invest New Drugs. 2004;22(3):343-9.
21. Grendys EC Jr, Blessing JA, Burger R, Hoffman J. A phase II evaluation of flavopiridol as second-line chemotherapy of endometrial carcinoma: a Gynecologic Oncology Group study. Gynecol Oncol. 2005;98(2):249-53.
22. Aghajanian C, Sill MW, Darcy KM, Greer B, McMeekin DS, Rose PG, et al. Phase II trial of bevacizumab in recurrent or persistent endometrial cancer: a Gynecologic Oncology Group study. J Clin Oncol. 2011;29(16):2259-65.
23. Slomovitz BM, Jiang Y, Yates MS, Soliman PT, Johnston T, Nowakowski M, et al. Phase II study of everolimus and letrozole in patients with recurrent endometrial carcinoma. J Clin Oncol. 2015;33(8):930-6.

24. Slomovitz BM, Filiaci VL, Coleman RL, Walker JL, Fleury AC, Holman LL, et al. GOG 3007, a randomized phase II (RP2) trial of everolimus and letrozole (EL) or hormonal therapy (medroxyprogesterone acetate/tamoxifen, PT) in women with advanced, persistent or recurrent endometrial carcinoma (EC): A GOG Foundation study. Gynecol Oncol. 2018;149(Suppl 1):2.
25. Howitt BE, Shukla SA, Sholl LM, Ritterhouse LL, Watkins JC, Rodig S, et al. Association of Polymerase e-Mutated and Microsatellite-Instable Endometrial Cancers With Neoantigen Load, Number of Tumor-Infiltrating Lymphocytes, and Expression of PD-1 and PD-L1. JAMA Oncol. 2015;1(9):1319-23.
26. Cancer Genome Atlas Research Network; Kandoth C, Schultz N, Cherniack AD, Akbani R, Liu Y, Shen H, et al. Integrated genomic characterization of endometrial carcinoma. Nature. 2013;497(7447):67-73.
27. Halle MK, Tangen IL, Berg HF, Hoivik EA, Mauland KK, Kusonmano K, et al. HER2 expression patterns in paired primary and metastatic endometrial cancer lesions. Br J Cancer. 2018;118(3):378-87.
28. De Grève J, Teugels E, Geers C, Decoster L, Galdermans D, De Mey J, et al. Clinical activity of afatinib (BIBW 2992) in patients with lung adenocarcinoma with mutations in the kinase domain of HER2/neu. Lung Cancer. 2012;76(1):123-7.
29. Geyer CE, Forster J, Lindquist D, Chan S, Romieu CG, Pienkowski T, et al. Lapatinib plus capecitabine for HER2-positive advanced breast cancer. N Engl J Med. 2006;355(26):2733-43.
30. Chambers JT, MacLusky N, Eisenfield A, Kohorn EI, Lawrence R, Schwartz PE. Estrogen and progestin receptor levels as prognosticators for survival in endometrial cancer. Gynecol Oncol. 1988;31(1):65-77.
31. Thigpen JT, Brady MF, Alvarez RD, Adelson MD, Homesley HD, Manetta A, et al. Oral medroxyprogesterone acetate in the treatment of advanced or recurrent endometrial carcinoma: a dose-response study by the Gynecologic Oncology Group. J Clin Oncol. 1999;17(6):1736-44.
32. Stelloo E, Nout RA, Osse EM, ulz IJ, Jobsen JJ, Lutgens LC, et al. Improved Risk Assessment by Integrating Molecular and Clinicopathological Factors in Early-stage Endometrial Cancer-Combined Analysis of the PORTEC Cohorts. Clin Cancer Res. 2016;22(16):4215-24.
33. Said R, Hong DS, Warneke CL, Lee JJ, Wheler JJ, Janku F, et al. P53 mutations in advanced cancers: clinical characteristics, outcomes, and correlation between progression-free survival and bevacizumab-containing therapy. Oncotarget. 2013;4(5):705-14.
34. Wheler JJ, Janku F, Naing A, Li Y, Stephen B, Zinner R, et al. TP53 Alterations Correlate with Response to VEGF/VEGFR Inhibitors: Implications for Targeted Therapeutics. Mol Cancer Ther. 2016;15(10):2475-85.
35. Schwaederlé M, Lazar V, Validire P, Hansson J, Lacroix L, Soria JC, et al. VEGF-A Expression Correlates with TP53 Mutations in Non-Small Cell Lung Cancer: Implications for Antiangiogenesis Therapy. Cancer Res. 2015;75(7):1187-90.
36. Mallen AR, Filiaci VL, Levine DA, Fowler JM, Dewdney SB, Leslie KK, et al. Evidence for synthetic lethality between bevacizumab and chemotherapy in advanced, p53 null endometrial cancers. Gynecol Oncol. 2018;149:29-30.

37. Mjos S, Werner HMJ, Birkeland E, Holst F, Berg A, Halle MK, et al. PIK3CA exon9 mutations associate with reduced survival and are highly concordant between matching primary tumors and metastases in endometrial cancer. Sci Rep. 2017;7(1):10240.
38. Janku F, Wheler JJ, Westin SN, Moulder SL, Naing A, Tsimberidou AM, et al. PI3K/AKT/mTOR inhibitors in patients with breast and gynecologic malignancies harboring PIK3CA mutations. J Clin Oncol. 2012;30(8):777-82.
39. Janku F, Hong DS, Fu S, Piha-Paul SA, Naing A, Falchook GS, et al. Assessing PIK3CA and PTEN in early-phase trials with PI3K/AKT/mTOR inhibitors. Cell Rep. 2014;6(2):377-87.
40. Oza AM, Elit L, Tsao MS, Kamel-Reid S, Biagi J, Provencher DM, et al. Phase II study of temsirolimus in women with recurrent or metastatic endometrial cancer: a trial of the NCIC Clinical Trials Group. J Clin Oncol. 2011;29(24):3278-85.
41. Athanassiadou P, Athanassiades P, Grapsa D, Gonidi M, Athanassiadou AM, Stamati PN, et al. The prognostic value of PTEN, p53, and beta-catenin in endometrial carcinoma: a prospective immunocytochemical study. Int J Gynecol Cancer. 2007;17(3):697-704.
42. Terakawa N, Kanamori Y, Yoshida S. Loss of PTEN expression followed by Akt phosphorylation is a poor prognostic factor for patients with endometrial cancer. Endocr Relat Cancer. 2003;10(2):203-8.
43. Salvesen HB, MacDonald N, Ryan A, Jacobs IJ, Lynch ED, Akslen LA, et al. PTEN methylation is associated with advanced stage and microsatellite instability in endometrial carcinoma. Int J Cancer. 2001;91(1):22-6.
44. Bachmann IM, Halvorsen OJ, Collett K, Stefansson IM, Straume O, Haukaas SA, et al. EZH2 expression is associated with high proliferation rate and aggressive tumor subgroups in cutaneous melanoma and cancers of the endometrium, prostate, and breast. J Clin Oncol. 2006;24(2):268-73.
45. Mizuuchi H, Nasim S, Kudo R, Silverberg SG, Greenhouse S, Garrett CT. Clinical implications of K-ras mutations in malignant epithelial tumors of the endometrium. Cancer Res. 1992;52(10):2777-81.
46. Falchook GS, Lewis KD, Infante JR, Gordon MS, Vogelzang NJ, DeMarini DJ, et al. Activity of the oral MEK inhibitor trametinib in patients with advanced melanoma: a phase 1 dose-escalation trial. Lancet Oncol. 2012;13(8):782-9.
47. Cox AD, Fesik SW, Kimmelman AC, Luo J, Der CJ. Drugging the undruggable RAS: Mission possible? Nat Rev Drug Discov. 2014;13(11):828-51.
48. Zighelboim I, Goodfellow PJ, Gao F, Gibb RK, Powell MA, Rader JS, et al. Microsatellite instability and epigenetic inactivation of MLH1 and outcome of patients with endometrial carcinomas of the endometrioid type. J Clin Oncol. 2007;25(15):2042-8.
49. Piulats JM, Matias-Guiu X. Immunotherapy in Endometrial Cancer: In the Nick of Time. Clin Cancer Res. 2016;22(23):5623-5.
50. Hampel H, Frankel W, Panescu J, Lockman J, Sotamaa K, Fix D, et al. Screening for Lynch syndrome (hereditary nonpolyposis colorectal cancer) among endometrial cancer patients. Cancer Res. 2006;66(15):7810-7.

51. Mo Z, Liu J, Zhang Q, Chen Z, Mei J, Liu L, et al. Expression of PD-1, PD-L1 and PD-L2 is associated with differentiation status and histological type of endometrial cancer. Oncol Lett. 2016;12(2):944-50.
52. Vanderstraeten A, Luyten C, Verbist G, Tuyaerts S, Amant F. Mapping the immunosuppressive environment in uterine tumors: Implications for immunotherapy. Cancer Immunol Immunother. 2014;63(6):545-57.
53. Ott PA, Bang YJ, Berton-Rigaud D, Elez E, Pishvaian MJ, Rugo HS, et al. Safety and Antitumor Activity of Pembrolizumab in Advanced Programmed Death Ligand 1-Positive Endometrial Cancer: Results From the KEYNOTE-028 Study. J Clin Oncol. 2017;35(22):2535-41.

14 Genitourinary Syndrome of Menopause

CHAPTER

Suvarna Khadilkar

■ INTRODUCTION

Menopause has a significant impact on various aspects of one's well-being, and maintaining urogenital health is crucial for preserving a good quality of life post-menopause. The National Academy of Medical Sciences (NMAS) and the International Society for the Study of Women's Sexual Health introduced the term "genitourinary syndrome of menopause" in 2014. This term refers to a condition previously known as vaginal atrophy, vulvovaginal atrophy, urogenital atrophy, or atrophic vaginitis. It is characterized by dryness, inflammation, and thinning of the epithelial lining of the vagina and lower urinary tract. These symptoms occur as a result of decreased estrogen levels.

The term "Genitourinary syndrome of menopause (GSM)" was coined to describe the condition of vaginal atrophy, which commonly affects the vulva and lower urinary tract.

Genitourinary syndrome of menopause, or GSM, is a persistent and advancing disorder that necessitates prompt identification and suitable treatment in order to maintain urogenital well-being. Despite the crucial significance of early detection and intervention, the condition is persistently undervalued in terms of diagnosis and therapy.

Genitourinary syndrome of menopause, or genitourinary syndrome of menopause, is a broader and more neutral word used to refer to the various consequences of low estrogen levels during menopause. It is preferred because it avoids the negative societal associations and allows women to discuss the condition more openly.

▌GENITOURINARY SYNDROME OF MENOPAUSE: PREVALENCE

More than 80% of women going through menopause encounter vulvovaginal discomfort.

▌GENITOURINARY SYNDROME OF MENOPAUSE: DIAGNOSTIC CHALLENGES

The condition of GSM is often not properly recognized and treated due to the presence of societal stigma and limited access to healthcare professionals in specific regions. Approximately 70% of women experiencing symptoms of vaginal atrophy refrain from discussing their condition with their gynecologists. Certain individuals hold the belief that their symptoms are a predictable and important component of the natural aging phenomenon.

Women may have discomfort in addressing genitourinary difficulties due to the influence of cultural, religious, and societal views.

Furthermore, a significant number of women lack knowledge regarding available treatment alternatives. Instead of pursuing medical intervention, women frequently choose for modifying their lifestyle to manage their symptoms. For instance, individuals may cease engaging in sexual activity as a result of dyspareunia triggered by vaginal dryness.

GENITOURINARY SYNDROME OF MENOPAUSE: UNDERSTANDING THE CONDITION

The genitourinary syndrome of menopause is a long-lasting and advancing condition affecting the vulvovaginal, sexual, and lower urinary tract. It is characterized by many symptoms that occur as a result of a clinical state of low estrogen levels, which often happens around or after menopause.

Physiological Role of Estrogen

The symptoms of GSM occur due to a decrease in the levels of estrogen and androgen, as well as a decrease in the number of their receptors in the genitourinary tract.

Postmenopausal women rely only on dehydroepiandrosterone (DHEA) for intracellular estrogen and androgen, as the production of sex hormones decreases considerably after menopause. The production of DHEA decreases by up to 60% as a person ages, leading to a deficiency in accessible estrogen.

Estrogen stimulation is the cause of maintaining a well-epithelialized vaginal vault during the reproductive years. Estrogen exerts its effects on the receptors located in the vagina, vulva, urethra, and trigone of the bladder to preserve the collagen content of the epithelium. This, in turn, influences the thickness and suppleness of the epithelium.

Acid mucopolysaccharides and hyaluronic acid maintain moisture on epithelial surfaces and ideal circulation of blood in the vaginal area.

Consequently, the vaginal epithelium, which is composed of nonkeratinized stratified squamous cells, becomes thick, folded, and contains a high amount of glycogen due to the influence of estrogen. The sloughed cells provide glycogen as a substrate for Döderlein's lactobacilli. These lactobacilli convert glucose into lactic acid, resulting in the formation of an acidic vaginal environment with a pH range of 3.5–4.5.

The vaginal acidity has a crucial role in preserving the natural vaginal microbiota and safeguarding the urogenital region against infections of the vagina and urinary system.

Moreover, the existence of lactobacilli exhibits a reciprocal correlation with vaginal dryness.

The decreased glycogen levels in the thinned epithelium cause a decline in lactic acid generation by lactobacilli, leading to an elevation in vaginal pH. The alterations in the vaginal environment promote the excessive growth of non-acidophilic coliforms and the depletion of *Lactobacillus* species, making women more susceptible to infection by skin and rectal bacteria (such as streptococci, staphylococci, coliforms, diphtheroids, Candidiasis, bacterial vaginosis, and *Trichomonas* species).

The urinary tract structures share the same embryologic genesis as the genital system and likewise possess estrogen receptors. Consequently, a decrease in estrogen levels has an impact on the bladder, urethra, pelvic floor muscles, and endopelvic fascia.

Menopause causes a significant decrease in the production of estrogen, resulting in a roughly 95% drop in estradiol levels from the premenopausal to postmenopausal stage. Following menopause, the levels of estradiol stabilize and remain at an average concentration of 5 pg/mL.[1]

Hypoestrogenic alterations encompass the following:
- Thinning of the outermost layer of superficial epithelial cells, which may be completely absent in women with severe atrophy.
- Vaginal epithelium experiencing reduced elasticity
- Subepithelial connective tissue undergoing increased growth
- Rugae atrophy
- Vaginal canal undergoes reduction in length and width, resulting in decreased elasticity
- There was a decrease in the amount of vaginal secretions from 3 to 4 g per 4 hours to 1.7 g per 4 hours.
- The vaginal pH increased to a level of 5 or higher.
- Decreased collagen concentration in the bladder trigone
- Reduced strength and elasticity of the muscles of the pelvic floor.
- Diminished responsiveness of alpha-adrenergic receptors in the bladder neck and urethral sphincter.

RISK FACTORS FOR GENITOURINARY SYNDROME OF MENOPAUSE

- Menopause
- Premature ovarian failure
- Abstinence or decreased frequency of sexual intercourse
- Absence of vaginal childbirth

- Lack of exercise
- Smoking/alcohol abuse
- Relative hypoestrogenism due to:
  - *Systemic:*
    - Postpartum estrogen deficiency
    - Prolactinemia during breastfeeding
    - Autoimmune disorders of thyroid
    - Pituitary tumors
  - *Pharmacological:*
    - High-dose oral contraceptive use
    - Danazol
    - Aromatase inhibitors
    - Selective estrogen receptor modulators (tamoxifen)
    - Gonadotropin-releasing hormone agonists (leuprolide/nafarelin)
  - *Iatrogenic:*
    - Surgical menopause (bilateral oophorectomy)
    - Post-radiation ovarian failure
    - Chemotherapy

CLINICAL FEATURES AND SEQUELAE OF GENITOURINARY SYNDROME OF MENOPAUSE

Genitourinary syndrome of menopause symptoms are present in nearly 50% of postmenopausal and 15% of premenopausal women **(Tables 1 to 3)**.[2]

TABLE 1: Clinical features and sequelae of genitourinary syndrome of menopause.

Symptoms	Signs	Sequelae
• Vaginal/vulvar pain and pressure • Dryness • Irritation • Burning • Itching	• Tenderness • Pruritus vulvae • Decreased turgor/elasticity • Leukorrhea • Ecchymosis/petechiae • Erythema • Thinning/graying of pubic hair • Thinning/pallor of vaginal epithelium • Fusion of labia minora • Labial shrinking • Leukoplakic patches • Fewer vaginal rugae • Increased vaginal friability/fissures • Clitoral hood retraction	• Labial atrophy • Vulvar atrophy and lesions • Atrophy of Bartholin glands • Alkaline vaginal pH (5–7) • Reduced vaginal and cervical secretions • Pelvic organ prolapse • Vaginal vault prolapse • Vaginal stenosis and shortening • Introital stenosis

TABLE 2: Clinical features and sequelae of genitourinary syndrome of menopause.

Symptoms	Signs	Sequelae
• Frequency • Urgency • Post-void dribbling • Nocturia • Dysuria • Hematuria • Bacteriuria • Post-void pain	• Stress incontinence • Prominent/retracted urethral meatus • Urethral polyp/caruncle • Ischemia of vesical trigone • Thinning of urethral mucosa	• Cystocele • Meatal stenosis • Urethral prolapse/atrophy • Recurrent UTI

TABLE 3: Clinical features and sequelae of genitourinary syndrome of menopause.

Signs/Symptoms
- Pelvic/suprapubic pain
- Decreased arousal/orgasm/desire
- Lack of lubrication
- Dyspareunia
- Dysorgasmia
- Postcoital bleeding
- Hypertonic pelvic floor

DIFFERENTIAL DIAGNOSIS OF GENITOURINARY SYNDROME OF MENOPAUSE

- Vaginal infections such as candidiasis, bacterial vaginosis, trichomoniasis, desquamative inflammatory vaginitis
- Irritant dermatitis in response to soaps, lubricants, spermicides, pads, panty liners
- Vulvar lichen sclerosus/lichen planus/lichen simplex chronicus
- Vulvodynia
- Herpes
- Vulvovaginal malignancy

Efficient Genitourinary Syndrome of Menopause

Diagnosis

The diagnosis of GSM is predominantly made by clinical means, relying on distinct symptoms and observations obtained from the patient's medical history and physical examination. Although laboratory tests to verify hypoestrogenic observations are accessible, they are generally deemed unnecessary.

History

- During regular clinical visits, it is important to inquire about symptoms of urogenital atrophy in women who are peri- or postmenopausal or who have other causes of hypoestrogenism.
- Obtain information about the user's menstrual and medication history in order to determine their menopausal status and identify potential causes of low estrogen that are not related to menopause.
- The healthcare provider should inquire about symptoms that could be indicative of infection or inflammatory conditions, as well as inquire about the use of products that may cause irritation or allergic reactions (such as perfumes, powders, panty liners, soaps, deodorants, spermicides, lubricants, and tight clothing).
- Is there any record of previous pelvic radiation treatment?
- A comprehensive assessment of the patient's sexual history is necessary to determine if the symptoms are related to sexual activity.

On Inspection

An external visual assessment is required, and the following factors must be evaluated:
- The symmetry and size of genital tissues
- Signs of vaginal shrinkage, stenosis, or dermatological changes to the vulvar vestibule
- Observable lesions such as urethral caruncle, suburethral tumors, excoriations resulting from itching, or scars from previous procedures.
- Existence of POPs

Pelvic Examination

Exercise caution while conducting speculum and bimanual examinations in women with severe atrophic alterations, since even gentle contact may elicit discomfort and bleeding.

The following factors must be evaluated:
- Areas of induced pain
- Pelvic floor muscle tone and voluntary control
- Presence and character of vaginal discharge
- Classical findings of vaginal atrophy include pale, dry vaginal epithelium that is smooth, shiny with loss of rugae.
- Signs of inflammation—patchy erythema, petechiae, friability, and bleeding
- Vagina may be short, narrow, and poorly distensible.
- Cervix may become flush with obliterated fornices.

Laboratory Evaluation

Laboratory tests are usually not necessary, other than for exclusion of other etiologies under consideration **(Table 4)**. These include:

TABLE 4: Laboratory evaluations.

Tests	Findings
Vaginal pH	*Symptomatic pH: 5–7 (Normal pH: 3.5–4.5)*
Maturation index	Basal epithelial cells predominate and decreased percentage of superficial cells 65:35:5–100:0:0 (Normal—predominance of intermediate and superficial cells, 40–70:30–60:0)
Microscopic examination of vaginal smear	Loss of superficial cells associated with atrophy, while at the same time, rules out the possibility of infection
Cervical cytology	Findings on cervical cytology in women with atrophic vaginitis can mimic those observed in women with squamous intraepithelial lesions and can even be confused with cancer. Atrophic epithelium is often characterized by nuclear enlargement, which meets one of the pathologic criteria for atypical squamous cells and low-grade squamous intraepithelial lesions. For this reason, hypoestrogenic women with atypical squamous cells and low-grade squamous intraepithelial lesions may be treated with topical estrogen before further cytological follow-up
Serum estradiol levels	<20 pg/mL support a clinical diagnosis of a hypoestrogenic state
Ultrasonography	A thin endometrial strip, measuring <4–5 mm on TVS suggests a hypoestrogenic state and supports the clinical diagnosis of vaginal atrophy

Endoscopy (Table 5): Endoscopy is depicted as:

TABLE 5: Findings in endoscopy.

Cystoscopy	Laparoscopy
• Squamous metaplasia of trigone • Shortening of urethra • Pale urethral mucous membrane • Urinary sphincter dysfunction (e.g., decreased contractility) • Compliance • Pale trigone	• Atrophic uterus, fallopian tubes and ovaries • Supporting lax ligaments

TABLE 6: Vaginal health index.

Parameters	1	2	3
pH	>6.5	5–6.5	<5
Moisture/consistency	No moisture	Minimal/superficial layer of scanty mucous	Normal/floccluent fluid
Rugosity	None	Minimal	Good
Elasticity	Poor	Fair	Excellent
Length of vagina	<4 cm	4–6 cm	>6 cm
Epithelial integrity	Petechiae+	Petechiae after scraping	Normal, not friable
Vascularity	Minimal	Fair	Good

Others

Vaginal Health Index (VHI) and Vulvar Health Index provide standardized measure of reported physical examination findings with score given between 5 and 25 **(Table 6)**. Lower scores correspond to greater severity of GSM.[4]

GENITOURINARY SYNDROME OF MENOPAUSE

Whom to Treat?

Prior to starting treatment evaluate her for:
- Any endometrial hyperplasia or carcinoma
- Evaluate the women with urinary tract symptoms for presence of UTI or cystitis, or in case of hematuria for any bladder malignancy.

When to Treat?

- When the symptoms cause distress to a woman and hinder her normal day-to-day life.
- In case of an asymptomatic woman, we might like to treat her also:
  - Prior to a vulvovaginal surgery
  - Pelvic organ prolapse or urinary incontinence (benefit uncertain)
  - Therapy is considered a reasonable option in appropriately screened women following treatment for endometrial or ovarian cancer.
  - Controversial in women with breast cancer

TREATMENT MODALITIES FOR GENITOURINARY SYNDROME OF MENOPAUSE

The principal purpose of treatment is to resolve symptoms, restore vaginal pH and prevent recurrent UTI **(Table 7)**.

TABLE 7: Treatment modalities.

Nonhormonal therapy (for non-severe symptoms)	Lifestyle changes (maintenance of sexual activity, smoking cessation)	
	Vaginal lubricants	
	Vaginal moisturizers	
	Liquid lidocaine compresses to the vulvar vestibule	
	Microablative fractional CO_2 laser	
	Non-ablative photothermal erbium: Erbium:yttrium aluminum garnet (YAG) laser	
	Oral ospemifene (SERM)	
	Nutraceuticals (phytoestrogens)	
	Alternative and complementary therapies	Oral vitamin D
		Vaginal vitamin E
		Probiotics
Hormonal therapy (for moderate-severe dyspareunia with GSM)	Estrogen systemic	Oral estrogen
		Transdermally (patch or gel)
		Subcutaneously (estrogen implant)
		Vaginally-creams, tablets, rings
	DHEA (prasterone)	
	Testosterone	
Others	Pelvic floor physical therapy (PFPT)	
Lifestyle modifications	• Cessation of smoking • Wearing looser undergarments and legwear may improve air circulation (reduces microorganisms) • Stress reduction therapy and psychological counseling in nonorganic causes of vaginal dryness • Increased sexual activity is advised for maintaining robust vaginal muscle condition/lubrication/elasticity	

Nonhormonal Treatment

Water-based personal lubricants can alleviate mild vulvovaginal symptoms during sexual intercourse, while regular use of long-acting vaginal moisturizers can provide relief as well. They offer temporary alleviation of symptoms but do not reverse the alterations linked with GSM **(Table 8)**.[5]

Local Vaginal Estrogen Treatment

The initial and most efficacious treatment for GSM is the first-line therapy. Formulations such as creams, pills, and rings are equally successful in treating feelings of vaginal dryness and dyspareunia. They also minimize the

TABLE 8: Non-hormonal treatment.

Treatment	Use	Symptom relief	Considerations
Vaginal moisturizers have high content of hyaluronic acid	Routinely 2–3 days/week, not just during sexual activity	Mild-to-moderate symptoms, improve coital comfort, increase, vaginal moisture, but do not reverse most atrophic vaginal changes	Some have bacteriocidal properties that disrupt vagina microbiome
Vaginal lubricants—silicone/water/oil-based	Use as needed, before intercourse	Relieve discomfort during intercourse, reduce friction and trauma to tissues	• Silicone—main ingredient glycol, and its metabolite glycerine degraded into sugar can predispose to candidial growth. Water-based, evaporate quickly and require reapplication • Oil-based can cause breakdown of condom
Pelvic floor muscle training	As needed for patients with contraindication to hormonal therapy and women with high-tone pelvic floor dysfunction	Improve vaginal blood flow parameter, increased muscle strength and improve vaginal atrophy index	
Vaginal dilators	Consistent use	Increase in vaginal elasticity, decrease dyspareunia, stimulate blood flow, and preserve vaginal function	Vaginal shortening and stenosis does not improve

occurrence of recurrent urinary tract infections, relieve lower urinary tract symptoms, increase the presence of lactobacilli, and decrease vaginal pH.

A systematic analysis conducted in 2006 by Cochrane, which compared 19 studies assessing the effectiveness of various medications, found that all examined products provided relief from symptoms with comparable efficacy. Moreover, there have been seven trials that have demonstrated a decrease in the occurrence of recurring urinary tract infections.

After 2–4 weeks of usage, symptoms show improvement and can be sustained for a maximum duration of 1 year. Given that these estrogens are administered at modest doses, there is no need for concurrent progesterone therapy.

Although local estrogen therapy does not have a higher risk of endometrial cancer, it is not recommended for patients with hormone-sensitive breast cancer due to insufficient safety data in this specific group **(Table 9)**.[3,6,7]

Advantages

A more favorable risk profile than systemic ET because:
- Estrogen doses are significantly lower
- Minimal systemic absorption
- Absence of a hepatic first-pass effect

TABLE 9: Estrogen therapy.

Treatment	Initial dose	Maintenance dose
Vaginal cream		
Estradiol-17β	0.5 g nightly × 2 weeks	0.5 g, 1–3 times/week
Conjugated estrogens (Premarin)	625 mg conjugated estrogen per 1 g cream 0.5 g nightly × 2 weeks	0.5 g, 1–3 times/week
Vaginal insert		
Estradiol hemihydrate	10 µg, nightly × 2 weeks	One insert, twice weekly
Estradiol-17β	4 µg, nightly × 2 weeks	One insert, twice weekly
DHEA (Prasterone)—especially for moderate–severe dyspareunia in menopausal women	6.5 mg, once nightly	6.5 mg, once nightly
Vaginal ring		
Estradiol-17β	Insert for 90 days (2 mg releases, approximately 7.5 µg/day)	Change every 90 days
Estradiol acetate	Insert for 90 days (12.4 mg or 24.8 mg releases, 0.05–0.1 µg/day respectively)	Change every 90 days
Selective estrogen receptor modulator		
Ospemifene—for women who have contraindication/no effect to local estrogen. Decreased risk breast cancer and its recurrence	60 mg, daily	60 mg, daily
Tamoxifen and raloxifen are no effective for GSM		
Bazedoxifene combined with conjugated estrogens improves vasomotor and vulvovaginal symptoms, dyspareunia, while preventing bone loss and being safe for endometrium and breast		

- Minimal, if any, effect on prothrombotic factors
- Serum estrogen levels with use of low-dose vaginal ET remain within the post-menopause range
- May have protective effect on bone turnover

Contraindications

Women with:
- Undiagnosed uterine/vaginal bleeding
- Estrogen-dependent neoplasia

Side Effects

- *Genital:* Vulvovaginal pruritus, candidiasis, leukorrhea, vaginitis, vaginal discomfort, vaginal pain, asymptomatic bacterial vaginosis, vaginal hemorrhage, and UTI
- *Systemic:* Headache, nausea, vomiting, bloating, weight gain, and stomach upset
- Breast tenderness
- Hot flushes is common with use of Ospemifene.

Absorption by Sexual Partner

The NAMS recommends administering the medication at least 12 hours before engaging in sexual activity in order to prevent the absorption of estrogen by a sexual partner. Nevertheless, there is insufficient evidence to suggest abstaining from sexual intercourse for a certain duration as a means of safeguarding a partner from potential exposure to the minimal dosage of vaginal estrogen being administered.[9]

Topical Testosterone

- Topical testosterone cream has been utilized to treat vulvovaginal diseases, such as lichen sclerosus and vestibulodynia, despite the scarcity of data supporting its effectiveness.
- While not officially endorsed by the government for this specific purpose, there is little evidence to support the use of vaginal testosterone cream as a therapy for GSM.
- A 4-week pilot experiment was conducted on postmenopausal women with breast cancer to assess the effects of vaginal testosterone (150 mg and 300 mg). The trial indicated that vaginal testosterone improved symptoms such as dyspareunia, vaginal dryness, and vaginal maturation index. Importantly, the increase in testosterone levels did not lead to an increase in estradiol levels. Specifically, the median testosterone level went from 15.5 to 21.5 ng/dL.

Genitourinary Syndrome of Menopause

- The current clinical trial data is inadequate to support the recommendation of using vaginal testosterone for GSM.
- Additional research of greater duration and scope is required to evaluate the safety and effectiveness.

Systemic Hormonal Therapy

- Estrogen-only and estrogen-progestin formulations can be beneficial in treating vulvovaginal symptoms when there is a vasomotor component, but it is important to use them for the shortest duration possible.
- These are accessible in the form of oral tablets or transdermal patches.
- For women who have a uterus, it is necessary to utilize a combination of estrogen and progestin in order to protect the lining of the uterus.
- Estrogen-only treatment is suitable for women who do not have a uterus.

Contraindications

Women with liver disease, endometrial cancer, history of breast cancer, stroke, VTE, coronary artery disease, and history of smoking.

Non-pharmacological Treatment

- Fractional microablative CO_2 laser or erbium:yttrium aluminum garnet (YAG) laser[8]
- *Emission wavelength:* 1,064 nm
- Laser energy stimulates collagen synthesis, elastin production, vasodilation, and angiogenesis of vaginal tissues.
- Not Food and Drug Administration (FDA)-approved and costly
- Effectiveness and safety of the devices have not yet been established
- *Side-effects:*
  - Discomfort during treatments, vaginal scarring
  - Vaginal lacerations on resumption of intercourse
  - Persistent and/or worsening dyspareunia.

WOMEN WITH BREAST CANCER AND GENITOURINARY SYNDROME OF MENOPAUSE

Sexually active women with breast cancer, especially those taking tamoxifen, frequently have symptoms of vaginal atrophy. Tamoxifen has anti-estrogenic effects on the vagina in premenopausal women and modest estrogenic effects in postmenopausal women. However, some women treated with tamoxifen still have signs of urogenital atrophy.[3]

Management

First line: Use of nonhormonal treatment modalities

Second line: Vaginal DHEA are preferred. They can be used with tamoxifen but not with aromatase inhibitors.

Third line: Laser therapy

■ CONCLUSION

Genitourinary syndrome of menopause refers to a persistent and advancing disorder characterized by a range of symptoms related to the genitals, sexuality, and urinary system. It is crucial to identify this condition early on and provide suitable treatment. Patients exhibiting symptoms of GSM should be provided with ongoing treatment and frequent clinical assessment to address symptom resolution. Nonhormonal treatment options should be considered initially, with hormonal options being included if symptom resolution is insufficient or urinary tract infections continue.

■ REFERENCES

1. Gandhi J, Chen A, Dagur G, Suh Y, Smith N, Cali B, et al. Genitourinary syndrome of menopause: an overview of clinical manifestations, pathophysiology, etiology, evaluation, and management. Am J Obstet Gynecol. 2016;215(6):704-11.
2. The NAMS 2020 GSM Position Statement Editorial Panel. The 2020 genitourinary syndrome of menopause position statement of the North American Menopause Society. Menopause. 2020;27(9):976-92.
3. Loibl S, Lintermans A, Dieudonné AS, Neven P. Management of menopausal symptoms in breast cancer patients. Maturitas. 2011;68(2):148-54.
4. Management of symptomatic vulvovaginal atrophy: 2013 position statement of the North American Menopause Society. Menopause. 2013;20(9):888-902.
5. Farrell Am E. Genitourinary syndrome of menopause. Aust Fam Physician. 2017;46(7):481-4.
6. Ferri FF. Genitourinary syndrome of menopause. In: Ferri's Clinical Advisor 2024. 1st edition. New Delhi: Elsevier; 2023.
7. Cox S, Nasseri R, Rubin RS, Santiago-Lastra Y. Genitourinary syndrome of menopause. Med Clin North Am. 2023;107(2):357-69.
8. Perino A, Calligaro A, Forlani F, Tiberio C, Cucinella G, Svelato A, et al. Vulvo-vaginal atrophy: a new treatment modality using thermo-ablative fractional CO_2 laser. Maturitas. 2015;80(3):296-301.
9. Shindel AW, Goldstein I. Sexual function and dysfunction in the female. In: McDougal WS, Wein AJ, Kavoussi LR, Partin AW, Peters CA (Eds). Campbell-Walsh Wein Urology. 11th edition. New Delhi: Elsevier; 2016. pp. 749-64.

CHAPTER 15

Total Laparoscopic Hysterectomy

Sunita Tandulwadkar, Rashmika Gandhi, Vatsla Vats

■ INTRODUCTION

Hysterectomy is the most common surgery performed by the gynecologist, which has evolved over the years ever since Harry Reich performed the first laparoscopic hysterectomy in 1988. With technological advances and standardization of surgical techniques, laparoscopic approach for hysterectomy has replaced abdominal hysterectomy due to its varied benefits.[1-4] Three different laparoscopic techniques for hysterectomy have been described by Harry Reich in 1988.[5]

1. *Laparoscopic-assisted vaginal hysterectomy (LAVH):* The ovarian or infundibulopelvic ligament and the round ligament are dealt with laparoscopically, whereas the uterine artery ligation and subsequent steps are done vaginally.
2. *Laparoscopic supracervical hysterectomy (LSH):* Laparoscopic hysterectomy is performed leaving behind the cervix, cardinal ligaments, and uterosacral ligaments.
3. *Total laparoscopic hysterectomy (TLH):* All the steps of the hysterectomy are performed laparoscopically including closure of the vault.

■ INDICATIONS

The indications for laparoscopic hysterectomy are similar to that of abdominal or vaginal hysterectomy. They include:
- Symptomatic fibroid
- Adenomyosis refractory to medical management
- Abnormal uterine bleeding (AUB) refractory to medical management
- Pelvic organ prolapse along with concomitant uterine pathology
- Concomitant adnexal pathology
- Chronic pelvic pain
- Severe endometriosis not desiring fertility
- Endometrial hyperplasia with atypia
- Benign ovarian tumor in postmenopausal woman
- Early stages of malignancies—endometrial, ovarian, and cervical.

CONTRAINDICATIONS

There are no absolute contraindications for laparoscopic approach in benign gynecological disease. However, certain medical conditions such as severe cardiovascular or pulmonary disease which are high risk for creation of pneumoperitoneum are absolute anesthetic contraindications. The relative contraindications include distorted pelvic anatomy, severe adhesions, large uterus or large fibroid, and suspicious pelvic masses. With recent introduction of novel tissue retrieval techniques, laparoscopic hysterectomy is feasible in cases of large fibroid and suspicious masses as well. Above all, the surgeons' skill and experience remains the limiting factor for TLH. In fact, all the relative contraindications have now become the indication with the expertise of the surgeon and the technological advances.

PREOPERATIVE EVALUATION

All patients should be thoroughly evaluated prior to the surgery and it is similar to any other major surgery. Detailed history to be taken and complete general and gynecological examination should be performed. All baseline investigations and pelvic ultrasonography are done for all patients. If indicated, computed tomography (CT), magnetic resonance imaging (MRI), or endometrial biopsy can be done.

PREOPERATIVE PREPARATION

Detailed informed consent is obtained. Patients are kept nil per os (NPO) for 8 hours prior to surgery. Bowel preparation with exelyte enema is given if adhesions are anticipated. Patients with deep infiltrating endometriosis are kept on a liquid diet the previous day and nil oral for 12 hours. Preparation of parts and vaginal douching is performed prior to surgery. Prophylactic intravenous (IV) antibiotic is given 60 minutes prior to the surgery.

SURGICAL PROCEDURE

Anesthesia

All laparoscopic hysterectomies are performed under general endotracheal anesthesia.

Positioning

Patient is positioned in modified dorsal lithotomy position. This will enable easy movement of the uterine manipulator and the lower accessory instruments. Patient is laid flat on the table with arms tucked by the sides and legs supported by the stirrups in slight flexion (30°), abduction, and external rotation. The thigh should be at the same level as the abdomen and this will permit the ease of movement of the lower accessory instruments without hitting the thigh. Buttocks are placed slightly below the edge of the table as this will facilitate easy movement of the uterine manipulator. After primary trocar insertion, the patient is put in the Trendelenburg position.

The laparoscopic tower is placed near the patient's right leg or in between the legs, which allows the surgeon and assistant surgeon to have a clear view and an ergonomic neck position (at the angle of resting eye, i.e., 30°). The second assistant standing in between the legs and manipulating the uterine manipulator also should have good access to the monitor.

The table is kept in a low position to enable wrist movements for intracorporeal knotting. The height of the table should be about the half of surgeon's height to enable wrist movements.

Trocar Placement

Trocar placement can vary in different cases and is determined by factors such as surgeon's preference, uterine size, and previous surgeries in view of adhesions.

- In ideal conditions, the 10 mm camera port is placed supraumbilical. If the size of the uterus is large, the palm is placed above the topmost part of the uterus and the port is inserted just above the palm.
- In case of adhesions, the first port is placed at palmer point and after insufflation, the 10 mm trocar is introduced under vision. We prefer to use the EndoTIP entry, where one can enter under vision seeing all the layers, and thereby avoid injury to the underlying structures.
- The site of the 10 mm port can be placed more cephalad to umbilicus, depending upon the size of the uterus or fibroid.
- The accessory trocars should be placed always under vision and lateral to inferior epigastric artery or lateral to the lateral border of the rectus.

This 10 mm port is utilized for the camera and other accessory trocars are inserted under vision. Three or four accessory trocars of 5 mm are used. The lower ports are placed 2 cm superior and medial to the anterior superior iliac spine. The upper ports are placed in the paramedian region at the level of umbilicus. The distance between the two accessory ports should be at least 4 cm to prevent clashing and crowding of the instruments. If the pathology is large, the accessory ports are placed slightly cephalad (baseball diamond concept) with a distance of 4 cm from the uppermost portion of the pathology. Trocar placement in ergonomic situation will allow an optimal triangulation and free movement of instruments. General rule for trocar placement is high and lateral. After inserting the ports, the trocars are withdrawn and instruments are inserted. Half of the instrument should be in and half out so that elevation angle is 60°.

■ SURGICAL STEPS

After creation of pneumoperitoneum and port insertion, the patient is put in the Trendelenburg position. Laparoscope is introduced and anatomy is inspected by panoramic view and the surgery is planned. The patient is placed in 15° head low position to move the bowel loops away from pelvis. The small intestine loops are mobilized upward to visualize the uterus and adnexa and the pathology is confirmed. Adhesiolysis is performed, if necessary. Uterine manipulator is inserted by an assistant and the uterine mobility is noted. One can also do the surgery without using uterine manipulator as well, by just using the myoma screw for traction.

The steps of TLH are mentioned in **Box 1**.

1. *Division of the round ligaments:* The uterus is pushed to the opposite side with the help of the uterine manipulator and the round ligament is put to stretch. The round ligaments are coagulated and cut away from the uterus, around 2–3 cm at the avascular triangle of the broad ligament, limited laterally by the iliac vessels and medially by the adnexal vessels. This will prevent bleeding from the medial side of the uterus **(Figs. 1A to D)**.

2. *Division of infundibulopelvic ligament/tuboovarian* **(Figs. 2A to C)**: The infundibulopelvic ligament is lifted up by the assistant and it is coagulated and cut if the ovary is to be removed. Care is taken to identify the ureter before ligating the infundibulopelvic ligament as the ureter runs very close to it and is prone to thermal injury. The coagulation and sectioning of the ligament should be progressive, plane to plane (peritoneum, followed by the vessels, and connective tissue). One can anticipate bleeding while ligating the infundibulopelvic ligament and should ensure proper precautions to tackle the ovarian artery which lies in the ligament. The bleeding can at times be torrential as it is a branch of abdominal aorta.

   If the ovary is to be preserved, one needs to take the tuboovarian ligament slightly away from the uterus to prevent backflow from the uterus. There is a chance of bleeding from the Sampson artery while

---

BOX 1: Steps of total laparoscopic hysterectomy.

1. Division of the round ligaments
2. Division of infundibulopelvic ligament if adnexa is to be removed
3. Opening of anterior leaf of broad ligament and opening of uterovaginal fascia
4. Opening of posterior leaf of broad ligament and opening the rectovaginal fascia
5. Uterine vessel ligation
6. Colpotomy
7. Uterus retrieval
8. Vault closure
9. Checking and confirming hemostasis
10. Trocar removal and skin suturing

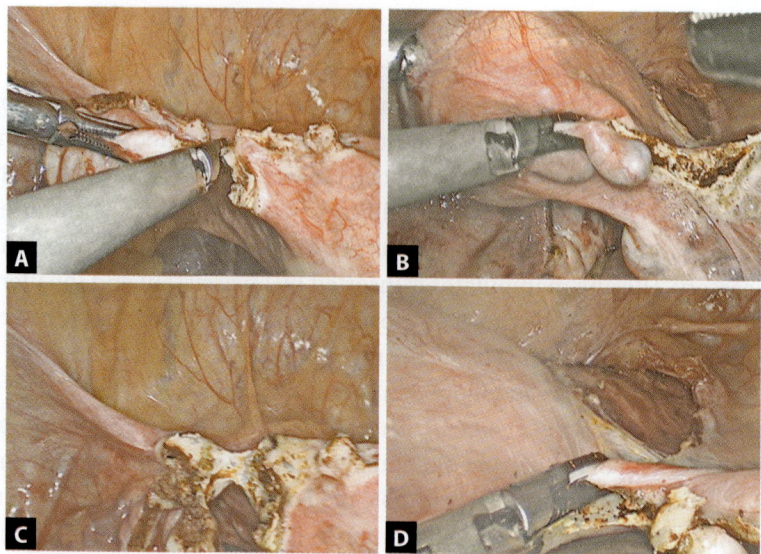

Figs. 1A to D: Division of the round ligaments.

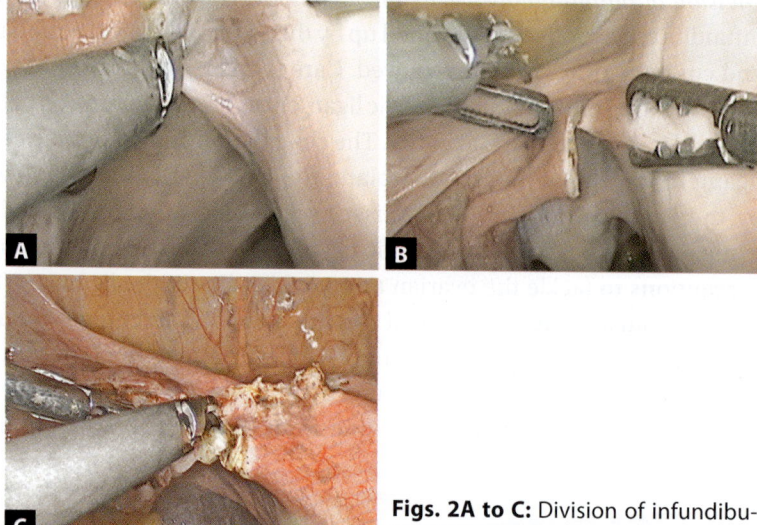

Figs. 2A to C: Division of infundibulopelvic ligament/tuboovarian.

ligating the tuboovarian ligament, so necessary precautions should be taken like coagulation close to the ovary to prevent injury.

3. *Opening of anterior leaf of broad ligament and separating the uterovesical fascia* **(Fig. 3)**: The anterior leaf of the broad ligament is opened and coagulated and cut toward the medial vesical line. This facilitates movement of the ureter well away from the uterine artery. Now, the dissection is done caudal to the white line adherent to uterus,

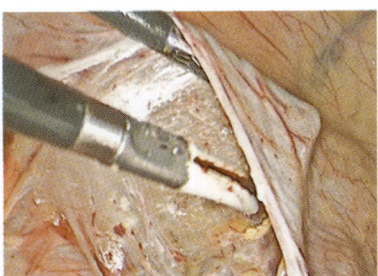

Fig. 3: Opening of anterior leaf of broad ligament and separating the uterovesical fascia.

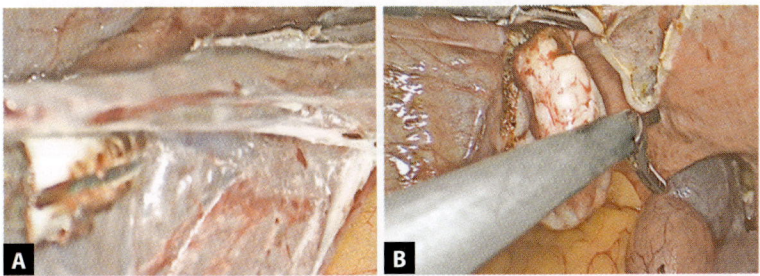

Figs. 4A and B: Opening of posterior leaf of broad ligament and separating the rectovaginal fascia.

which is 2-3 cm between the bladder and the uterus and it represents the vesicouterine junction. The same dissection is carried out to the contralateral side. During this dissection, the uterus is kept central and pushed cephalad by the vaginal assistant. The dictum, that the fat belongs to the bladder, is to be followed and the dissection is done above this layer. In case of previous lower segment cesarean section (LSCS), the dome of the bladder is found to be densely adherent in the central portion to the lower uterine segment; hence, lateral window technique is to be followed where the bladder is less densely adherent.

4. *Opening of posterior leaf of broad ligament and separating the rectovaginal fascia (**Figs. 4A and B**):* The posterior leaf of broad ligament is dissected up to the level of uterosacral ligament and the uterine vascular pedicles can be identified in between the leaves of the broad ligament. This ensures that the ureter has moved well away from the uterine artery. Dissection of the rectovaginal fascia is done next and it is extended to the opposite side.

5. *Uterine vessel ligation (**Figs. 5A to F**):* Having separated both the leaves of broad ligaments, uterine vascular pedicle is skeletonized and ligation of uterine artery can be done safely either by using bipolar energy source and cutting with scissors or by using vessel sealers. Uterine artery should always be ligated perpendicular to the vessel and not in an angle

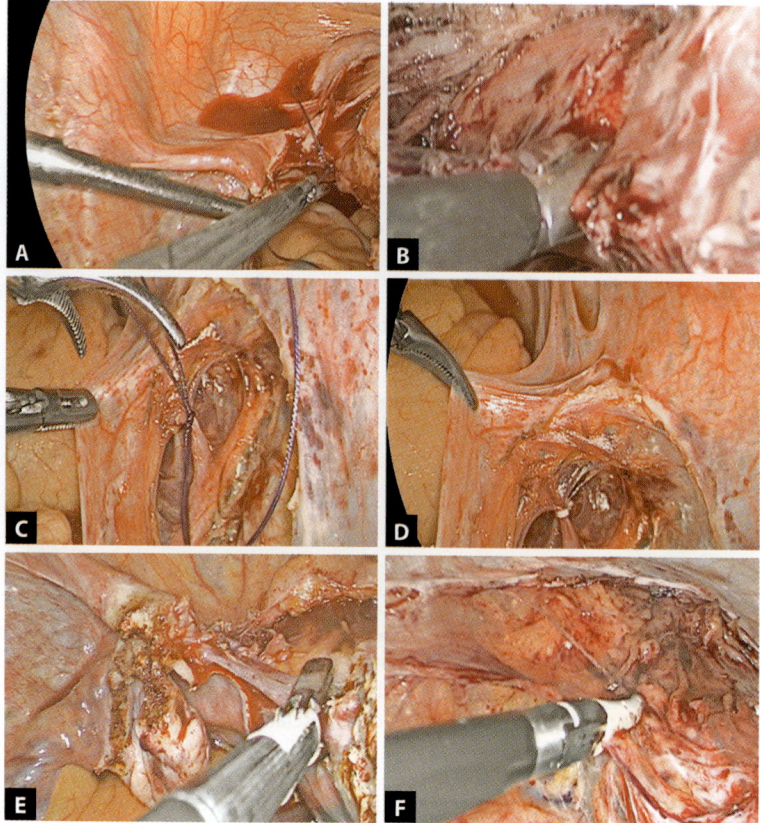

Figs. 5A to F: Uterine vessel ligation.

to maintain the same diameter of the vessel. Uterine artery can also be sutured instead of coagulation if the need arises. The medial end of the uterine artery is always cauterized using a bipolar along the ascending branch to prevent the backflow. Uterine artery can also be ligated at origin or can be clipped as an alternative when there are dense adhesions and in case of altered pelvic anatomy.

6. *Colpotomy (Figs. 6A to F):* Now that the bladder is pushed down and the uterine artery is cauterized and cut, the tube of the uterine manipulator is pushed up and fornices can be well visualized and a platform has now been created to safely perform the colpotomy. Either a monopolar hook or harmonic scalpel can be used to cut along the rim of the vaginal tube and it can be extended laterally. Care is taken near the lateral fornices, as one can encounter descending vaginal artery which needs to be cauterized and cut. The colpotomy is now extended posteriorly by acutely anteverting the uterus and the entire uterus is now detached. Care is taken not to cut the uterosacral ligament and to detach above the ligament to

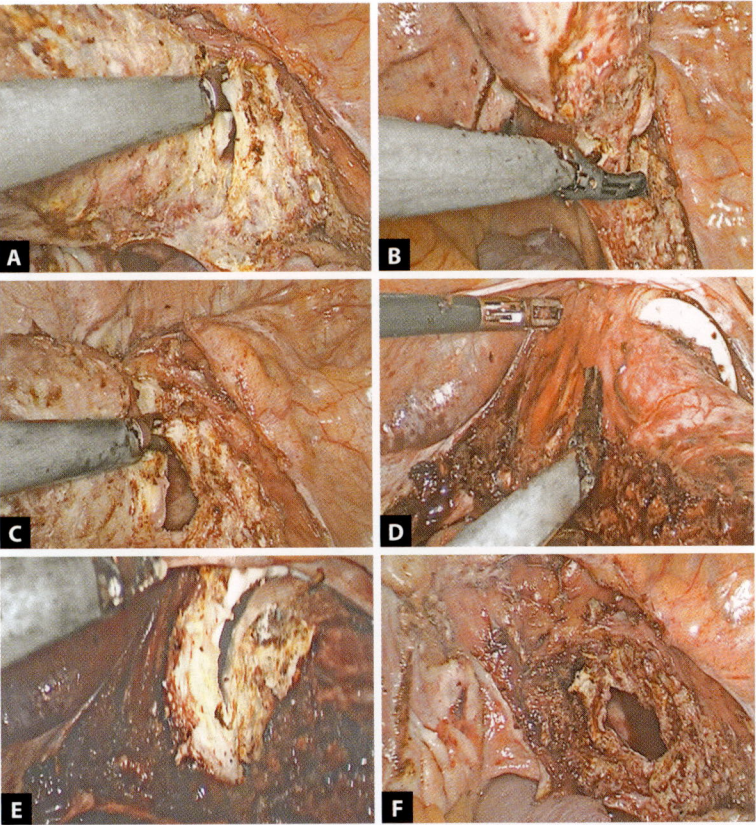

Figs. 6A to F: Colpotomy.

give support to the vault. Colpotomy can also be done without the use of uterine manipulator by plugging the vagina and opening the lateral fornices.

7. *Uterus retrieval* **(Figs. 7A to C)**: The specimen is retrieved vaginally, either by coring the uterus laterally or if the uterus is large, then by power morcellation and in-bag morcellation is done in suspicious cases or by mini-laparotomy if morcellation is not feasible.
8. *Vault closure* **(Figs. 8A to E)**: Vault should be closed laparoscopically to complete the definition of TLH. Suturing can be done with smooth sutures such as Vicryl (polyglactin) or using barbed sutures. While suturing the vault one needs to include the uterosacral ligament, rectovaginal fascia, and uterovesical fascia to make it an intrafascial hysterectomy and recreate the pericervical ring and give additional support to the vault. Either intermittent or continuous suturing of the vault can be done. The advantage of barbed suture is that as there are no knots, there is uniform tension on the suture line with less foreign body reaction due to the absence of the knot.

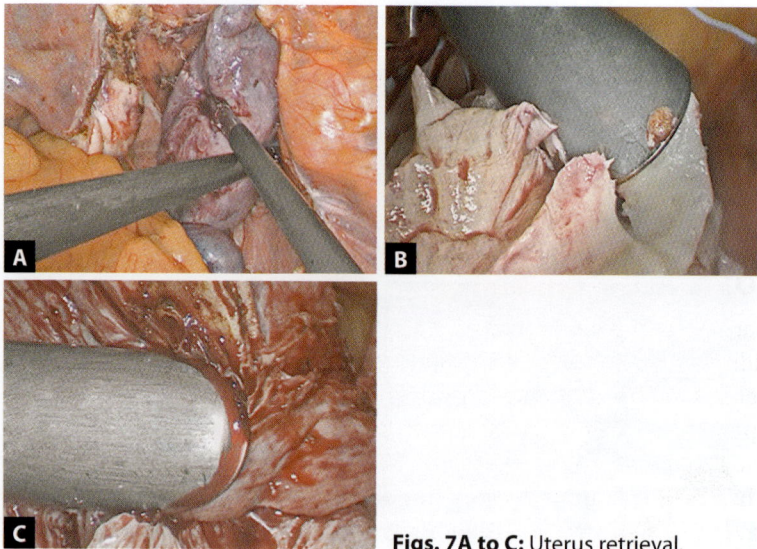

Figs. 7A to C: Uterus retrieval.

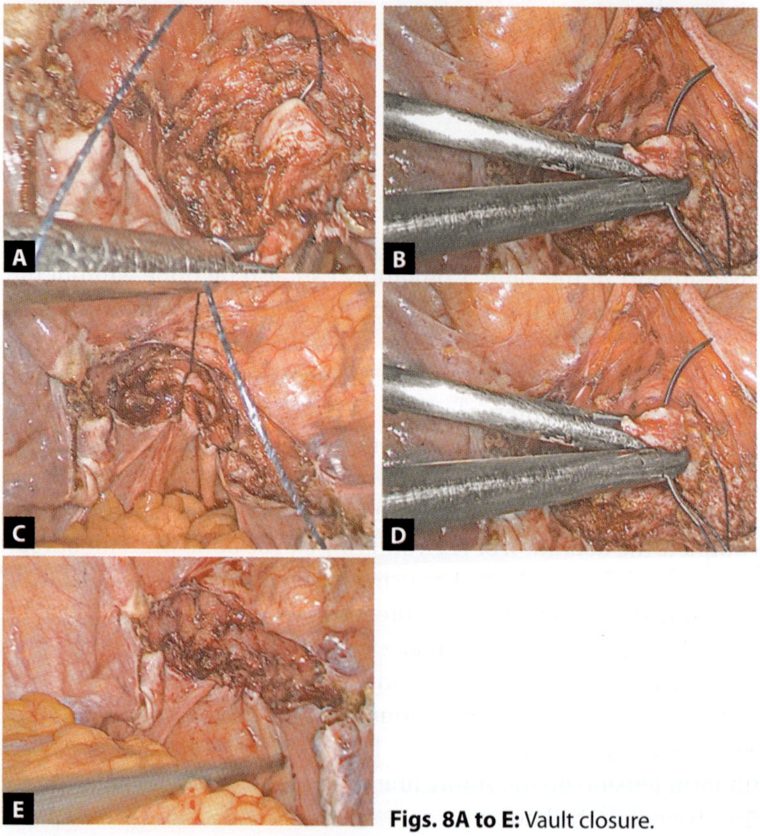

Figs. 8A to E: Vault closure.

9. *Checking and confirming hemostasis:* Vault and all vascular pedicles should be inspected for any bleeding. Underwater check can be done to detect small bleeders. Cystoscopy can be performed in cases of dense bladder adhesions to check for any injury to the bladder.
10. *Trocar removal and skin suturing:* Trocar should be removed always under vision. Pneumoperitoneum is let out. Port site is closed. Sensorcaine is injected at the port site to give postoperative analgesia.

■ POSTOPERATIVE CARE

All patients are given antibiotics, analgesics, and antiemetics. They are given liquids first, followed by semisolids. Patients are encouraged to walk and catheter is removed 12 hours postoperatively. Routine wound care is advised and patients are discharged the next day following surgery. They can resume their daily activities; however, they are advised to avoid strenuous activities and heavy lifting for 6 weeks. They should review a week later for suture removal and then 4 weeks later for postoperative follow-up.

■ COMPLICATIONS

Like any other surgery, laparoscopic hysterectomy is associated with certain complications **(Box 2)**. However with novel techniques, technological advances, and more surgical expertise, the reported incidence of these complications has been decreasing over the years. Most of the studies suggest that over 50% of the injuries occur at the time of entry. Techniques such as open Hasson's method, EndoTIP trocar entry, or optical

---

BOX 2: Complications of laparoscopic hysterectomy.

Anesthesia related:
- Metabolic acidosis
- Pneumothorax
- Pulmonary embolism
- Cardiovascular complications—arrhythmia and cardiac arrest

Operative:
- Entry-related complications
- Bowel and omental injury
- Urological injury
- Vascular injury
- Hemorrhage

Postoperative:
- Paralytic ileus
- Wound infection
- Postop hemorrhage/hematoma
- Pelvic infection
- Sepsis
- Port site hernia
- Vault prolapse

trocars were introduced to overcome this; however, it has been suggested that the entry technique with which the surgeon is most well versed and confident should be used to minimize these complications.

Urological Injuries

Bladder Injury

- *Incidence:* 0.05–0.06%[6]
    - Most commonly occurs at the dome of the bladder
- *Cause:* Most of the bladder injuries occur during suprapubic port insertion or during dissection of uterovesical fold of peritoneum, where the bladder is densely adherent to the uterus.
- *Risk factors:* Previous cesarean section, dense adhesions following previous laparotomy[7]
- *Prevention:*
    - Catheterization at the beginning of surgery
    - Direct suprapubic trocar away from retropubic space
    - Careful dissection of the bladder by lateral window technique
- *Management (Flowchart 1):*[8-10]

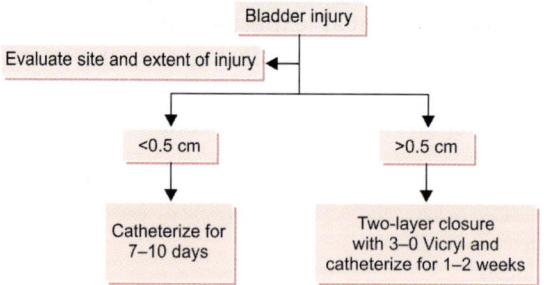

Flowchart 1: Management of bladder injury.

Ureteric Injury

- *Incidence:* 0.02–0.4%[6]
    - Most commonly occurs at the lower one-third part of ureter
- *Risk factors:* Cervical or broad ligament fibroid distorting the anatomy, endometriosis, dense adhesions, large ovarian cyst, and malignancy[11]
- *Possible site of ureteric injury:* Pelvic brim, traversing the base of infundibulopelvic ligament at the level of crossing of uterine artery, tunnel of cardinal ligament, and the lateral vaginal fornix, as ureter enters the bladder
- *Prevention:*[12]
    - Infundibulopelvic and cardinal ligament to be coagulated as medial as possible
    - Uterine artery to be skeletonized and coagulated only after pushing the bladder down

- While suturing vaginal vault, do not go beyond the limit of uterosacral ligaments.
- In high-risk cases, ureters should be dissected by doing ureterolysis or can be stented preoperatively[13]
■ *Management (Flowchart 2):*[14,15]

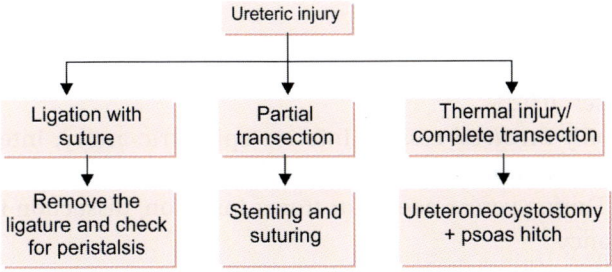

Flowchart 2: Management of ureteric injury.

Bowel Injury

- *Incidence:* 0.5–2.2%
  - Small bowel is affected more often than the large bowel.[16]
- *Cause:*[17] Injury can occur during verses needle or trocar insertion, during adhesiolysis, thermal injury, or during dissection.
- *Risk factors:* Previous laparotomies, dense adhesions, endometriosis, bowel distension
- *Prevention:*[18]
  - Preoperative bowel preparation
  - Palmer point entry or open or entry under vision technique in high-risk patients
  - Using electrosurgery with less thermal spread
  - Using rectal probes in cases of deep infiltrating endometriosis to identify the limits of the bladder
- *Management (Flowchart 3):*[18-20]

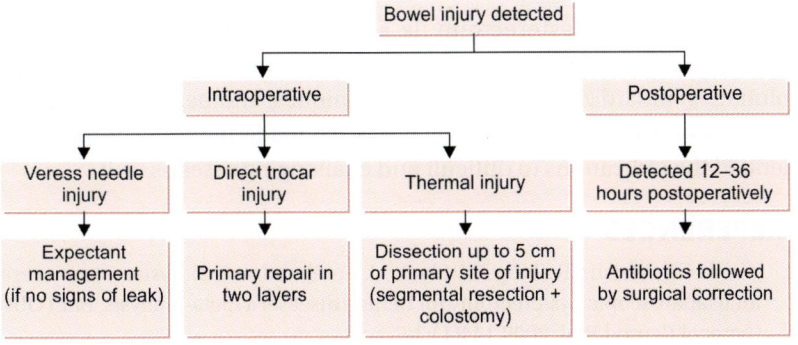

Flowchart 3: Management of bowel injury.

Omental Injury

- *Cause:* Veress needle, trocar, thermal injury
- *Risk factors:* Previous laparotomies, dense adhesions, endometriosis
- *Prevention:* Palmer point entry, entry under vision or open technique
- *Management:* Expectant management is done in cases of small injury without any active bleeding. In case bleeding is noted, coagulation is done.

Vascular Injuries

- *Incidence:*[21] 0.02%
- *Commonly involved vessels:* Inferior epigastric artery, internal iliac, inferior vena cava, and rarely aorta
- *Cause:* During veress needle or trocar insertion, dissection in cases of malignancy[22]
- *Prevention:*
  - Transillumination while accessory trocar placement is done
  - Careful dissection on vascular structures
- *Management (**Box 3**):*[23]

BOX 3: Management of vascular injuries.

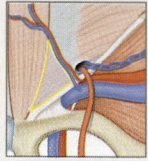

Abdominal wall vessels:
- Coagulation
- Suturing
- Tamponade effect by Foley's catheter

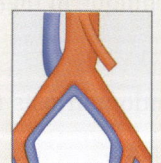

Major vessels:
- Pressure
- Arrange blood call for help [cardiothoracic and cascular surgery (CTVS)]
- Suturing

■ CONCLUSION

Total laparoscopic hysterectomy is a procedure with low incidence of complications if proper surgical techniques are adhered to. The technological evolution, standardization of surgical techniques, and better understanding of the anatomy of the lateral pelvic wall have made the procedure safe and extended the indications to difficult and challenging cases as well.

■ REFERENCES

1. Walsh CA, Walsh SR, Tang TY, Slack M. Total abdominal hysterectomy versus total laparoscopic hysterectomy for benign disease: a meta-analysis. Eur J Obstet Gynecol Reprod Biol. 2009;144(1):3-7.

2. Aarts JW, Nieboer TE, Johnson N, Tavender E, Garry R, Mol BW, et al. Surgical approach to hysterectomy for benign gynaecological disease. Cochrane Database Syst Rev. 2015;8:CD003677.
3. Sutasanasuang S. Laparoscopic hysterectomy versus total abdominal hysterectomy: a retrospective comparative study. J Med Assoc Thai. 2011; 94(1):8-16.
4. Olsson JH, Ellström M, Hahlin M. A randomised prospective trial comparing laparoscopic and abdominal hysterectomy. BJOG Int J Obstet Gynaecol. 1996;103(4):345-50.
5. Reich H, DeCaprio JO, McGlynn FR. Laparoscopic hysterectomy. J Gynecol Surg. 1989;5(2):213-6.
6. Adelman MR, Bardsley TR, Sharp HT. Urinary tract injuries in laparoscopic hysterectomy: a systematic review. J Minim Invasive Gynecol. 2014;21(4):558-66.
7. Lafay Pillet MC, Leonard F, Chopin N, Malaret JM, Borghese B, Foulot H, et al. Incidence and risk factors of bladder injuries during laparoscopic hysterectomy indicated for benign uterine pathologies: a 14.5 years experience in a continuous series of 1501 procedures. Hum Reprod. 2009;24(4):842-9.
8. Aydin C, Mercimek MN. Laparoscopic management of bladder injury during total laparoscopic hysterectomy. Int J Clin Pract. 2020;74(6):e13507.
9. Wohlrab KJ, Sung VW, Rardin CR. Management of laparoscopic bladder injuries. J Minim Invasive Gynecol. 2011;18(1):4-8.
10. Mat E, Yıldız G, Basol G, Kurt D, Kuru B, Gundogdu EC, et al. Laparoscopic Management of Bladder Injury During Total Laparoscopic Hysterectomy. South Clin Ist Euras. 2021;32(2).
11. Rovner ES. Urinary tract fistulae. In: Wein AJ, Kavoussi LR, Novick AC, Partin AW, Peters CA (Eds). Campbell-Walsh Urology, 10th edition. Philadelphia: Elsevier Saunders; 2012. pp. 2242-6.
12. Cirstoiu M, Munteanu O. Strategies of preventing ureteral iatrogenic injuries in obstetrics-gynecology. J Med Life. 2012;5(3):277.
13. Kuno K, Menzin A, Kauder HH, Sion C, Gal D. Prophylactic ureteral catheterization in gynecologic surgery. Urology. 1998;52:1004-8.
14. Brandes S, Coburn M, Armenakas N, McAninch J. Diagnosis and management of ureteric injury: an evidence-based analysis. BJU Int. 2004;94(3):277-89.
15. Burks FN, Santucci RA. Management of iatrogenic ureteral injury. Ther Adv Urol. 2014;6(3):115-24.
16. Llarena NC, Shah AB, Milad MP. Bowel injury in gynecologic laparoscopy: a systematic review. Obstet Gynecol. 2015;125(6):1407-17.
17. Zhu CR, Mallick R, Singh SS, Auer R, Solnik J, Choudhry AJ, et al. Risk factors for bowel injury in hysterectomy for benign indications. Obstet Gynecol. 2020;136:803.
18. Elbiss HM, Abu-Zidan FM. Bowel injury following gynecological laparoscopic surgery. Afr Health Sci. 2017;17(4):1237-45.
19. Birns MT. Inadvertent instrumental perforation of the colon during laparoscopy: nonsurgical repair. Gastrointest Endosc. 1989;35(1):54-6.
20. Gomel V, Taylor PJ (Eds). Complications and their management. Diagnostic and Operative Gynecologic Laparoscopy. St Louis: Mosby; 1995. pp. 299-308.

21. King N, Friedman J, Lin E, Traylor J, Wong J, Tsai S, et al. Systematic review of major vascular injuries (MVI) during gynecologic laparoscopy for benign indications. Am J Obstet Gynecol. 2019;220(3):S766.
22. Buras AL, Chern JY, Chon HS, Shahzad MM, Wenham RM, Hoffman MS. Major vascular injury during gynecologic cancer surgery. Gynecol Oncol Reps. 2021;37:100815.
23. Brierley G, Arshad I, Shakir F, Visvathanan D, Arambage K. Vascular injury during laparoscopic gynaecological surgery: a methodological approach for prevention and management. Obstet Gynaecol. 2020;22(3):191-8.

16 Decreased Fetal Movements

CHAPTER

Parikshit Tank, Jaydeep Tank

■ INTRODUCTION

The simplest, but not the only, proof of life is to find something that is alive. There are only two properties that can determine if an object is alive, i.e., metabolism and motion.[1] Movement in all forms—microscopic or macroscopic—is perhaps the most convincing and visible indicator of life. For the fetus, movement has historically been regarded as the earliest sign of life. In fact, in days gone by, fetal movement was a method of diagnosing pregnancy. The first perception of fetal movement in pregnancy is called quickening. As pregnancy progresses, fetal movements have been looked upon as a sign of fetal health. A change in the pattern of fetal movements, especially a reduction or absence has been seen as a precedent of poor fetal outcomes, including fetal death.[2]

■ FETAL MOVEMENT PHYSIOLOGY

It is possible to see distinct gross body movements by the fetus as early as the seventh week of gestation by ultrasound. However, the mother usually perceives movements by 18-20 weeks (multigravidae) or 20-22 weeks (primigravidae). The earliest movements are usually described as a flutter or a brief vibratory sense by the mother. As pregnancy advances, movements become more distinct and the mother can usually describe the fetus to be kicking, punching (limb movements), and rolling or turning (trunk movements). Fetal movements follow a circadian pattern and movements are more in the late evenings. Fetal movements increase in frequency and force till 32-34 weeks of pregnancy. After this, there is gradual decrease in the perception of fetal movements. This has been attributed to improved fetal coordination, increased fetal size, and relatively less amniotic fluid.[3] Ultrasound studies suggest that there is no reduction in the actual number of fetal movements, but there is a change in the maternal perception.[4] There is great variability in the number of fetal movements and reports indicate that a healthy fetus may move between 4 and 100 times in an hour.[2] The difference in mean time to perceive 10 movements is between 21 minutes for focused counting to 162 minutes with unfocused perception of fetal movements.[3,5]

■ FACTORS AFFECTING FETAL MOVEMENT

Since fetal movement is a sign of fetal health, decreased movement is a cause for concern. Decreased fetal movements affect 5–15% of pregnancies.[6] A number of conditions are associated with reduced fetal movements. The one of primary concern is fetal hypoxia. The fetus responds to chronic hypoxia by conserving energy and the subsequent reduction of fetal movements is an adaptive mechanism to reduce oxygen consumption. 11–29% of women presenting with reduced fetal movements carry a small for gestational age (SGA) fetus with estimated weight and abdominal circumference below the 10th centile.[6,7] The diagnosis or suspicion of the growth restricted fetus is important so that further testing can be initiated and obstetric intervention can be appropriately planned. Decreased fetal movements are regarded as a marker for suboptimal intrauterine conditions as outlined in **Table 1**. Some of these are iatrogenic and should be kept in mind when assessing a woman presenting with a history of reduced fetal movements. In theory, it may be possible that centrally acting antihypertensive agents such as methyldopa may reduce fetal movement. However, in a clinical trial, there was no change in fetal movements with this agent.[8] In a situation where a hypertensive mother is on methyldopa, reduced fetal movements should not be ascribed to drugs and thorough fetal evaluation is warranted.

Fetal movement is a maternally perceived and reported symptom. Studies on the correlation between maternal perception of fetal movements and fetal movements concurrently detected on ultrasound scans show wide variation, with correlation ranging from 37 to 88% and large body movements and those lasting >7 seconds most likely to be felt.[9] Reduced fetal movement is usually a subjective evaluation by the mother. There is scope for perception

TABLE 1: Factors associated with reduction of fetal movements.

Actual reduction in fetal movements	*Maternal perception is reduced*
Fetal hypoxia	Obesity
Small for gestational age (SGA) or growth restricted fetus	Anteriorly located placenta
Oligohydramnios	Polyhydramnios
Fetus with major anomalies, central nervous system (CNS), and musculoskeletal anomalies	Fetal position—fetus with the back anterior
Fetal anemia	Maternal position—upright postures
Fetal infection	Attention on other activities over prolonged periods
Maternal habits—cigarette smoking, alcohol, and methadone use	
Iatrogenic—glucose, steroids, and sedatives	

to be affected by factors not related to the fetal condition. The factors which reduce the perception (and not the actual number of movements) are listed in **Table 1**. If these are present, it may be difficult for the mother and clinician to rely on fetal movements as a parameter of fetal health.

ASSESSING FETAL MOVEMENT

The advantage of fetal movement as a parameter of fetal health is that it does not involve any medical technology. There have been attempts to make an objective recording of the fetal movements by using a Doppler transducer attached to the maternal abdominal wall or even with ultrasound. However, these are cumbersome and come with the difficulties of access. In practice, maternal perception is the only technique that is used.

Informal evaluation of the fetal movements is done by routine enquiry at antenatal visits or when the mother may present to the clinician with other complaints. Formal fetal movement counting has been described. When counting fetal movements at rest, a woman may be asked to empty her bladder, lie on her side, relax, put her hand on her abdomen, and count the fetal movements over the period specified for the method used. It has been suggested that a clinician should go through the procedure with her and palpate her abdomen as she is counting fetal movements to see whether she can identify them.[2,10]

In the earliest studies, counting was performed as full "daily movement counts (DMCs)".[11] This methodology requires women to note fetal movements through both rest and daily activities over 12 hours. The actual studies were performed on high-risk hospitalized women. The correlation between perceptions of fetal movements of women at rest versus women involved in normal daily activities is not known, but it is expected to be significantly lower with activity. Later studies used "focused counting" for either a specific time or the time needed for a defined number of movements (e.g., Cardiff count to ten), while the mother is instructed to lie down and focus on fetal movements.[12]

The problem with the described methods is that at present, we do not have well-defined guidelines on what constitutes a basis for further testing. There is a range of "normal" fetal movements, leading to wide variability. Ideally, an alarm limit would be developed using the whole obstetric population and then be proved to reduce stillbirth rates in a prospective study. Currently, the best-founded definition of decreased fetal movements comes from the study by Moore and Piacquadio, who defined it as maternal perception of less than ten movements within 2 hours which is approximately five standard deviations from the mean counting time in normal pregnancies.[5] Kuwata et al. proposed decreased fetal movement as the maternal perception of <10 movements within 25 and 35 minutes before and after 37 weeks of gestation, respectively.[13]

IS THERE AN EVIDENCE BASE TO SUPPORT FORMAL FETAL MOVEMENT COUNTING?

In 2008, the National Institute for Health and Care Excellence (NICE) and the National Collaborating Centre for Women's and Children's Health renewed their guideline on the routine antenatal care of healthy pregnant women. They concluded that routine formal fetal movements counting should not be offered.[14] In contrast, the American College of Obstetricians and Gynecologists supports formal movement counting. In their bulletin on antepartum fetal surveillance, they instruct the woman to count ten movements, preferably after a meal, and to write down the hours this takes.[15] This variation in clinical guidance may result from different interpretation of the published data regarding reduced fetal movements. This difference in opinion also reflects the dilemma and controversy of the definition and management of reduced fetal movements.

A systematic review in the Cochrane database evaluated four studies involving 71,370 women. All the studies compared different modalities of formal fetal movement counting. There was a significantly higher compliance with Cardiff "count to ten" (once a day) method than the fetal movement counting method where women were counting 30 minutes before meals and at bedtime (more than once a day). All other outcomes reported were nonsignificant. In particular, no trials compared fetal movement counting with no fetal movement counting. Robust research is needed in this area.[2]

Therefore, even though fetal movement counting is simple, can be done at home, economical and does not involve medical resources directly, we must consider some potential downsides before prescribing it routinely. There is an intrusion on the woman's time, the chance that it may cause unnecessary maternal anxiety, and staff overload as additional investigations may have to be done to exclude fetal compromise. It could increase antenatal admissions, obstetric interventions, and prematurity.

APPROACH TO A WOMAN WITH REDUCED FETAL MOVEMENTS

Even in settings where clinical guidelines for the evaluation of women with reduced fetal movements have been in place, there is wide variation in practice.[16] The first step in a woman presenting with reduced fetal movements is to exclude fetal death. Fetal heartbeat can be confirmed by a handheld Doppler device in most pregnancies after 24 weeks of gestation. Hearing the fetal heartbeat is reassuring for the mother. The fetal and maternal heartbeat (uterine souffle) should be distinguished. If the fetal heartbeat is not confirmed, an ultrasound scan should be done immediately to ascertain fetal viability.

Flowchart 1: Approach to a woman with the first episode of reduced fetal movements.

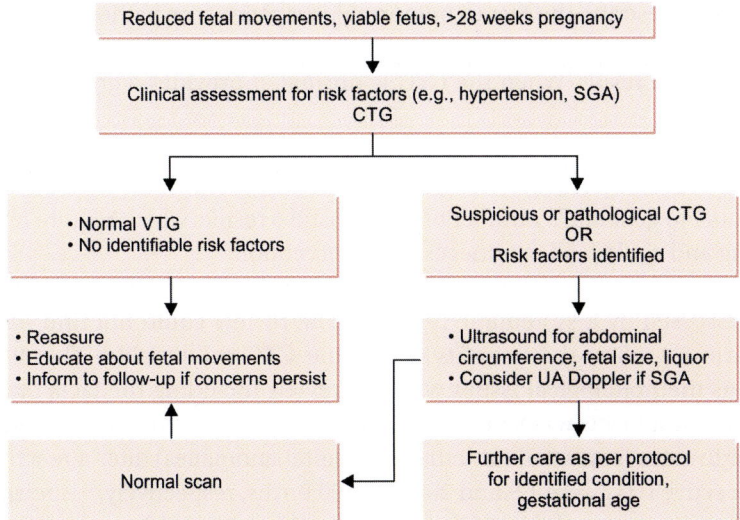

(CTG: cardiotocography; SGA: small for gestational age; UA: umbilical arterial)

Having established that the fetus is alive, the objectives of further evaluation are to assess the fetal growth and wellbeing. There should be documentation of the findings and of the "thought process" in the evaluation of the woman. The woman should be discharged from care only when the caregiver is satisfied that the risk to the fetus is low.

Clinical evaluation should be directed toward identifying the high-risk fetus. The history should include duration of the reduction or absence of fetal movements, repeat episodes, and access to care. Clinical examinations including measuring the blood pressure and urine albumin which can help to identify some of the factors associated with reduced fetal movements that are known to increase perinatal morbidity and mortality are listed in **Table 1**.

The approach to a woman with reduced fetal movements is represented in **Flowchart 1**. The basic testing modality is fetal cardiotocography (CTG) and assessment of the fetal size by clinical and ultrasound examination. Further management depends on identifiable risk factors, persistence of the complaints, and the gestational age.

FETAL CARDIOTOCOGRAPHY IN WOMEN WITH REDUCED FETAL MOVEMENTS

Cardiotocography is the first and almost universally performed fetal testing in a woman with reduced fetal movements. In a Norwegian study of over 3,000 women presenting with reduced fetal movements, it was reported that 97.5% had a CTG as a part of the assessment.[17] The reasons for the CTG being a popular test are that it can be performed readily and is not operator dependent. It is not expensive or time-consuming. There are well-established criteria to describe the test to be normal, suspicious, or pathological.[18] The initial test of 20 minutes may be extended to 80 minutes to achieve the criteria for a normal result. When the CTG is normal, it provides a great degree of reassurance.

However, the CTG may be misinterpreted by error. These errors can be reduced by the use of computerized analysis.[19] The CTG also has the potential to generate a number of false-positive results which require further testing and could lead to unnecessary intervention.

The evidence for the use of CTG in monitoring "high-risk pregnancies" was assessed by a systematic review.[20] The review could not find data to confirm or refute the benefits of routine CTG monitoring. There were serious methodological issues with the review including the facts that the number of subjects was small. Even among the studies from that period, the stillbirth rates (corrected for lethal congenital anomalies) after a reactive or nonreactive CTG were 1.9 and 26 per 1,000 births, respectively.[21] A relatively small study reported that 56% of women with a high-risk pregnancy who reported reduced fetal movement had an abnormal CTG. This was associated with an unfavorable perinatal outcome in nine out of ten cases.[22] A recent Cochrane review found that the consensus opinion was to use CTG as a first-line assessment tool for a woman presenting with reduced fetal movements. They also opined that computerized CTG assessment and fetal arousal tests should be prioritized as areas for further research.[23]

ASSESSING FETAL GROWTH IN WOMEN WITH REDUCED FETAL MOVEMENT

Women presenting with reduced fetal movements represent a population where the fetus is likely to be SGA or even growth restricted. Identifying such a pregnancy is important since it has implications for the management and outcome of the baby. An accurate assignment of the date and period of gestation at the time of presentation is mandatory in assessing fetal growth.

Despite the fact that abdominal palpation only detects 30% of small fetuses, symphysis fundal height (SFH) measurement has a positive predictive value of 60% and a negative predictive value of 76.8%.[24] This implies that if the SFH is within normal limits, fetal growth restriction or placental insufficiency are unlikely to be present. Fetal biometry assessment should be performed if SFH suggests a small fetus or if there is suspected oligohydramnios. It should also be considered for women with risk factors for growth restriction and on second and subsequent presentations of reduced fetal movements. Abdominal circumference and estimated fetal weight below the 10th centile should be used to predict the SGA fetus.[24] If an SGA fetus is identified, further testing and care should be instituted as per the protocol for the clinical situation.

ULTRASOUND IN WOMEN WITH REDUCED FETAL MOVEMENTS

Besides biometry, ultrasound can assess amniotic fluid status, biophysical profile, and blood flow in the uteroplacental and fetoplacental circulation by Doppler. Amniotic fluid assessment can be done by the deepest pocket technique or amniotic fluid index from four quadrants. Amniotic fluid volume and biophysical profile of the fetus have limited value in diagnosing the at-risk fetus.[24] However, they may be useful in monitoring the high-risk fetus at preterm gestations or to identify false-positive CTG. There are no studies specifically assessing the value of these parameters in a population of women presenting with reduced fetal movements. Doppler velocimetry of the umbilical artery has been compared to CTG in women presenting with reduced fetal movements. Dubiel et al. compared these techniques in the assessment of 599 women with low-risk pregnancies complaining of reduced fetal movements; both were normal in 93% of women. The overall perinatal mortality in their study was 3.8%. They found that the CTG seemed to be a better predictor of mortality and infant handicap than Doppler velocimetry.[25] A normal umbilical Doppler velocimetry may be reassuring to the clinician. It is however, of more value in monitoring the growth restricted fetus rather than diagnosing one.

SPECIAL CLINICAL SITUATIONS

Repeat Episodes of Reduced Fetal Movements Despite Normal Testing

About 5% of women may present with another episode of reduced movements.[7] A large proportion of them will have normal test results on CTG and ultrasound. There are some less common causes such as anomalies and anemia due to fetomaternal hemorrhage which can be sought but are difficult to diagnose. Further care depends on individual situations, since there is little evidence to base recommendations on. Having ruled out a growth restricted or SGA fetus, one could offer daily CTG testing. If the woman is worried about pregnancy outcome due to reasons other than purely medical ones, there may be some benefit from counseling. If the mother persists with the concerns of reduced movements at a gestational age when the fetus is mature, there should be a consideration for inducing labor and delivery.

Reduced Fetal Movement Before Obstetric Intervention can be Offered (24–26 Weeks)

The gestational age at which different obstetric units would offer delivery and neonatal care varies with the settings. However, this is usually at 24–26 weeks in most circumstances with access to advanced neonatal care. Before this gestational age, women presenting with reduced fetal movements are difficult to assess. Fetal heartbeat should be recorded but CTG interpretation may not be meaningful. An ultrasound to assess fetal structure should be performed if not already done.

No Fetal Movements Perceived Till 24 Weeks of Gestation

If fetal movements have never been perceived till 24 weeks of gestation, there could be a possibility of a fetus with abnormalities if fetal death is ruled out. The abnormality could be one which affects the fetal neuromuscular or skeletal system in the form of a congenital structural or metabolic disorder, or a chromosomal anomaly. A referral to a fetal medicine specialist should be made to assess such a pregnancy.

CONCLUSION

There is evidence that fetal movements reflect fetal conditions in utero. Reduced fetal movements are a coarse indicator of fetal wellbeing. At present, there is little evidence to recommend routine daily movement counting as a strategy to prevent poor perinatal outcomes in the general population. A woman presenting with reduced fetal movements should be screened for the fetus at risk of perinatal morbidity and mortality. A uniform protocol should be available at obstetric units so that assessment and interventions follow a logical pattern.

REFERENCES

1. McKay CP. What is life—and how do we search for it in other worlds? PLoS Biol. 2004;2(9):e302.
2. Mangesi L, Hofmeyr GJ, Smith V, Smyth RM; Cochrane Pregnancy and Childbirth Group. Fetal movement counting for assessment of fetal wellbeing. Cochrane Database Syst Rev. 2015;2015(10):CD004909.
3. Grant E, Elbourne D, Valentin L, Alexander S. Routine formal fetal movement counting and risk of antepartum late death in normally formed singletons. Lancet. 1989;2:345-9.
4. Unterscheider J, Horgan R, O'Donoghue K, Greene R. Reduced fetal movements. Obstet Gynaecol. 2009;11:245-51.
5. Moore TR, Piacquadio K. A prospective evaluation of fetal movement screening to reduce the incidence of antepartum fetal death. Am J Obstet Gynecol. 1989;160:1075-80.
6. Sergent F, Lefevre A, Verspyck E, Marpeau L. Decreased fetal movements in the third trimester: what to do? Gynecol Obstet Fertil. 2005;33:861-9.
7. Sinha D, Sharma A, Nallaswamy V, Jaygopal N, Bhatti N. Obstetric outcome in women complaining of reduced fetal movements. J Obstet Gynaecol. 2007;27:41-3.
8. Wide-Swensson D, Montan S, Arulkumaran S, Ingemarsson I, Ratnam SS. Effect of methyldopa and isradipine on fetal heart rate pattern assessed by

computerized cardiotocography in human pregnancy. Am J Obstet Gynecol. 1993;169:1581-5.
9. Royal College of Obstetricians and Gynecologists. Reduced Fetal Movements (Green-top Guideline No. 57). London: RCOG; 2011.
10. Tucker SM. Fetal Monitoring and Assessment. London: Mosby; 2000.
11. Sadovsky E, Yaffe H. Daily fetal movement recording and fetal prognosis. Obstet Gynecol. 1973;41:845-50.
12. Heazell AE, Frøen JF. Methods of fetal movement counting and the detection of fetal compromise. J Obstet Gynaecol. 2008;28:147-54.
13. Kuwata T, Matsubara S, Ohkusa T, Ohkuchi A, Izumi A, Watanabe T, et al. Establishing a reference value for the frequency of fetal movements using modified 'count to 10' method. J Obstet Gynaecol Res. 2008;34:318-23.
14. National Institute for Health and Clinical Excellence and National Collaborating Centre for Women's and Children's Health. Clinical Guideline CG62. Antenatal Care: Routine Care for the Healthy Pregnant Woman. London: NICE; 2008.
15. ACOG Practice Bulletin. Antepartum fetal surveillance. Antepartum fetal surveillance. Number 9, October 1999 (replaces Technical Bulletin Number 188, January 1994). Clinical Management Guidelines for Obstetrician-Gynecologists. Int J Gynaecol Obstet. 2000;68:175-85.
16. Heazell AE, Green M, Wright C, Flenady V, Frøen JF. Midwives and obstetricians knowledge and management of women presenting with decreased fetal movements. Acta Obstet Gynecol Scand. 2008;87:331-9.
17. Saastad E, Ahlborg T, Frøen JF. Low maternal awareness of fetal movement is associated with small for gestational age infants. J Midwifery Womens Health. 2008;53:345-52.
18. National Collaborating Centre for Women's and Children's Health. Intrapartum care. Care of healthy women and their babies during childbirth. London: RCOG; 2007.
19. Dawes GS, Moulden M, Redman CW. Improvements in computerized fetal heart rate analysis antepartum. J Perinat Med. 1996;24:25-36.
20. Pattison N, McCowan L. Cardiotocography for antepartum fetal assessment. Cochrane Database Syst Rev. 2000;(2):CD001068.
21. Freeman RK, Anderson G, Dorchester W. A prospective multi-institutional study of antepartum fetal heart rate monitoring. I. Risk of perinatal mortality and morbidity according to antepartum fetal heart rate test results. Am J Obstet Gynecol. 1982;143:771-7.
22. Rayburn WF. Clinical significance of perceptible fetal motion. Am J Obstet Gynecol. 1980;138:210-2.
23. Hofmeyr GJ, Novikova N. Management of reported decreased fetal movements for improving pregnancy outcomes. Cochrane Database Syst Rev. 2012;4:CD009148.
24. Royal College of Obstetricians and Gynecologists. The Investigation and Management of the Small-for-Gestational-Age Fetus. Green-top Guideline No. 31. London: RCOG; 2002.
25. Dubiel M, Gudmundsson S, Thuring-Jönsson A, Maesal A, Marsel K. Doppler velocimetry and nonstress test for predicting outcome of pregnancies with decreased fetal movements. Am J Perinatol. 1997;14:139-44.

CHAPTER 17

Insulin Sensitizers in Polycystic Ovary Syndrome

Rakhi Singh

■ INTRODUCTION

Polycystic ovary syndrome (PCOS) is the most common endocrine disorder affecting women of reproductive age group, prevalence of 4–12%, even up to 25% in some populations.[1,2]

Insulin resistance (IR) is defined clinically as the inability of a known quantity of exogenous or endogenous insulin to increase glucose uptake and utilization in an individual as much as it does in a normal population.

Insulin resistance can also be defined as a pathological condition characterized by a decreased responsiveness or sensitivity to the metabolic actions of insulin. It is an established predictor of a range of disorders. In women with PCOS, IR plays an important role in the development and persistence of this disorder[3,4] and is recognized to lead to many of the metabolic abnormalities associated with metabolic syndrome.

Polycystic ovary syndrome patients with IR are likely to have chronic subclinical inflammation and impaired fasting plasma glucose levels, which in turn enhance the prevalence of the more atherogenic, low-density cholesterol (LDL-C) particles.[5]

Given this high prevalence, the need for accurate screening of IR in women with PCOS is obvious. Early recognition and management of IR in women with PCOS would offer important preventive measures.[6]

Insulin resistance causes compensatory hyperinsulinemia, which in turn causes hyperandrogenism by following mechanism:
- Stimulating the ovary to release androgens.
- Increasing free androgen by suppressing liver production of sex hormone binding globulin.

Insulin resistance is present is both obese and nonobese women with PCOS. The severity of IR in women with PCOS is associated with the amount of abdominal obesity, even in lean women with PCOS.

Approximately 75% patients with PCOS are found to be insulin resistant. Insulin resistance is reported 40.2%, as high as 76.9% from India in women with PCOS.

Because insulin resistance with compensatory hyperinsulinemia is widely considered the pivotal feature of PCOS, insulin-sensitizing drugs (ISDs) are introduced for the treatment of these patients.

■ INSULIN SENSITIZING AGENTS

Metformin

Metformin (1,1-dimethylbuguanide hydrochloride) is a biguanide currently used as an oral antihyperglycemic agent. Metformin was introduced in 1957, but it only became available for use in the United States in 1995. To date, metformin administration is approved by the US Food and Drug Administration (USFDA) to treat type 2 diabetes mellitus (DM). Metformin, in fact, is the most extensively studied ISD in the treatment of the short- and long-term sequelae.

In 1994, Velazquez et al.[7] administered metformin in 26 obese PCOS women to investigate role of insulin resistance in pathogenesis of PCOS. Significant reduction in circulating androgen levels, significant weight loss, its role in inducing regular menstrual, and ovulatory cycles were demonstrated.

Azziz et al.[8] suggest that metformin should be used to treat and prevent progression to impaired glucose tolerance in PCO patients.

In Rotterdam consensus, they concluded that metformin should not be used as first-choice agents in ovulation induction of women with PCOS, and their use should be restricted to those patients with IGT.[9]

Metformin works by improving the sensitivity of peripheral tissues to insulin,[10,11] which results in a reduction of circulating insulin levels.

Metformin inhibits hepatic gluconeogenesis and it also increases the glucose uptake by peripheral tissues and reduces fatty acid oxidation.[12]

Metformin has a positive effect on the endothelium and adipose tissue independent of its action on insulin and glucose levels.[1]

Dose

Metformin is available in two formulations—immediate and extended-release. Metformin at immediate-release is commercialized as 500-, 850-, and 1,000-mg tablets, whereas the drug at extended-release is available as 1,000- and 2,000-mg tablets. Metformin is indicated in patients over the age of 10 years, and the extended-release preparation is indicated in those over the age of 17 years. An extremely variable target dose of 1,500–2,550 mg/day was proposed.[13]

It can be started with a daily dose of 500 mg and slowly increased every 2 weeks by 500 mg to build tolerance.[13] If increase in dose causes worsening of side effects, previous suitable dose can be continued.

In particular, the extended-release metformin administered at a daily dosage of 1,500 mg was similarly effective as the immediate-release metformin at a 500-mg dosage three times daily.

Almost all published studies including PCOS patients used metformin in immediate-release preparation; however, in a recent RCT, PCOS patients were treated with the extended-release formulation (1 g twice daily). In that trial, there were significant decreases in body mass index (BMI) and total testosterone levels and significant increases in sex hormone-binding globulin (SHBG) levels with extended-release metformin. No change in fasting markers of insulin resistance was observed.

Duration of therapy is not standardized. Usually 3-6 months therapy is advised.

After a long-term metformin treatment, drug suspension is related to a quick reversion of its beneficial effect on peripheral insulin sensitivity. In fact, a slightly, but significant, worsening of the insulin resistance and hyperandrogenic state was observed in comparison with baseline and with patients who received placebo. The quick loss of beneficial effects due to metformin on insulin resistance and subsequently on hyperandrogenism after metformin suspension seemed to be related to a worsening of menstrual cyclicity.

Side Effects

Common side effects—abdominal discomfort, bloating, constipation, diarrhea, flatulence, heartburn, indigestion, nausea, vomiting, slight/moderate chest pain, cough, mouth metallic taste, nail changes, rash, runny nose, sneezing, skin flushing, and alopecia.

Rare side effects—severe/serious, lactic acidosis, and liver failure.

To date, metformin is still found in the B classification for US-FDA pregnancy category. This means that no teratogenic effect was demonstrated in animal models, and human safety studies are not adequate.

Lord and colleagues compiled early studies of metformin and ovulation induction in a meta-analysis.[14]

Metformin as First-line of Therapy

It was concluded that metformin was an effective therapy to induce ovulation in PCOS women. They associated better outcomes when combined with lifestyle management whereas no change in live birth rate was demonstrated in women receiving metformin when compared to women receiving placebo or no treatment.

Metformin with Clomiphene Citrate

Better ovulation rates were demonstrated when metformin and clomiphene citrate (CC) were given in combination, compared to metformin alone or clomiphene citrate alone therapy. Palomba et al. in 2009 concluded that metformin with clomiphene citrate is not superior to clomiphene alone with regard to ovulation, pregnancy and live birth rates. In CC-resistant PCOS women, the addition of metformin was demonstrated to be effective in inducing ovulation in the two meta-analyses by Lord et al.

Metformin plus CC association was related to higher ovulation rates than LOD, even if no difference in the rates of pregnancies, live births and miscarriages were detected between two procedures.

Metformin with Gonadotropins for Ovulation Induction[15]

Due to the small number of studies included and small sample size in each study, a conclusion could not be reached on the efficacy of metformin as a coadjuvant to gonadotropins for ovulation induction in PCOS women. It seems, however, that the length of ovarian stimulation was shorter among those receiving a combination of gonadotropins and metformin.

Metformin and In Vitro Fertilization

Cochrane review has concluded that adding metformin to the ovarian stimulation protocol in PCOS undergoing in vitro fertilization (IVF) treatment had no impact on pregnancy or live birth rates. However, it reduced the risk of ovarian hyperstimulation syndrome (OHSS).[16]

In a small study, it was reported that the addition of metformin to an antagonist protocol improved the oocyte quality in PCOS patients undergoing IVF.[17] Others have also reported that the addition of metformin to their regular stimulation protocol had a positive effect on the quality of the oocytes and embryos.[18]

Metformin and Weight Loss

It was reported independently by two other groups that the combination of low-calorie diet and metformin led to a significant reduction in visceral fat.[19-21] In a recent meta-analysis, it was reported that metformin treatment was associated with a significant decrease in BMI compared with placebo.

Metformin and Pregnancy

Observational studies have suggested that metformin administration reduced the risk of miscarriage among PCOS sufferers.[22-24]

Metformin and Gestational Diabetes Mellitus

The continuation of metformin throughout pregnancy reduced the risk of GDM among PCOS women. Glueck and colleagues reported a prevalence of GDM of 7% among pregnant PCOS women who continued taking metformin throughout pregnancy compared with 30% among those who did not.

As for the safety profile, a study by Rowan and colleagues reported that the use of metformin in the treatment of GDM had no increased risk of perinatal complications.[25]

Metformin and Pregnancy-induced Hypertension

The evidence regarding the benefits of metformin in reducing the risk of pregnancy-induced hypertension (PIH) and preeclampsia (PE) is less clear.

The long-term use of metformin to prevent remote complications of PCOS is uncertain and a significant amount of work is needed before a decision can be made.

Inositols

Inositols belong to the vitamin B complex group, which is synthesized in the human body. There are nine stereoisomers, of which the most important ones are myoinositol and D-chiro-inositol. Inositols are considered insulin sensitizers, as they modulate the members of insulin signaling pathways. They positively influence menstrual cycle regularity, carbohydrate metabolism, and the clinical and laboratory symptoms of hyperandrogenism (e.g., free testosterone, total testosterone, SHBG).

Compared to metformin, cycle normalization and reduction in BMI are higher in Myo Inositol Group.

The inositol phosphoglycans (IPGs) are putative mediators in an on classic insulin signaling cascade for glucose uptake and use. Insulin-resistant women with PCOS display decreased insulin stimulated release of d-chiro-inositol (DCI)-containing IPGs (DCI-IPGs) during an oral glucose tolerance test (OGTT), compared with control women, which was related to impaired coupling between insulin action and the release of the DCI-IPG.

Oral nutritional supplementation with inositol, part of the vitamin B-complex and an intracellular second messenger, was demonstrated to enhance insulin sensitivity and improve the clinical and hormonal characteristics of patients with PCOS. In addition, inositol supplementation was shown to restore spontaneous ovulation with the consequent increase in conception, either alone or when combined with gonadotropin.

Myoinositol is the most abundant form of inositol in nature, while D-chiro-inositol is synthetized by an epimerase that convert MI to DCI. In particular, this reaction is insulin dependent.

Dose

- One gram of D-chiro-inositol and 400 μg of folic acid *per* day.
- Myo-inositol 2 g/day in divided doses.
- Better drug combination, available in ratio of 40:1.

Duration of Therapy

Minimum 3–6 months of therapy is needed for metabolic effects to get better.

Pretreatment with myo-inositol increased the clinical pregnancy rate by 6.13% and also reduced the miscarriage rate by 27.08%.

It was confirmed recently by a human study in PCOS women where the ratio 40:1 was most effective in restoring ovulation and normalizing important parameters in these patients while decreased activity was observed with other formulations (1:3.5; 2.5:1; 5:1; 20:1; 80:1), especially when the 40:1 ratio was modified in favor of DCI.[26] Some studies however show different results—the combination 550 mg MI + 150 mg DCI twice daily (3:1) showed higher pregnancy and live birth rates and lower risk of OHSS compared to the control group (CG) was administered 550 mg of MI + 13.8 mg of DCI twice daily (40:1).[27]

Side effects, if any, tend to be mild and may include nausea, stomach pain, tiredness, headache, and dizziness.

Thiazolidinediones (TZDs) are synthetic ligands also known as glitazones (troglitazone, rosiglitazone, or pioglitazone), which can bind and activate the nuclear receptor, peroxysome proliferator-activated receptor-gamma (PPAR-γ).

Activation of PPAR-γ by TZDs increases insulin sensitivity mainly in adipocytes and muscle cells, and also stimulates the differentiation of adipose cells.

Pioglitazone and rosiglitazone are both classified by the FDA as pregnancy category C and present potential teratogenic risks. PPARγ is important for embryonic development and TZDs can cause a decrease in fetal maturation.

Insulin sensitizers have a big impact on the outcome of metabolic and endocrinological functions in PCOS women. They also have benefits during fertility treatments, such as better ovulation rates, reduced miscarriage rates, reduced risks of developing GDM or PIH.

Metformin and inositols are most studied and routinely used insulin sensitizing drugs, metformin more commonly than inositols. Better patient selection and therapeutic doses can give better outcomes.

■ CONCLUSION

Insulin sensitizers play a crucial role in the management of PCOS. These medications, such as metformin and thiazolidinediones, address the underlying insulin resistance that often accompanies PCOS. By improving insulin sensitivity, they contribute to better metabolic health, hormonal balance, and fertility outcomes in individuals with PCOS. However, it is important to note that individual responses to these medications may vary, and their use should be guided by a healthcare professional. As research continues to explore the complexities of PCOS, insulin sensitizers remain a valuable component of the multifaceted approach to addressing this common endocrine disorder.

■ REFERENCES

1. Diamanti-Kandarakis E, Christakou CD, Kandaraki E, Economou FN. Metformin: an old medication of new fashion: evolving new molecular mechanisms

and clinical implications in polycystic ovary syndrome. Eur J Endocrinol. 2010;162(2):193-212.
2. Diamanti-Kandarakis E, Kouli CR, Bergiele AT, Filandra FA, Tsianateli TC, Spina GG, et al. A survey of the polycystic ovary syndrome in the Greek island of Lesbos: hormonal and metabolic profile. J Clin Endocrinol Metab. 1999;84(11):4006-11.
3. Polak K, Czyzyk A, Simoncini T, Meczekalski B. New markers of insulin resistance in polycystic ovary syndrome. J Endocrinol Invest. 2017;40:1-8.
4. Amato MC, Vesco R, Vigneri E, Ciresi A, Giordano C. Hyperinsulinism and Polycystic ovary syndrome (PCOS): role of insulin clearance. J Endocrinol Invest. 2015;38:1319-26.
5. Singh B, Saxena A. Surrogate markers of insulin resistance: a review. World J Diabetes. 2010;1:36-47.
6. Wild RA, Carmina E, Diamanti-Kandarakis E, Dokras A, Escobar-Morreale HF, Futterweit W, et al. Assessment of cardiovascular risk and prevention of cardiovascular disease in women with the polycystic ovary syndrome: a consensus statement by the Androgen Excess and Polycystic Ovary Syndrome (AE-PCOS) Society. J Clin Endocrinol Metab. 2010;95:2038-49.
7. Velazquez E, Mendoza S, Hamer T, Sosa F, Glueck C. Metformin therapy in polycystic ovarian syndrome reduces hyperinsulinema, insulin resistance, hyperandrogenemia, and systolic blood pressure, while facilitating normal menses and pregnancy. Metab Clin Exp. 1994;43:647-54.
8. Azziz R, Carmina E, Dewailly D, Diamanti-Kandarakis E, Escobar-Morreale HF, Futterweit W, et al. The Androgen Excess and PCOS Society criteria for the polycystic ovary syndrome: the complete task force report. Fertil Steril. 2009;91(2):456-88.
9. The Rotterdam ESHRE/ASRM-Sponsored PCOS Consensus Workshop Group. Revised 2003 consensus on diagnostic criteria and long-term health risks related to polycystic ovary syndrome. Fertil Steril. 2004;81(1):19-25.
10. Bailey CJ. Biguanides and NIDDM. Diabetes Care. 1992;15(6):755-72.
11. Bailey CJ, Turner RC. Metformin. 1996;334(9):574-9.
12. Kirpichnikov D, McFarlane SI, Sowers JR. Metformin: an update. Ann Intern Med. 2002;137(1): 25-33.
13. Nestler JE. Metformin for the treatment of the polycystic ovary syndrome. N Engl J Med. 2008;358:47-54.
14. Lord JM, Flight IH, Norman RJ. Insulin-sensitising drugs (metformin, troglitazone, rosiglitazone, pioglitazone, D-chiro-inositol) for polycystic ovary syndrome. Cochrane Database Syst Rev. 2003;3:CD003053.
15. Costello MF, Chapman M, Conway U. A systematic review and meta-analysis of randomized controlled trials on metformin co-administration during gonadotrophin ovulation induction or IVF in women with polycystic ovary syndrome. Hum Reprod. 2006;21(6):1387-99.
16. Tso LO, Costello MF, Albuquerque LE, Andriolo RB, Freitas V. Metformin treatment before and during IVF or ICSI in women with polycystic ovary syndrome. Cochrane Database Syst Rev. 2009;(2):CD006105.
17. Doldi N, Persico P, Di Sebastiano F, Marsiglio E, Ferrari A. Gonadotropin-releasing hormone antagonist and metformin for treatment of polycystic ovary syndrome patients undergoing in vitro fertilization-embryo transfer. Gynecol Endocrinol. 2006;22(5): 235-8.

18. Qublan HS, Al-Khaderei S, Abu-Salem AN, Al-Zpoon A, Al-Khateeb M, Al-Ibrahim N, et al. Metformin in the treatment of clomiphene citrate-resistant women with polycystic ovary syndrome undergoing in vitro fertilisation treatment: a randomised controlled trial. J Obstet Gynaecol. 2009;29(7): 651-5.
19. Gambineri A, Patton L, Vaccina A, Cacciari M, Morselli-Labate AM, Cavazza C, et al. Treatment with flutamide, metformin, and their combination added to a hypocaloric diet in overweight-obese women with polycystic ovary syndrome: a randomized, 12-month, placebo-controlled study. J Clin Endocrinol Metab. 2006;91(10): 3970-80.
20. Gambineri A, Pelusi C, Genghini S, Morselli-Labate AM, Cacciari M, Pagotto U, et al. Effect of flutamide and metformin administered alone or in combination in dieting obese women with polycystic ovary syndrome. Clin Endocrinol (Oxf). 2004;60(2): 241-9.
21. Pasquali R, Gambineri A, Biscotti D, Vicennati V, Gagliardi L, Colitta D, et al. Effect of long-term treatment with metformin added to hypocaloric diet on body composition, fat distribution, and androgen and insulin levels in abdominally obese women with and without the polycystic ovary syndrome. J Clin Endocrinol Metab. 2000;85(8):2767-74.
22. Thatcher SS, Jackson EM. Pregnancy outcome in infertile patients with polycystic ovary syndrome who were treated with metformin. Fertil Steril. 2006;85:1002-9.
23. Glueck CJ, Wang P, Goldenberg N, Sieve-Smith L. Pregnancy outcomes among women with polycystic ovary syndrome treated with metformin. Hum Reprod. 2002;17: 2858-64.
24. Jakubowicz DJ, Iuorno MJ, Jakubowicz S, Roberts KA, Nestler JE. Effects of metformin on early pregnancy loss in the polycystic ovary syndrome. J Clin Endocrinol Metab. 2002;87: 524-9.
25. Rowan JA, Hague WM, Gao W, Battin MR, Moore MP. Metformin versus insulin for the treatment of gestational diabetes. N Engl J Med. 2008;358: 2003-15.
26. Nordio M, Basciani S, Camajani E. The 40:1 myo-inositol/D-chiro-inositol plasma ratio is able to restore ovulation in PCOS patients: comparison with other ratios. Eur Rev Med Pharmacol Sci. 2019;23:5512-21.
27. Mendoza N, Diaz-Ropero MP, Aragon M, Maldonado V, Llaneza P, Lorente J, et al. Comparison of the effect of two combinations of myo-inositol and D-chiro-inositol in women with polycystic ovary syndrome undergoing ICSI: A randomized controlled trial. Gynecol Endocrinol. 2019;35(8):695-700.

18

Vaccination Against Cervical Cancer

CHAPTER

Neerja Bhatla

■ INTRODUCTION

Cervical cancer is the fourth leading cancer among women, following breast, colorectal, and lung cancer. Globally, more than six lakh cases of cervical cancer were reported in year 2020, with 342,000 deaths attributable to cancer cervix.[1] More than two-thirds of these occur in low-middle-income countries (LMIC). Cervical cancer is also the leading cause of cancer mortality in 33 developing countries and India contributes to 28% of cervical cancer deaths.[2,3] Risk of developing cancer cervix is about 1 in 70 for women.

The World Health Organization (WHO) recommended three strategic actions involving 90:70:90 rule for elimination of cervical cancer by the year 2030, as depicted in **Figure 1**. These three actions can achieve elimination of cancer cervix, i.e., achieving less than four cases per one lakh population.[4] Except few developed countries, most of LMICs are far behind the required target set by the WHO. Only 12.2% of eligible girls are vaccinated worldwide with human papillomavirus (HPV) vaccine and in India, only 3.1% are screened for cervical cancer, which calls for comprehensive policy actions against cancer cervix.[3,5] HPV vaccination in India is very low, except in few states such as New Delhi, Punjab, and Sikkim, where it is introduced as a part of immunization policy to adolescents.

Human papillomavirus is the necessary causative agent for development of cervical precancer and cancer. It accounts for 99% of cancer cervix. HPV also causes noncervical cancers and anogenital warts (AGW) in all genders

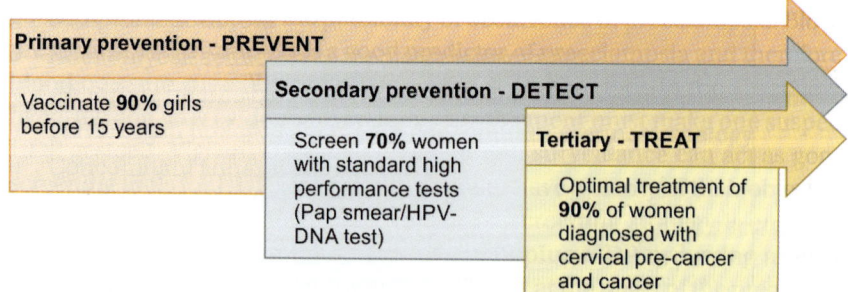

Fig. 1: WHO 90:70:90 strategy for elimination of cervical cancer. (HPV: human papillomavirus; WHO: World Health Organization)

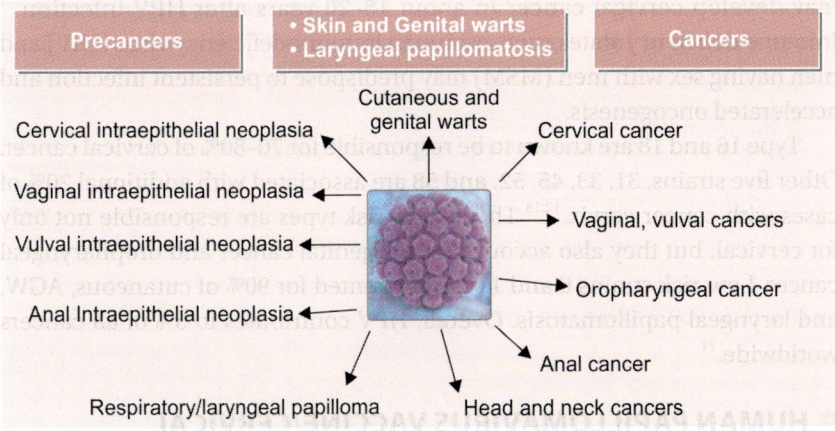

Fig. 2: Human papillomavirus (HPV)-related conditions.

including women and men, as shown in **Figure 2**. Cervical cancer vaccine directed against HPV is the primary prevention for cervical precancer, cancer, AGW, and other noncervical cancers for all genders.[3,6]

■ HUMAN PAPILLOMA VIRUS

Human papillomavirus is a small deoxyribonucleic acid (DNA) virus of *Papillomaviridae* family, infecting skin and mucus membrane. HPV infection is the most common condition acquired by sexual contact, 40% of women acquire HPV within 2 years of sexual activity.[7] It is also transmitted by intimate/close contact, resulting in AGW and oropharyngeal lesions. Autoinoculation is also reported as causing nongenital/oropharyngeal infection.[8,9]

More than 200 types of HPV have been described. They are classified as high and low risk based on malignant potential. High-risk types are associated with precancers and cancers (genital and nongenital), whereas low-risk types are associated with AGW, low-grade cervical lesions, and respiratory papillomatosis.[8,10] Low-risk types tend to be recurrent infections, causing recurrence of AGW and making management difficult.

High-risk types: 16, 18, 31, 33, 35, 39, 45, 51, 52, 56, 58, 59, 66, and 68

Low-risk types: 6, 11, 40, 42, 43, 44, 53, 54, 61, 72, 73, and 81

Prevalence of HPV varies among countries (2–42%), highest in sub-Saharan Africa—about 24%. Prevalence is more in young women aged <22 years. Type 16 is the most common type. Men have more prevalence of HPV across all age groups. Majority of these HPV infections, up to 75–100% clear spontaneously, but persistent infection with high-risk HPV type accounts for oncogenesis over prolonged time. Women with good immunological status may develop cervical cancer in about 15–20 years after HPV infection.[11] Immune deficiency states such as human immunodeficiency virus (HIV) and men having sex with men (MSM) may predispose to persistent infection and accelerated oncogenesis.

Type 16 and 18 are known to be responsible for 70–80% of cervical cancer. Other five strains, 31, 33, 45, 52, and 58 are associated with additional 20% of cases with cancer cervix.[12,13] These high-risk types are responsible not only for cervical, but they also account for anogenital cancer and oropharyngeal cancer. Low-risk strains 6 and 11 are accounted for 90% of cutaneous, AGW, and laryngeal papillomatosis. Overall, HPV contributes to 5% of all cancers worldwide.[14]

HUMAN PAPILLOMAVIRUS VACCINE/CERVICAL CANCER VACCINE[13-20]

Human papillomavirus vaccines contain virus-like particles (VLP), which are noninfectious particles made by recombinant technology resembling major capsid protein L1 of specific types of HPV. Vaccines were introduced in the year 2006 (Gardasil). VLP are 50–55 nm in size, which are optimal for pick up by lymphatics and generate strong cellular immunity and neutralizing antibody response, unlike natural infection.

Human papillomavirus vaccines are highly immunogenic and elicit strong antibody response compared to natural infection, with antibody levels being 1–4 logs higher than the natural infection. Chances of reinfection or breakthrough clinical infection are extremely rare after HPV vaccine administration, unlike natural infection where chance of reinfection is still higher with similar serotype. Studies have shown nearly 100% seroconversion for HPV vaccination type-specific virus. Efficacy trials have shown reduction in clinical outcomes such as HPV-related AGW and in-situ carcinoma. More than 85% reduction in cancer cervix is seen in countries with early implementation of routine HPV vaccination of children (Sweden and United Kingdom).[21] However, cut-off antibody titer levels for prevention of clinical endpoints like carcinoma cervix are not known.

There are three types of vaccines available for vaccination based on content of vaccine (number of HPV strains). Though at least 12 types have been implicated in cancers, the available vaccines cover either two or four or nine types of HPV. The strains included in the vaccine account for majority of cancers and protection cover based on epidemiological data as depicted in **Table 1**.[15-17]

- Bivalent vaccines contain two strains—16 and 18, responsible for 70–80% of cancer cervix, with trade names—Cervarix, Cecolin, and Walrinvax. Cervarix was available in India till 2022, but the manufacturer has discontinued the vaccine in India with the arrival of cost-effective quadrivalent vaccine by the Serum Institute of India.

TABLE 1: Percentage of vaccine-type coverage against human papillomavirus (HPV) diseases.

Disease	Bivalent vaccine—16, 18	Quadrivalent vaccine—16, 18, 6, 11	Nonavalent vaccine—6, 11, 16, 18, 31, 33, 45, 52, 58
Cervical cancer	70%	70%	90%
Vulval cancer	75%	70–75%	85–90%
Vaginal cancer	65%	65%	80–85%
Anal cancer	85–90%	85–90%	90–95%
Penile cancer	75–80%	75–80%	85%
Oropharyngeal cancer	85%	85%	>90%
Anogenital and cutaneous warts	Not covered	90%	90%
Respiratory papillomatosis	Not covered	90%	90%

- Quadrivalent vaccines have four strains—16, 18, 6, and 11, which provide protection against genital-cutaneous warts along with protection for cervical cancer. Trade names are Cervavac and Gardasil. Both are available in India.
- Nonavalent vaccine contains nine strains—16, 18, 31, 33, 45, 52, 58, 6, and 11. These vaccines have additional protection and more efficacy for cancer cervix prevention. Contribution of types include type 45—6%, 31—4%, 33—4%, 52—3%, and 58—2% of cervical cancer.[22] Trade name includes Gardasil 9. Nonavalent vaccine is available in India since 2022.

Available vaccine, content, dosage, and gender-specific use as per manufacturer instructions are summarized in **Table 2**.

■ FEATURES OF HUMAN PAPILLOMAVIRUS VACCINE

The salient features of human papillomavirus vaccine are:[13-18]
- It is the most effective and safe vaccine. Number of deaths reduced by vaccines is highest for HPV as compared to any vaccine, with about 20 deaths averted for one thousand vaccinations, as depicted in **Figure 3**.
- *Safety and efficacy data:* All available HPV vaccines are safe and are well studied with good amount of evidence in support of routine vaccination. More than 100 countries have implemented as a part of childhood vaccination and till now >300 million doses have been administered. Efficacy trials have shown 100% seroconversion with 96–100% reduction in vaccine-type-specific clinical infections, dysplasia, and in-situ carcinoma. Some amount of cross-protection is seen among HPV viruses

TABLE 2: HPV vaccines—types, content, and use.

	Bivalent vaccines (Cervarix)	Quadrivalent vaccines (Cervavac, Gardasil)	Nonavalent vaccines (Gardasil 9)
HPV types	16, 18	High risk: 16, 18 Low risk: 6, 11	High: 16, 18, 31, 33, 45, 52, 58 Low: 6, 11
Licensed since	2009	Cervavac: 2023 Gardasil: 2009	2014
Production	Trichoplusia ni insect cell	Cervavac: Hansenula polymorpha Gardasil: Saccharomyces cerevisiae	Saccharomyces cerevisiae
Adjuvant	Aluminum hydroxide	Cervavac: Aluminum hydroxide Gardasil: Aluminum hydroxy phosphate sulfate	Aluminum hydroxy phosphate sulfate
Gender	Female	Cervavac: GNV Gardasil: Licensed in India for females	GNV
Volume per dose	0.5 mL, single-dose vial	Cervavac: 0.5 mL single-dose vial and 1 mL multi-dose vial Gardasil: 0.5 mL, single-dose vial	0.5 mL, single-dose vial
Schedule	Two doses: 0, 6–12 months for 9–14 years Three doses: • 0, 2, and 6 months (all to be completed within 1 year) for age ≥15 years, up to 26 years • 27–45 years: After discussing with woman (shared clinical decision) • For immune compromised (HIV or organ transplant)		

(GNV: gender-neutral vaccine; HIV: human immunodeficiency virus; HPV: human papillomavirus)

which are phylogenetically similar but antibody levels to these viruses after vaccination are not statistically significant.

- *Age:* Recommended for 9–14 years of age, vaccines can be used by all genders (except bivalent vaccines). They can also be given after 15 years up to the age of 26 years, as catch-up vaccination. After 26 years, women may receive after shared clinical decision. Immunogenicity is higher when given to sexually naïve women. However, as all women may not be exposed to the HPV types in a given vaccine, benefits of vaccination are still higher among women in reproductive age group.
- *Dosage:* Vaccine contains 0.5 mL of solution given as intramuscular injection to deltoid or anterolateral part of thigh. Cervavac is available as 1 mL two doses vial. Vial is agitated well to mix contents before injection.

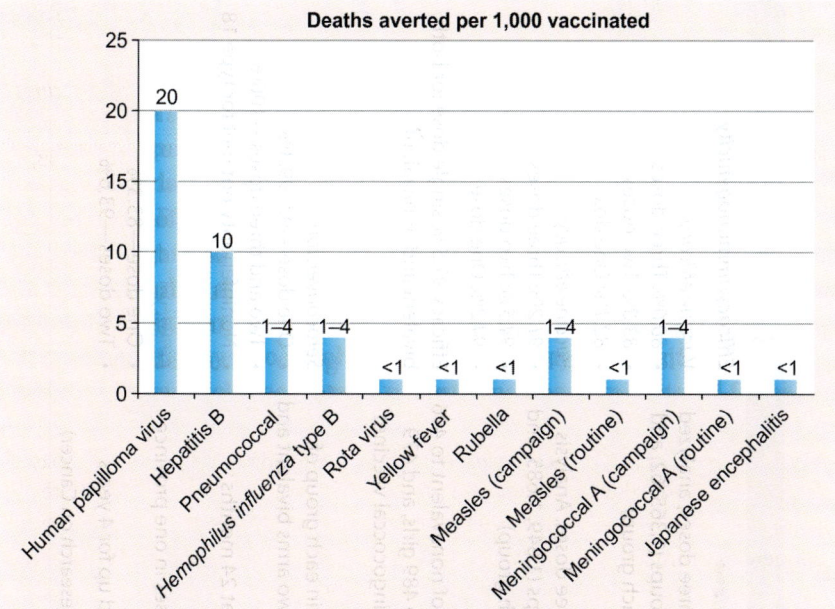

Fig. 3: Prevention of deaths—human papillomavirus (HPV) vaccine versus other vaccines.

All vaccines are initially licensed as three-dose injections. Later, two doses were approved between the ages of 9 and 14 years based on immunogenicity and efficacy data.[23-27] However, three doses are required when the target group individuals are ≥15 years and ≤26 years. Three doses are also given in immune-compromised status such as HIV, organ transplant groups, and in MSM as seroconversion and antibody titer are lower in these groups.

Single-dose recommendation: Strategic Group of Experts on Immunization (SAGE) from the WHO recommended single-dose vaccine based on well-designed randomized case-controlled trials (RCTs), which are elaborated in **Table 3**. Single-dose-elicited immune response was noninferior to the responses seen after two or three doses. Hence, the WHO (2022) updated its position paper on HPV vaccine with dosage as follows:

- One or two doses for girls aged 9–20 years
- Two doses at 6 months gap for women >20 years
- Three doses in HIV-infected individuals and immune-compromised status

This off-label recommendation by the WHO–SAGE was based on cost-effectiveness, flexibility of program, and to improve implementation of vaccination as national program for public health. Whenever possible, two doses should be given.[17] If scheduled

TABLE 3: Studies supporting single-dose HPV vaccination.[23-27]

Trial	Vaccine type	Age of female	Type of study	Efficacy/Immunogenicity
CVT—Costa Rica	Bivalent	18–25 years	• Post-hoc analysis. Started as three doses, analyzed as one, two, and three dose groups (1,365, 62, and 112 women, respectively, in each group) • Follow-up—11 years	*Vaccine efficacy:* • 80.0%: Three doses • 83.8%: Two doses • 82.1%: One dose
India IARC	Quadrivalent (Gardasil)	10–18 years	• Post-hoc. Started as two or three doses. Analysis one, two, and three dose groups (1,649, 1,685, and 2,454 girls, respectively, in each group) • Follow-up—10 years	*Vaccine efficacy:* • 91.2%: Three doses • 94.5%: Two doses • 94.2%: One dose
Ken She—Kenya	Bivalent and nonavalent	15–20 years	• Randomized trial (single dose of nonavalent to 496 girls, single dose of bivalent to 489 girls, and 479 girls in control group got meningococcal vaccine) • Follow-up—18 months	Efficacy 97.5%, single dose for both bivalent and nonavalent
DoRIS (Dose Reduction Immunobridging and Safety Study) Tanzania	Bivalent and nonavalent	9–14 years	• Randomized trial (around 140 in each group of one, two, and three doses of two arms bivalent and nonavalent) • Follow-up for seroconversion at 24 months	*Seroconversion:* • One dose—97–99.3% • Two and three doses—100% • Noninferiority not met for type 18
Thailand Impact Study	Bivalent	Grade 8 (<15 years)	• Observational study—two doses in one province versus one dose in another • One versus two doses followed up for 4 years	*Efficacy:* • One dose—83.3% • Two doses—93.6%

(CVT: Costa Rica vaccine trial; HPV: human papillomavirus; IARC: International Agency for Research on Cancer) vaccination (second or third dose) is interrupted or delayed, vaccination schedule need not be restarted. The next dose can be given as soon as possible.[17] Antibody titers remain high up to 10–12 years after vaccination. No booster dose is recommended as of now, but long-term data is awaited for recommendation.

The Centers for Disease Control and Prevention (CDC) recommends primary vaccination from 11 and 13 years, catch-up vaccination between 13 and 26 years of age, and vaccinating women after 26 years up to 45 years after discussing the benefits and importance of screening with women (shared clinical decision group).

- Approved for use by all standard organizations including the WHO, CDC, American College of Obstetricians and Gynecologists (ACOG), and Royal College of Obstetricians and Gynaecologists (RCOG) with proven safety record. Common adverse effects include local injection site pain and redness. Transient headache and giddiness are systemic side effects. Myalgia, body pain, and fever is uncommon. Adverse effects and adverse events due to HPV vaccination are similar to other injectable vaccines.
- *Gender-neutral vaccination (GNV):* Vaccination is approved for use in all genders (including male) except bivalent vaccine. GNV has advantage of improved acceptability during immunization programs at schools and contributes to herd immunity. Purpose of GNV is shown in **Figure 4**. Modeling studies reported herd immunity and drastic reduction in the HPV prevalence with GNV, as depicted in **Table 4**.[28,29]
- *Storage:* Stored at 2°–8°; should not be frozen. Kept away from light
- *Administration:* Injection is given in sitting position to avoid giddiness or syncopal attacks (0.1%). Syncopal attacks are similarly seen with any vaccination, not typical for HPV vaccination. Children are observed for 30 minutes after vaccination.
- *Coadministration:* Vaccine can be administered with other immunization like DPT (diphtheria, tetanus, and pertussis) or pneumococcal or

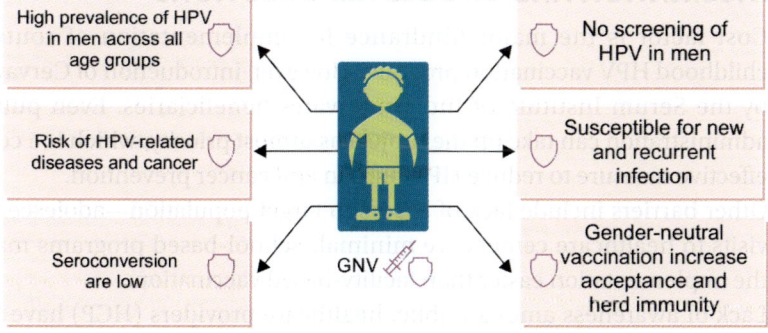

Fig. 4: Importance of GNV. (GNV: gender-neutral vaccination; HPV: human papillomavirus)

TABLE 4: Herd immunity—female only versus gender-neutral vaccination (GNV).

Vaccination type	Coverage	Expected drop in HPV prevalence
Female only	40%	Females—53%, males—36%
Female only	80%	Females—93%, males—83%
GNV	40%	Females—71%, males—71%
GNV	80%	Females—100%, males—99%

meningococcal vaccine. They need to be given at different sites with separate syringe and needle. There is no increased risk of adverse events with coadministration.

- *Pregnancy and lactation:* HPV vaccines are not to be given in pregnancy. Inadvertent use has not resulted in anomalies. Lactation/breastfeeding are not contraindications for HPV vaccination. Lactation period can be used as a window of opportunity for catch-up vaccination.
- *Contraindications:* Pregnancy—vaccine administration may be delayed in case of any acute illness. Hypersensitivity to any of the components of vaccines (yeast) is a contraindication.
- Currently, all available HPV vaccines are recommended for prophylaxis, i.e., highly effective before exposure to the HPV. Hence, adolescent girls are the main target group before sexual debut.[13,15] However, prior testing for HPV is not necessary before vaccination. Therapeutic vaccines which can be used among population treated for precancers are under trial, which prevent reinfection with high-risk HPV strain.[30]
- HPV vaccination does not eliminate screening for cervical cancer. Vaccinated individuals need to undergo screening as per local guidelines as all oncogenic 12 strains are not covered and to detect breakthrough clinical infections which is extremely rare.

BARRIERS FOR IMPLEMENTATION OF ROUTINE HPV VACCINATION AND SUGGESTED SOLUTIONS

- Cost factor is the major hindrance for implementation of routine childhood HPV vaccination program. However, introduction of Cervavac by the Serum Institute of India motivates beneficiaries. Even public administration can take up the project as utmost priority, which is a cost-effective measure to reduce HPV burden and cancer prevention.
- Other barriers include lack of access to target population—adolescent's visits to healthcare centers are minimal. School-based programs make the implementation easier than facility-based vaccination.
- Lack of awareness among public, healthcare providers (HCP) have led to decreased utilization of HPV vaccines. Awareness and educational activities for HCP and public is important.

- Fear about vaccine safety and vaccine misinformation has colluded the thought process of vaccination. Health awareness programs using media, nongovernment organization (NGO), and school education can resolve these issues.

  Talking about HPV vaccination as "cancer prevention" rather than as sexually transmitted disease (STD) prevention increases acceptance. Vaccine eliminates six cancers, namely cervical, vulval, vaginal, male genital, anal, and oral cavity cancers.
- Window of opportunity—pediatricians and gynecologists to utilize the adolescent healthcare visits to provide vaccination.
- Simple, quick, and nontechnical counseling by HCP improves acceptance. *"Vaccine before teen"* as the theme for adolescent health shall be the priority.
- Maintain vaccination registries and audit of parent's and HCP feedback enhances acceptability and uniform implementation.

CONCLUSION

- HPV-related diseases are high, more so in LMI countries. Two-thirds of cervical cancer is reported from the countries where there are no HPV vaccination programs. HPV causes not only cervical cancers in women, it also causes anogenital cancer, oropharyngeal cancer, AGW, condyloma, and respiratory papillomatosis in all genders.
- Though majority of HPV infections clear spontaneously, persistent infection with high-risk HPV leads to precancer and cancer.
- The WHO recommends 90:70:90 policy to prevent, detect, and treat cervical cancer, with a goal of eliminating cervical cancer by 2030. 90% vaccination of target population will eliminate cancer-related deaths.
- HPV vaccinations are highly immunogenic, safe, and effective against vaccine-specific HPV diseases.
- Recommended dose schedule is two doses for 9–14 years; three doses for ≥15 years and immune-compromised individuals. WHO–SAGES has recommended off-label use of *single dose* of vaccination from 9–21 years as a cost-effective measure for implementation by LMIC countries based on high-quality evidence.
- Adverse effects of HPV vaccination are comparable to other vaccinations. Coadministration with other vaccines can be done in the same sitting without increase in the adverse effects.
- GNV improves acceptance and herd immunity. However, female vaccination in the target age of ≤15 years should be the first priority. Catch-up vaccination should be considered whenever women visit facility for healthcare visits. School-based vaccination programs are known to improve vaccination rather than facility-based vaccination.

- Seroconversion and immunogenicity data suggest good efficacy of vaccines against vaccine-type HPV diseases. Antibody levels remain higher up to 10–12 years. Booster dose is not recommended till further data is available.
- As HPV vaccines are prophylactic, best efficacy is seen before sexual debut.
- Though there is 80% reduction in cancer cervix risk after vaccination, screening programs should be continued as per the standard protocols as all high-risk types are not covered in the vaccine.

REFERENCES

1. Sung H, Ferlay J, Siegel RL, Laversanne M, Soerjomataram I, Jemal A, et al. Global Cancer Statistics 2020: GLOBOCAN Estimates of Incidence and Mortality Worldwide for 36 Cancers in 185 Countries. CA Cancer J Clin. 2021;71(3):209-49.
2. Bray F, Ren JS, Masuyer E, Ferlay J. Global estimates of cancer prevalence for 27 sites in the adult population in 2008. Int J Cancer. 2013;132(5):1133-45.
3. Bruni L, Albero G, Serrano B, Mena M, Collado J, Gomez D, et al. (2021). ICO/IARC Information Centre on HPV and Cancer (HPV Information Centre). Human Papillomavirus and Related Diseases in Africa. Human Papillomavirus and Related Diseases in India. Summary Report 2021. [online] Available from https://hpvcentre.net/statistics/reports/XFX.pdf [Last accessed December, 2023].
4. World Health Organization. Global strategy to accelerate the elimination of cervical cancer as a public health problem. Geneva: World Health Organization; 2020.
5. Spayne J, Hesketh T. Estimate of global human papillomavirus vaccination coverage: analysis of country-level indicators. BMJ Open. 2021;11(9):e052016.
6. Forman D, de Martel C, Lacey CJ, Soerjomataram I, Lortet-Tieulent J, Bruni L, et al. Global burden of human papillomavirus and related diseases. Vaccine. 2012;30 (Suppl 5):F12-23.
7. UK Health Security. (2013). Human papillomavirus (HPV): the green book, chapter 18a. [online] Available from https://www.gov.uk/government/publications/human-papillomavirus-hpv-the-green-book-chapter-18a [Last accessed December, 2023].
8. Bernard HU, Burk RD, Chen Z, van Doorslaer K, zur Hausen H, de Villiers EM. Classification of papillomaviruses (PVs) based on 189 PV types and proposal of taxonomic amendments. Virology. 2010;401:70-9.
9. Cossellu G, Fedele L, Badaoui B, Angiero F, Farronato G, Monti E, et al. Prevalence and concordance of oral and genital HPV in women positive for cervical HPV infection and in their sexual stable partners: An Italian screening study. PLoS One. 2018;13(10):e0205574.
10. Baseman JG, Koutsky LA. The epidemiology of human papillomavirus infections. J Clin Virol. 2005;32 (Suppl 1):S16-24.
11. Erickson BK, Alvarez RD, Huh WK. Human papillomavirus: what every provider should know. Am J Obstet Gynecol. 2013;208(3):169-75.

12. Zhang Z, Zhang J, Xia N, Zhao Q. Expanded strain coverage for a highly successful public health tool: Prophylactic 9-valent human papillomavirus vaccine. Hum Vaccin Immunother. 2017;13(10):2280-91.
13. Centers for Disease Control and Prevention. Hamborsky J, Kroeger A, Wolfe S (Eds). Epidemiology and prevention of vaccine-preventable diseases: The Pink Book, 13th edition. USA: Public Health Foundation; 2015. pp. 376.
14. World Health Organization. (2023). Immunization coverage. [online] Available from https://www.who.int/news-room/fact-sheets/detail/immunization-coverage [Last accessed December, 2023].
15. World Health Organization (WHO) vaccine position papers. (2022). Weekly epidemiological record. [online] Available from https://iris.who.int/bitstream/handle/10665/365350/WER9750-eng-fre.pdf?sequence=1 [Last accessed December, 2023].
16. WHO newsletter. Recommendations to assure the quality, safety and efficacy of recombinant human papillomavirus virus-like particle vaccines, Annex 4, TRS No 999. Available from https://www.who.int/publications/m/item/recombinant-hpv-like-particle-vaccines-annex-4-trs-no-999 [Last accessed December, 2023].
17. Meites E, Szilagyi PG, Chesson HW, Unger ER, Romero JR, Markowitz LE. Human Papillomavirus Vaccination for Adults: Updated Recommendations of the Advisory Committee on Immunization Practices. MMWR Morb Mortal Wkly Rep. 2019;68:698-702.
18. WHO. (2016). Guide to introducing HPV vaccine into National Immunization Programmes. [online] Available from https://www.who.int/publications/i/item/9789241549769 [Last accessed December, 2023].
19. American College of Obstetricians and Gynecologists' Committee on Adolescent Health Care, American College of Obstetricians and Gynecologists' Immunization, Infectious Disease, and Public Health Preparedness Expert Work Group. Human Papillomavirus vaccination: ACOG Committee Opinion, Number 809. Obstet Gynecol. 2020;136(2):e15-21.
20. FOGSI Gynaecologic Oncology Committee. (2018). FOGSI GCPR Screening and Management of Preinvasive Lesions of Cervix and HPV Vaccination. [online] Available from https://www.fogsi.org/wp-content/uploads/2018/03/FOGSI-GCPR-March-2018-final.pdf [Last accessed December, 2023].
21. Falcaro M, Castañón A, Ndlela B, Checchi M, Soldan K, Lopez-Bernal J, et al. The effects of the national HPV vaccination programme in England, UK, on cervical cancer and grade 3 cervical intraepithelial neoplasia incidence: a register-based observational study. Lancet. 2021;398(10316):2084-92.
22. Serrano B, de Sanjosé S, Tous S, Quiros B, Muñoz N, Bosch X, et al. Human papillomavirus genotype attribution for HPVs 6, 11, 16, 18, 31, 33, 45, 52 and 58 in female anogenital lesions. Eur J Cancer. 2015;51(13):1732-41.
23. Porras C, Tsang SH, Herrero R, Guillén D, Darragh TM, Stoler MH, et al.; Costa Rica Vaccine Trial Group. Efficacy of the bivalent HPV vaccine against HPV 16/18-associated precancer: long-term follow-up results from the Costa Rica Vaccine Trial. Lancet Oncol. 2020;21(12):1643-52.
24. Basu P, Malvi SG, Joshi S, Bhatla N, Muwonge R, Lucas E, et al. Vaccine efficacy against persistent human papillomavirus (HPV) 16/18 infection at 10 years after one, two, and three doses of quadrivalent HPV vaccine in girls in India: a multicentre, prospective, cohort study. Lancet Oncol. 2021;22(11):1518-29.

25. Barnabas RV, Brown ER, Onono MA, Bukusi EA, Njoroge B, Winer RL, et al. Efficacy of single-dose HPV vaccination among young African women. NEJM Evid. 2022;1(5):EVIDoa2100056.
26. Watson-Jones D, Changalucha J, Whitworth H, Pinto L, Mutani P, Indangasi J, et al. Immunogenicity and safety of one-dose human papillomavirus vaccine compared with two or three doses in Tanzanian girls (DoRIS): an open-label, randomised, non-inferiority trial. Lancet Glob Health. 2022;10(10):e1473-84.
27. Jiamsiri S, Rhee C, Ahn HS, Poudyal N, Seo HW, Klinsupa W, et al. A community intervention effectiveness study of single dose or two doses of bivalent HPV vaccine (CERVARIX®) in female school students in Thailand. PLoS One. 2022;17(4):e0267294.
28. Kahn JA, Brown DR, Ding L, Widdice LE, Shew ML, Glynn S, et al. Vaccine-type human papillomavirus and evidence of herd protection after vaccine introduction. Pediatrics. 2012;130(2):e249-56.
29. Brisson M, Bénard É, Drolet M, Bogaards JA, Baussano I, Vänskä S, et al. Population-level impact, herd immunity, and elimination after human papillomavirus vaccination: a systematic review and meta-analysis of predictions from transmission-dynamic models. Lancet Public Health. 2016;1(1):e8-17.
30. WHO. (2023). WHO preferred product characteristics for therapeutic HPV vaccines. [online] Available from https://cdn.who.int/media/docs/default-source/reproductive-health/cervical-cancer/who-ppc-therapeutic-hpv-vaccines-public-comment.pdf?sfvrsn=dccee58_3 [Last accessed December, 2023].

CHAPTER 19

Recurrent Urinary Tract Infections

JB Sharma, Mohini Agrawal

■ INTRODUCTION

Urinary tract infections (UTIs) are one of the most common bacterial infections in women and account for a significant number of office and emergency department visits per year. UTI symptoms include suprapubic pain, acute dysuria, worsened urinary urgency, frequency and urinary incontinence, fever and fatigue. 60% of women will experience symptomatic acute bacterial cystitis in their lifetime. The risk of UTI recurrence has been shown to be between 20 and 30% after one infection. Of which, 25–50% will experience multiple recurrent episodes.[1]

Uncomplicated UTI is one of the most common indications for antimicrobial exposure in otherwise healthy women. Overuse of antibiotics leads to collateral damage. Antimicrobial resistance among uropathogens has increased dramatically over two decades.

Collateral damage from antibiotic therapy; leads to the selection of drug-resistant organisms and the unwanted development of colonization or infection with multidrug resistant organisms.[3] The US FDA has announced a black box warning against the use of fluoroquinolones for adverse effects such as tendon ruptures, irreversible nerve damage, chronic pain (fluoroquinolone associated disability) and risk of aortic dissection **(Tables 1 and 2)**. Unnecessary use of antibiotics puts a health and economic

TABLE 1: Definitions.

Terms	Definition
Asymptomatic bacteriuria	Presence of bacteria in the urine that causes no illness or symptoms (patient is asymptomatic)
Acute bacterial cystitis	A culture-proven infection of the urinary tract with a bacterial pathogen associated with acute-onset symptoms such as dysuria in conjunction with variable degrees of increased urinary urgency and frequency, suprapubic pain, hematuria, and new or worsening incontinence
Recurrent UTI	Two urine culture-proven UTIs within 6 months, or three within 1 year with associated symptom[2]

TABLE 2: Definitions.

Terms	Definition
Uncomplicated UTI	An infection of the urinary tract in a healthy patient with an anatomically and functionally normal urinary tract and no known factors susceptible to develop a UTI
Complicated UTI	An infection in a patient with one or more complicating factors that increases the risk for development of a UTI and potentially decrease efficacy of therapy. Such factors include the following: • Anatomic or functional abnormality of the urinary tract (e.g., stone disease, diverticulum, fistula, neurogenic bladder) • Immunocompromised host, pregnancy, elderly patient • Symptoms for >7 days at presentation • Childhood urinary tract infection • Indwelling catheter • Urinary tract instrumentation • Multidrug-resistant bacteria

burden to the society and thus treatment of recurrent urinary tract infection presents a challenge for treating clinician and patient. Here, comes the role of Antibiotic Stewardship.

Antibiotic Stewardship refers to a set of coordinated strategies to improve the use of antimicrobial medications with the goal of enhancing patient health outcomes, reducing resistance to antibiotics, and reducing unnecessary cost and health burden.[4]

Differentiation between uncomplicated and complicated UTIs is important because the risks of complications, long treatment, or treatment failure are increased for patients with a complicated UTI.

Considering the magnitude and occurrence of urinary tract infection, recurrent urinary tract infection is underdiagnosed at times, overdiagnoses at times, misdiagnoses at times, and has its aftereffects on society in terms of growing antimicrobial resistance, cost, and systemic exposure to multiple antibiotics increasing morbidity and affecting quality of life. Diagnosis, investigation, management, and prevention of recurrent urinary tract infection (rUTI) are a challenge to a clinician and patient as well.

■ ETIOLOGY

The underlying etiology of rUTI is unknown; however, the cyclic nature of this condition suggests that uropathogens may persist within the bladder between UTI episodes but often standard method of urine culture does not detect them.[5] Recurrent infections are hypothesized to be secondary to either bacterial persistence within urinary tract or, more commonly, novel reinfection. Persistence caused by the same bacterial strain, usually leads to recurrent infections in a short time frame, whereas reinfections generally occur over a more remote period. Reinfection is likely secondary to ascent of uropathogens from fecal flora into the urinary tract or from reemergence of bacteria from urothelial intracellular colonies.

Recent evidence suggests that the urinary tract harbors a variety of bacterial species, known collectively as the urinary microbiome, even when clinical cultures are negative. Negative urine cultures despite lower urinary tract symptoms (LUTS) may be due to atypical anaerobic bacteria or polymicrobial infection. Differences between the urinary microbiome of healthy populations and women with chronic urological diseases, such as overactive bladder (OAB), have been reported.

■ RISK FACTORS (TABLE 3)

TABLE 3: Factors predisposing to UTI.[3]

Urinary tract anatomic abnormality	Polycystic kidneys, cystocele, paraurethral cyst, diverticulum, fistula, and pelvic organ prolapse
Urinary tract obstruction	Bladder outflow obstruction, congenital abnormality, post-sling surgeries ureteral/urethral stricture, and urolithiasis
Voiding dysfunction	Vesicoureteric reflux, neurological disease, i.e., multiple sclerosis, Parkinsonism, high post-void residual volume, and incontinence
Iatrogenic	Indwelling catheter, long-term catheterization, ureteral stent, prolonged hospitalization leading to nosocomial infections, surgery, and prior augmentation cystoplasty
Genital anatomical variation	Shorter urethra-vagina (U-V) distance, shorter urethra-anus (U-A) distance, type 3 labia minora[6]
Genetic	Non-secretors of ABH blood group antigens, history of urinary tract infection in first degree female relative, P-blood group
Hypoestrogenic state	Menopause (presence of opportunistic uropathogen—Finegoldia magna)
Sexual intercourse	• Trauma and disruption of uroepithelial cells • Introduction of rectal and vaginal flora
Spermicides diaphragm	Alteration of vaginal flora
Past history	Previous history of surgery on urinary tract, previous urinary tract trauma, previous urinary calculi, and previous abdominopelvic malignancy
Others	Immunosuppressive medications, unstable diabetes, pregnancy, renal failure, high BMI, low serum level of vitamin D, fecal incontinence, dehydration (reduced fluid intake), urea-splitting bacteria on culture

PATHOGENESIS

The ability of bacteria to adhere to uroepithelial cells is a prerequisite for infection to occur. Factors that typically help deter the development of a urinary tract infection include acidic vaginal secretions, acidic urine, periodic voiding, the glycosaminoglycan (GAG) layer of the bladder, and immunoglobulins in the urine. Tamm–Horsfall proteins secreted by the loop of Henle may also inhibit bacterial adherence to the urothelial cells. Any factor leading to disruption of urothelium barrier predisposes to UTI. And persistent adherence or repeated adherence of bacteria to uroepithelial cells leads to recurrent UTI.

CLINICAL PRESENTATION

Urinary symptoms are central to the diagnosis of UTI. Acute onset dysuria is a highly specific symptom, with >90% accuracy for UTI in young women in the absence of concomitant vaginal irritation or increased vaginal discharge. Other symptoms are urinary urgency and frequency, nocturia, hematuria, pneumaturia, fecaluria, suprapubic pain and new or worsening incontinence.

Whether a patient receives no treatment or short-term, long-term, or prophylactic antimicrobial treatment, the risk of recurrent bacteriuria remains the same; antimicrobial treatment appears to alter only the time until recurrence.

DIFFERENTIAL DIAGNOSIS

- The differential diagnosis of a urinary tract infection includes candidiasis, trichomonal vaginitis, and other sexually transmitted diseases.
- Bladder pain syndrome (interstitial cystitis) and urethral syndrome should also be considered, because they are pain disorders of the urinary tract characterized by lower urinary tract symptoms despite negative urine, vaginal, and urethral cultures.
- Overactive bladder and urinary tract infection both may lead to each other's misdiagnosis.

HISTORY AND EXAMINATION

Patients with recurrent UTI should have a complete history obtained with emphasis of all the risk factors described above. Baseline genitourinary symptoms between infections should be derived. Any symptoms of incontinence, systemic symptoms, risk factor evaluation, high-risk behavior, and any associated comorbid conditions should be looked for.

A physical examination including the pelvic examination should be performed to look for any structural or functional abnormalities, to look for distance between urethra and vagina, urethra and anus, to observe for types of labia minora. Evaluation for incomplete bladder emptying to rule out occult retention, obstruction should be done in all patients with suspicion of incomplete emptying and voiding dysfunction.

■ INVESTIGATIONS

Urine Dipstick

It is a simple, cheap, easy to access, useful screening tool to detect urine nitrites and leukocyte esterase. Gram-negative bacteria convert nitrates to nitrites. False negatives can occur with Gram-positive infection. False positive can occur with urine contamination. Leukocyte esterase correlates to pyuria and indicates infection. Though dipstick provides clinical value, it cannot be used as a diagnostic test.

Microscopic Urinalysis

Microscopic urinalysis detects the presence of epithelial cells, leukocytes, bacteria, and red blood cells. Pyuria is defined as ≥10 leukocytes/mL or ≥3 leukocytes/hpf of unspun urine. Pyuria signifies infection, though sterile pyuria does not rule out urinary tract infection. Causes of sterile pyuria are tuberculosis, mesh or suture in the bladder, painful bladder syndrome, chlamydia or ureaplasma urethritis, after initiating antimicrobial therapy. Hematuria is defined as 3–5 RBC/hpf, though negative microscopic urinalysis does not rule out urinary tract infection.

Urine Culture

Microbial confirmation at the time of acute-onset urinary tract-associated symptoms and signs is an important component to establish a diagnosis of recurrent UTI. Typically, the culture technique used to confirm the diagnosis of UTI is by standard urine culture (SUC) laboratory technique originally designed to culture *Escherichia coli* (*E. coli*). This method preferentially grows Enterobacteriaceae, most often *E. coli*. *Expanded quantitative urine culture (EQUC)* is an enhanced urine culture technique shown to reproducibly detect more uropathogens than SUC in symptomatic populations.[7] This is because EQUC utilizes larger urine volumes, more diverse growth conditions, and longer incubation times than SUC.

Recent evidence suggests that the urinary tract harbors a variety of bacterial species, known collectively as the urinary microbiome, even when clinical cultures are negative. *Urine, as such, is not sterile.* The female urinary microbiome has been identified using RNA sequencing techniques, and knowledge of these microbiota should inform UTI management and interpretation of novel culture techniques such as the expanded quantitative urine culture (EQUC) protocol.[8]

Imaging
- Measurement of *post-void residual* for detection of high post-residual urine volume, in case of patients with voiding dysfunction
- Renal ultrasound to look for upper and lower urinary tract and standing voiding cystourethrogram should be done in complicated UTI.
- Non-contrast CT scan for diagnosis of urinary calculi

Cystoscopy
- In the evaluation of complicated UTI to assess for anatomical or structural abnormalities.
- In patients with previous pelvic surgery, cystoscopy can be helpful to assess for anatomic abnormalities from the previous surgery, including urethra stricture or obstruction, foreign body such as mesh, bladder stones, fistula, or urethral/bladder diverticulum.
- In search for inflammatory sites (cystitis), small waxy-yellow raised areas of microabscess, as part of "cystitis cystica" appearance.
- In all cases of hematuria, imaging, and cystoscopy to be considered in patients with risk factors for a complicated UTI.

■ INTERPRETATION OF URINE ANALYSIS AND APPROACH
- Urine collected for analysis should be clean-catch or a catheterized specimen. Catheterized sample, samples bladder directly, while voided urine represents whole lower urogenital tract, moreover vulvovaginal skin. To minimize the contamination and to detect bladder samples, collect a mid-stream urine sample. The bacterial count is likely to be highest if the urine has been in the bladder for over 4 hours, such as with the first void of the day, hence avoid first void sample
- Urinalysis can determine the presence of epithelial cells suggesting contamination. Growth of organisms such as *Lactobacilli*, *Streptococci*, *Corynebacteria*, and *Staphylococci* are thought to be contaminants and generally do not require treatment. In either of above case, obtaining catheterized sample for urinalysis is desired to accurately evaluate the culture results.[9]
- Without symptoms, bacteriuria of any magnitude is considered "asymptomatic bacteriuria". One should omit surveillance urine testing, including urine culture, in asymptomatic patients with recurrent UTIs. Asymptomatic bacteriuria should be treated in pregnant women and in patients undergoing procedures where transmucosal bleeding is expected. In asymptomatic bacteriuria patient, no evaluation is needed with exception of asymptomatic microhematuria, which needs evaluation after resolution of infection.

- After resolution of episode of UTI, as a test of cure, urine culture should not be performed. Symptomatic cure is sufficient. Only if symptoms persist beyond 7 days, urinalysis may be considered to guide further management following antimicrobial therapy.

■ TREATMENT

Other antibiotics:
- Pivmecillinam 400 mg BD for 5 days, to be avoided if early pyelonephritis suspected (availability limited to some European countries).
- Beta-lactams can also be given (avoid ampicillin and ampicillin), though lower efficacy is described.
- Fluoroquinolones should be reserved as antibiotic of last resort in agreement with FDA warning.

The choice between the antibiotics depends upon patient profile including history, allergy, cost, compliance, availability, and local community resistance prevalence **(Table 4)**.

Since women with confirmed clinical history of rUTI are frequently exposed to antibiotic treatment without complete disease resolution, the role of specific uropathogen identification is critical and adherence to the principles of antibiotic stewardship. Continued documentation of cultures during symptomatic periods prior to prescribing antibiotics therapy helps to plan further treatment.

Recurrent UTI patients should be treated for short duration of antibiotics as possible generally no longer than 7 days. In patient with rUTIs associated with urine culture resistant to antimicrobial therapy, these cases should be treated with parenteral antibiotics as per culture sensitivity for a short course possible. These organisms should be specifically tested for susceptibility with Fosfomycin, as many drug-resistant bacteria are susceptible to Fosfomycin.

TABLE 4: First-line therapy for the treatment of uncomplicated symptomatic UTI.			
Treatment effects	TMP and TMP-SMX	Nitrofurantoin	Fosfomycin
Efficacy	90–94%	88–93%	83–94%
Antimicrobial spectrum	Typical uropathogens	Narrow spectrum	Typical uropathogen and antibiotic resistant bacteria
Resistance	High	Low	Low
Strength and duration	One DS BID × 3 days	100 mg BID × 5/7 days	3 g single dose at night time
Collateral damage	Low	No	No

Women diagnosed with antibiotic-recalcitrant rUTIs and concurrent inflammatory bladder lesions on cystoscopy responds to electrofulguration over time.[10] Regular intravesical instillations of gentamicin may reduce the frequency of recurrent UTI.[11] Intravesical sodium hyaluronate reduces severity, frequency and improves quality of life in recurrent UTI.[12]

Nonantibiotic Interventions for Urinary Tract Infection

- D-mannose—more studies are needed to validate its use.
- Methenamine salts (hippurate and mandelate) are bacteriostatic, with a dose of 1 g twice daily, based on the evidence available its use cannot be recommended.
- Cranberry contains proanthocyanidin-A, it has antibacterial activity, has some role in prevention of recurrence of UTI, though evidence does not support its use. Large randomized controlled trials are required to prove its long-term benefits and role.[13]
- *Intravesical glycosaminoglycan layer:*
  - The hypothesis is infection causes damage to bladder mucosa and loss of protective layer. By replenishing the GAG layer, it prevents bacterial adherence to urothelium.
  - Hyaluronic acid and chondroitin sulfate appear to reduce the rate of UTI and increase the time to recurrence in women with recurrent UTI.[14]
- Probiotics like *Lactobacilli*, at present based on data available, it is not recommended.
- Vitamin supplements—vitamin C and vitamin D supplements are used to prevent recurrences of UTI, though limited evidence is available.
- Maintain hydration—increased water intake >1.5 L of water per day in RCT conducted has shown to have fewer UTI episodes and greater interval between the UTI episodes.[15]
- Local estrogen therapy **(Table 5)** in perimenopausal and postmenopausal women is supposed to be best non-antibiotic treatment for UTIs, provided there are no contraindications. Local estrogen therapy appears

TABLE 5: Local estrogen therapy protocols.

Formulation	Composition	Dose and duration
Vaginal cream	17β-estradiol	2 g daily for 2 weeks, then 1 g 2–3 times/week for 3 months
	Conjugate equine estrogen	0.5 g daily for 2–3 weeks, then 0.5 g twice a weekly for 3 months
Vaginal tablet	Estradiol hemihydrate	10 μg/day for 2 weeks, then 10 μg 2–3 times weekly for 3 months
Vaginal ring	17β-estradiol	2 mg ring releases 7.5 μg/day for 3 months

to be benefit in case of atrophic vaginitis with UTI. Systemic estrogen does not reduce the risk of recurrent UTIs. Those women who are on systemic estrogen therapy and presents with recurrent UTI should be prescribed vaginal estrogen. The beneficial effect may take around 12 weeks to manifest.

A combination of these agents might be the treatment and prevention strategy for reducing the rate of recurrent UTI without resorting to antimicrobial use.[16]

PREVENTION

- Behavioral and dietary modifications can be recommended to decrease the risk of UTI.
- Voiding immediately before and after sexual activity and avoiding spermicide use and diaphragm may reduce UTI risk.
- Staying hydrated, timed, or frequent voiding may also be beneficial.
- Vulvovaginal hygiene measures such as refraining from douching and using hygiene products in the vulvovaginal area, wiping from front to back after urination and defecation, and limiting pad use should be emphasized.
- Screening for and addressing concomitant fecal incontinence if present will be helpful.[17]
- Antibiotic prophylaxis remains the mainstay for prevention and management.[2] The aim of treatment is to eradicate urinary bacteria without affecting the healthy flora of the bowel and vagina or causing the development of resistant strains. Sterile urine culture is a prerequisite to start prophylaxis. The antibiotics preferred are trimethoprim, trimethoprim, and sulfamethoxazole, nitrofurantoin, Fosfomycin, nalidixic acid, and cephalexin. The drugs for low dose continuous prophylaxis are:
  - Trimethoprim 100 mg once daily
  - Trimethoprim-sulfamethoxazole 40 mg/200 mg once daily or 40 mg/200 mg thrice weekly
  - Fosfomycin 3 g every 10 days
  - Nitrofurantoin 50 mg daily or 100 mg daily
  - Cephalexin 125 or 250 mg once daily
- Four vaccines have been tested in human clinical trials, Uro-Vaxom, Urovac, ExPEC4V, and Uromune. Widespread use of vaccine has been limited because of its toxic, adverse effects and cost.[18]

COMPLICATIONS

The long-term effects of uncomplicated recurrent UTIs are not completely known, but so far, no clear association between recurrent infections and renal scarring, hypertension, or progressive renal insufficiency has been established.

CONCLUSION

- Clinical history with emphasis on past and present risk factors is important.
- The clinical applications, efficacy, long-term safety, and cost factors of these new strategies for prevention and treatment of recurrent UTI are still unclear. Each case should be individualized.
- With the better understanding of recurrent UTI, with its causative and predisposing factors, enhanced prevention and treatment are likely to improve targeted therapy.
- For prevention of recurrent UTI, nonantibiotics measures should be preferred.

REFERENCES

1. Geerlings SE. Clinical presentations and epidemiology of urinary tract infections. Microbiol Spectr. 2016;4(5).
2. Anger J, Lee U, Ackerman AL, Chou R, Chughtai B, Clemens JQ, et al. Recurrent uncomplicated urinary tract infections in women: AUA/CUA/SUFU Guideline. J Urol. 2019;202(2):282-9.
3. Paterson DL. "Collateral damage" from cephalosporin or quinolone antibiotic therapy. Clin Infect Dis Off Publ Infect Dis Soc Am. 2004;38 (Suppl 4):S341-5.
4. Shrestha J, Zahra F, Cannady Jr P. Antimicrobial Stewardship. 2023. In: StatPearls. Treasure Island (FL): StatPearls Publishing; 2023.
5. McLellan LK, Hunstad DA. Urinary tract infection: pathogenesis and outlook. Trends Mol Med. 2016;22(11):946-57.
6. Aydın A, Atılgan AE, Sönmez MG. "Do labial anatomic variations have an effect on recurrent urinary tract infection?" Letter to the editor. Int Urogynecology J. 2021;32(3):747-8.
7. Price TK, Hilt EE, Dune TJ, Mueller ER, Wolfe AJ, Brubaker L. Urine trouble: should we think differently about UTI? Int Urogynecology J. 2018;29(2):205-10.
8. Mueller ER, Wolfe AJ, Brubaker L. The female urinary microbiota. Curr Opin Urol. 2017;27(3):282-6.
9. Kline KA, Lewis AL. Gram-positive uropathogens, polymicrobial urinary tract infection, and the emerging microbiota of the urinary tract. Microbiol Spectr. 2016;4(2):10.
10. Ma R, Chavez JA, Christie AL, Zimmern PE. Electro-fulguration for extensive inflammatory bladder lesions in post-menopausal women with antibiotic-recalcitrant recurrent urinary tract infections. Int Urogynecology J. 2023;34(7):1415-22.
11. Sidaway P. Intravesical gentamicin ameliorates recurrent UTI. Nat Rev Urol. 2017;14(7):391.
12. Batura D, Warden R, Hashemzehi T, Figaszewska MJ. Correction to: intravesical sodium hyaluronate reduces severity, frequency and improves quality of life in recurrent UTI. Int Urol Nephrol. 2020;52(3):495.
13. Singh I, Gautam LK, Kaur IR. Effect of oral cranberry extract (standardized proanthocyanidin-A) in patients with recurrent UTI by pathogenic *E. coli*: a randomized placebo-controlled clinical research study. Int Urol Nephrol. 2016;48(9):1379-86.

14. Goddard JC, Janssen DAW. Intravesical hyaluronic acid and chondroitin sulfate for recurrent urinary tract infections: systematic review and meta-analysis. Int Urogynecology J. 2018;29(7):933-42.
15. Scott AM, Clark J, Mar CD, Glasziou P. Increased fluid intake to prevent urinary tract infections: systematic review and meta-analysis. Br J Gen Pract. 2020;70(692):e200-7.
16. Sihra N, Goodman A, Zakri R, Sahai A, Malde S. Nonantibiotic prevention and management of recurrent urinary tract infection. Nat Rev Urol. 2018;15(12):750-76.
17. Miranne JM. Recurrent urinary tract infection in women. Curr Obstet Gynecol Rep. 2017;6(4):282-9.
18. Butler D, Ambite I, Wan MLY, Tran TH, Wullt B, Svanborg C. Immunomodulation therapy offers new molecular strategies to treat UTI. Nat Rev Urol. 2022;19(7):419-37.

20. Fourth Degree Perineal Tear

Gaurav S Desai, Shyam V Desai

■ INTRODUCTION

Fourth degree or complete perineal tear occurs when the layers of tissue between the vagina and the rectum, i.e., the muscle, sphincter, vaginal mucosa, forchette, perineal skin, and rectal mucosa are torn. It constitutes the acronym OASI or obstetric anal sphincter injury. A fourth degree perineal tear is uncommon in today's obstetric practice. The application of perineal support has greatly reduced the incidence of injury to the rectum. However, the reasons for its occurrence and management are of importance to a practicing obstetrician.

■ PREVALENCE

Most perineal tears are first or second degree in severity and these occur in a majority of women during a vaginal delivery. Fourth degree tears are however very rare occurring in <1% of cases of vaginal deliveries.[1] They differ however from a buttonhole tear in which rectal contents can enter the vaginal passage, however, the sphincter is intact **(Fig. 1)**.

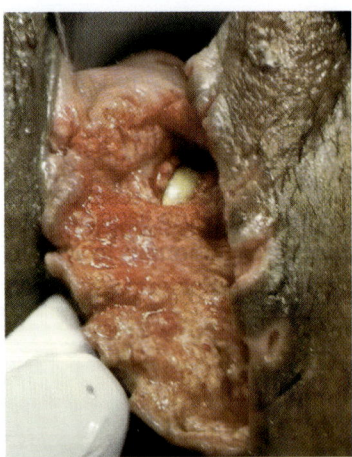

Fig. 1: Button-hole tear demonstrated by a finger placed within rectum. A 28-year-old primigravida complained of passage of stool from the episiotomy site and nonhealing of the episiotomy site 2 weeks after precipitate vaginal delivery. Tear was sutured after separating and suturing vagina and rectum.

■ CAUSES

- Childbirth is the leading cause of complete perineal tears especially when delivery of the fetus is done without perineal support. Additional reasons for fourth degree tears include a large fetus, e.g., in gestational diabetes, or when the passage, i.e., the vaginal canal is narrow as in the case of primigravidae or in cases of vaginal birth after cesarean section (VBAC). More specifically complete perineal tears have a higher propensity to occur if there is a disparity between the passenger, passage, and the force (uterine contraction) as in cases of precipitate labor.
- Fourth degree tears can also occur due to uncontrolled or incorrect application of obstetric forceps. They may also take place due to excessive force in pulling and downward traction with obstetric forceps in delivery of fetus in difficult labor.
- Iatrogenic reasons for complete tears include an overzealous episiotomy or an extension of a midline episiotomy. Complete perineal tears are however distinguishable from an episiotomy per se which is an intentional cut made on the perineal tissue to facilitate childbirth.
- A prolonged second stage of labor and shoulder dystocia can also lead to total perineal tears.
- Excessive scarring due to previous surgeries on the perineum, friability and edema of the perineum can reduce elasticity and lead to a breach in tissue.
- Complete perineal tears are also seen in victims of sexual violence and rape and result from excessive force during sexual intercourse as well as the voluntary or involuntary use of objects in the vagina or rectum.[2,3]

■ PREVENTION

Perineal support has become a mainstay in the conduct of a vaginal delivery. It should be taught in all residency programs and should be routinely practiced for all vaginal deliveries. This act prevents a large tear of the perineal tissue which during the final stages of labor and crowing get thinned out. In this method one hand of the accoucheur or obstetrician is placed over the rectum with a mop or towel while two fingers of the other hand are used to support the urinary bladder. They are released once the fetal body is born.

Avoidance of excessive uterine stimulation thereby reducing the incidence of precipitate labor and uncontrolled delivery of the fetus also reduces the chance of a complete tear. A good pelvic and vaginal examination of the pregnant woman during the antenatal period and in the course of labor will help determine whether she has a high chance of perineal tear and if she might need obstetric forceps application. Perineal massage and using an all fours birthing position have also been suggested to reduce risk of a complete tear.

■ MANAGEMENT

Superficial perineal tears involving just the vaginal mucosa or underlying muscle can heal if left alone (secondary intention). However complete perineal tears require to be treated surgically. The diagnosis and isolation of the perineal tear is essential. Both halves of torn perineal tissue need to be grasped with allis forceps. The vagina and rectum is then cleaned with povidone iodine. Pivotal to the repair of a complete perineal tear is the approximation and suturing of the rectal sphincter which helps in continence of stool. Both internal and external anal sphincter need to be approximated and sutured with interrupted suture. Two methods to suturing of complete perineal tear are end-to-end anastomosis and overlapping technique.[4] The vaginal mucosa is separated off and the rectal mucosa is sutured. The perineal muscle (levator ani) is then sutured followed by the vaginal mucosa with continuous polyfilament suture material, e.g., vicryl 1 or 1-0 rapid vicryl. Catgut is an alternative to vicryl.

The patient with complete perineal tear is kept nil by mouth for 3-5 days after which liquids are started followed by semi-solid and solid foods over the next 3-5 days. Antibiotic coverage with broad spectrum and against anaerobic bacteria is vital. Patient is discharged on stool softeners. Bowel continence is evaluated over the course of 2-3 weeks. Additionally, formation of fistula or communication between rectum and vagina is also a possibility and should be looked out for. Most complete perineal tears heal well and few persist 6-12 months after their occurrence. Sexual intercourse and vaginal manipulation is to be avoided for 2-3 months. It is recommended to have cesarean delivery hereafter.

■ COMPLICATIONS

Complete perineal tears can lead to significant morbidity for the woman if not managed effectively. Complications include fecal incontinence and soiling of inner wear, fistula formation and vaginal infection. Complications can also result from the correction of the tear and include non-approximation of the real sphincter as well as overcorrection of the tear leading to a narrow vagina and dyspareunia.

■ CONCLUSION

The exploration of 4th-degree perineal tears underscores the need for a comprehensive and empathetic approach to maternal care. Understanding the anatomical complexities, risk factors, and emotional impact is essential. Collaboration among healthcare professionals, ongoing research, and patient-centered support are vital in improving prevention, diagnosis, and treatment strategies. By prioritizing education and awareness, we can contribute to a more responsive and compassionate healthcare environment for women affected by 4th-degree perineal tears.

REFERENCES

1. Toglia MR. Repair of episiotomy and perineal lacerations associated with childbirth. UpToDate. Version 19.3. 2011.
2. Rosenberg K, Trevathan W. Birth, obstetrics and human evolution. BJOG. 2002;109(11):1199-206.
3. Eskandar O, Shet D. Risk factors for 3rd and 4th degree perineal tear. J Obstet Gynaecol. 2009;29(2):119-22.
4. Cunningham FG, Leveno KJ, Bloom SL, Spong CY, Dashe JS, Hoffman BL, et al. Wiliams Obstetrics. 24th edition. New York: McGraw Hill Publication; 2014. pp. 548-52.

Index

Page numbers followed by *b* refer to box, *f* refer to figure, *fc* refer to flowchart, and *t* refer to table.

A

Abdomen 140
Abdominal discomfort 206
Abdominal pain, acute 23
Abdominal palpation 200
Abdominal wall vessels 192
Acid mucopolysaccharides 167
Acidic vaginal
　environment 167
　secretions 228
Adenomyosis 144, 146*f*
　diagnosis of 143
　focal posterior-wall 146*f*
Adhesions, severe 181
Adipose tissue 205
Adnexa 153
Adnexal mass 140
Adnexal tumor 134, 135, 140
Adrenocorticotrophic hormone 61
Airway 94
Albumin 56
Alemtuzumab 49
Allograft
　function 45, 46
　patients 47
Alpha-methyldopa 46
Amiodarone 60
Amniocentesis 106
Amniotic fluid embolism 88, 90, 93
Anal cancer 215
Anaphylaxis 90, 93
　treatment for 91
Anemia 98
　maternal 21
Anesthesia 181
Anogenital cancer 214
Anogenital warts 212, 215
Antenatal care 22
Antenatal corticosteroid 37*t*
Antibiotic 39, 69, 117
　parenteral 231
　therapy 225
Antibody 55
　maternal 98

Anti-D immunoglobulin, dosage of 114
Antihypertensive medication doses 26*t*
Antihypertensive medications 27
Antihypertensive treatment 25
Antimicrobial therapy 231
Antiphospholipid syndrome 21
Antiretroviral therapy 21
Antithymocyte globulin 47, 49
Aortic compression, external 73
Aortic dissection 92
Aortic isthmus 5
Arrhythmia 189
Arterial pressure, mean 18, 22
Ascites 140
　causes of 103
Aspirin, low-dose 24
Assisted reproductive technology 120
Atheromatous 92
Autoimmune
　thyroid, indicator of 57
　thyroiditis 58
Azathioprine 49, 50

B

Bacteria, ability of 228
Bacterial cystitis, acute 225
Bacterial infections 58
Bacterial vaginosis 168
　asymptomatic 177
Bacteriuria, asymptomatic 225, 230
Bakri balloon 73*f*
Basiliximab 49
Bazedoxifene 176
Bed rest 39
Belatacept 49
Besides biometry 201
Beta-blockers 46
Beta-lactams 231
Betamethasone 37
Biophysical profile 31
Biopsy 152
Biotin, high-dose 60
Bivalent vaccines 214

Index

Bladder 168
  injury 190
    management of 190*fc*
  pain syndrome 228
Bloating 177, 206
Blood
  collection of 94
  group 107
  pressure 17*f*, 22, 31, 72, 82
    diastolic 23, 27
    raised 17
    systolic 23, 27
  urea 94
Body mass index 21
Bones 155
Bowel 189
Bowel injury 191
  management of 191*fc*
Breast cancer 130, 178
  history of 178
Breastfeeding 58
Breath, shortness of 23
Breathing, assessment of 95
Broad ligament 184
  posterior leaf of 185*f*

C

C cells 58
Calcineurin inhibitors 49
Calcitonin 58
  estimation 58
Cancer
  cervix 214
  leading 212
  patients 134
  prevent 153
  type of 148
Candidiasis 168, 177
Carcinoma
  cervix 214
  endometrium 146*f*
Carcinosarcoma 154
Cardiac arrest 189
Cardiac arrhythmia 90
Cardiac causes 99
Cardiac diseases 88, 89
Cardiac dysfunction 110
Cardiac rhythm, assess 95
Cardiopulmonary resuscitation 95
Cardiotocography 199
Cardiovascular abnormalities 102
Cardiovascular complications 189
Cardiovascular disease, family history of 21
Cardiovascular profile score 111*t*
Care bundles, advantages of 75
Cellular senescence, ischemia-induced 20
Central nervous system, tumors of 135
Cephalexin 47, 233
Cerebroplacental ratio 12, 12*f*
Cervical
  cytology 172
  stroma 145
  tumors 136
Cervical cancer 145, 215
  elimination of 212*f*
  vaccination against 212
  vaccine 214
Cervix, absence of 143
Cesarean section, perimortem 96
Chemotherapy 132, 152, 154
Chest pain, moderate 206
Chromosomal aneuploidy 102
Chromosomal anomaly 202
Chronic kidney disease 44
Circle of Willis 114
Circulatory disorders 103
Cisplatin 154
Cleft palate 50
Clomiphene 206
  citrate 206
Cochrane 207
Coliforms 168
Color Doppler, utility of 1
Colpotomy 186, 187*f*
Common bacterial infections 225
Competitive immunoassays 57
Complete blood count 31
Concurrent medications 60
Congenital abnormalities 136
Congenital anomalies 48
Congenital diaphragmatic hernias 50
Congenital heart
  disease 17*f*
  problems 50
Congestive cardiac failure 113
Constipation 206
Contralateral ovary 134
Coombs test
  direct 106, 106*t*, 107
  indirect 106, 106*t*
Cord clamping for preterm babies, timing of 42

Cord insertion 117
Cord lesions 101
Cord prolapse algorithm 86*f*
Coronary artery
   dissection 92
   spasm 92
Correctable disorder 110*f*
Corticosteroids 37, 50
Cortisol 61
   deficiency 93
Corynebacteria 230
Costa Rica vaccine trial 218
Cough 206
Critical care unit 29
Cryopreserved oocytes 123, 125
Cryopreserved ovarian tissue 137
Cutaneous warts 215
Cyclosporine 49
Cystic lesions, formation of 18
Cystitis 230
   cystica 230
Cystoscopy 230
Cytomegalovirus 106

D

D-chiro-inositol 208
Deaths, prevention of 217*f*
Delivery decision 31
Deoxyribonucleic acid 160, 213
Dermoid cysts 141
Dexamethasone 37
Diabetes mellitus
   gestational 21, 207
   type 2 205
Diarrhea 206
Diphtheria 219
Diphtheroids 168
Distal ureter 143
Diverticulum 226
Dizziness 209
D-mannose 232
Docosahexaenoic acid 22
Döderlein's lactobacilli 167
Doppler ultrasound 1
Drug overdose 90
Ductus venosus 5, 7, 12
   Doppler 1, 5, 12, 13, 13*f*
Dysorgasmia 170
Dyspareunia 170, 174
   moderate-severe 174
Dysplasia 215

E

Early-stage disease 130
Eclampsia 28*t*, 89-91
   management 30, 82*fc*
      algorithm 30*t*
Edema
   generalized 102*f*
   prenasal 103*f*
   pulmonary 27
   scalp 103*f*
   skin 102, 116
Egg freezing 121
   elective 121
   medical 121
   method for 121
   nonmedical 121
   optimal number of 123
Embryo
   cryopreservation 130
   culture 122
   transfer 122
Emergency department 83
End diastolic flow, reversal of 111
Endocrine resumption 138
Endometrial biopsy 181
Endometrial cancer 143, 154, 155, 157, 158, 159*t*, 178
   classification of 156*t*
   high-risk 152*b*, 158
   low-risk 152*b*
   management of 148, 161
   recurrent 154
   treatment of 148, 149*fc*
      recurrent 157
   types of stage I 152
Endometrial carcinoma 144, 148*f*, 150*t*, 156*f*, 157*f*, 173
   immunology of 157*f*
Endometrial hyperplasia 173
Endometrial malignancies, majority of 155
Endometrial polyp 144
Endometrioid cancers 151
Endometrioid tumors 151
Endometriosis
   implants 144
   infiltrating 181
Endopelvic fascia 168
Endoscopy 172, 172*t*
Endothelium tissue 205
Epigastric artery, inferior 192
Episiotomy 236*f*

Ergonomic neck position 182
Escherichia coli 229
Estradiol 61
    acetate 176
    hemihydrate 176
Estrogen
    levels 130
    physiological role of 167
    receptor 160
        blocker 130
        modulator, selective 176
    stimulation 167
    therapy 176*t*
Estrogen-progestin formulations 178
Extrapulmonary sequestration 110*f*

F

Fallopian tube 153
    abnormalities 140
Fattly liver, acute 17
Fertility
    preservation, female 130
    restoration of 138
Fetal abdomen 115
Fetal adrenal immunosuppression 50
Fetal anatomy 8
Fetal anemia 115, 115*f*, 116
    diagnosis of severe 114
    noninvasive diagnosis of 114
Fetal ascites 113
Fetal blood sampling 116
Fetal cardiotocography 199
Fetal cerebral vessel vasodilator 38
Fetal circulation 8*f*
Fetal complications 47
Fetal cord blood sampling 106
Fetal Doppler, multivessel 4
Fetal echocardiography 14*f*
Fetal erythrocytes, destroy 112
Fetal growth 8
    assessing 200
    restriction 2*t*, 3*f*, 17*f*, 22, 23
        classification of 4*f*
        fetuses, deliver 3*fc*
Fetal health
    parameter of 197
    sign of 196
Fetal heart 13
    changes in 116
    examination 14
Fetal heartbeat 198

Fetal hemoglobin 107
Fetal hemolysis 113, 115
Fetal hydrops 104
    maternal effects of 104
Fetal infection 104*f*
Fetal lung maturity 37*t*
Fetal monitoring, modes of 8, 8*t*
Fetal movement 195
    actual reduction in 196
    assessing 197
    decreased 195
    factors affecting 196
    perception of 195
    physiology 195
    reduced 196*t*, 198, 199, 199*fc*, 200, 201
Fetal red blood cells 98
Fetal side effects 37
Fetal therapy 107
Fetal weight, estimation of 31
Fetal wellbeing, indicator of 202
Fetomaternal bleed 113
Fetus
    delivery, course of 51
    growth restricted 201
    small 4*fc*
Fibroid
    large 181
    multiple 157*f*
    symptomatic 180
Fibromas 141, 144
Fibrothecoma 141, 144
First trimester, Doppler in 5*f*, 15
Fistula 226
Flash-freezing technique 121*f*
Fluid collection 116
Fluoroquinolone associated disability 225
Follicles, number of 120
Follicle-stimulating hormone 56, 61, 122
Fosfomycin 233
Free thyroid hormone, extraction of 57
Full blood count 82

G

Gadolinium 139
Gender-neutral
    vaccination 219, 219*f*
    vaccine 216
Genetic disorders 106
Genital anatomical variation 227
Genitourinary syndrome 179
    efficient 170

Genitourinary syndrome of menopause 166, 167, 169, 173, 178
   diagnosis of 170
   differential diagnosis of 170
   risk factors for 168
   sequelae of 169t, 170t
   symptoms of 167, 169
   treatment for 173
Gestational age 201, 202
   small for 199
Gestational hypertension 16, 17f
Gestosis
   pathogenesis with 18
   score application 22fc
Ghost cells 114
Glucose tolerance test 31
Glycosaminoglycan 228
Gonadotoxicity 129f
Gonadotropin 207
   releasing hormone 121
Gram-negative bacteria 229
Graves'
   disease 63
   illness 58
   ophthalmopathy 58
Growth hormone 61
Gynecological malignancies 130

H

Harmonic scalpel 186
Headache 177, 209
Heartburn 206
Hematologic disorders 131
Hematological abnormalities 102
Hematological malignancies 131
Hematoma, postoperatve 189
Hemolytic antibodies 98
Hemorrhage 75, 89, 189
   causes of postpartum 68
   fetomaternal 105
   incidence of postpartum 67
   intracranial 89-91
   postoperatve 189
   vaginal 177
Hemorrhagic cyst 140, 144, 145f
Hemostasis, confirming 189
Heparin 60
Hepatic rupture 93
Hepatitis B 106
Hepatosplenomegaly 98, 113
Herd immunity 220t
Hernia, port site 189

Herpes simplex 106
   infection 47
Hodgkin's lymphoma 135
Hormonal therapy 174
Hospitalized women, high-risk 197
Human anti-animal antibodies 60
Human chorionic gonadotrophin 56
Human epidermal growth 148
   factor receptor 160
Human immunodeficiency virus 214, 216
Human papillomavirus 212, 212f, 213, 213f, 216, 218, 219f
   diseases 215t
   infections, majority of 221
   vaccine 214, 215, 216t, 217f
Hyaluronic acid 167
Hydralazine 46
Hydronephrosis, moderate 47
Hydrops
   antenatal treatment of 104
   cases of 112
   etiology of 109t
   special category of 112
   treatment algorithm for 108fc
Hydrops fetalis 98, 102, 110, 113, 118
   diagnosis of 107
   management of 107
   prevalence of 98
   prognosis of 110
Hydrosalpinx 141f
Hypercalcemia 58
Hyperimmunoglobulin 47
Hyperinsulinemia 204
Hyperkalemia 91
Hypernatremia 91
Hypertension 16, 17, 21, 31, 45
   chronic 16, 17f
Hypertensive crisis 26
   management of 27t
Hypertensive disorders 16, 18, 21, 21t, 23, 32
   classification of 16
   diagnosis of 23
   in pregnancy
      gestosis, pathogenesis of 19f
      prediction of 22
   modern management of 16
Hyperuricemia 45
Hypoestrogenic state 227
Hypokalemia 91
Hyponatremia 91
Hypoproteinemia 113

Hypotension 93
Hypothermia 86, 91
Hypothyroidism 60
    temporary 59
Hypovolemia 88, 91
Hypoxia 86, 91, 93
Hysterectomy 153

I

Ice crystals, creation of 121
Ifosfamide 154
Immune hydrops 98, 105, 112, 115
    development of 116
    pathophysiology of 112
    treatment of 116
Immunosuppressant drugs 49t
Immunotherapy 148, 158
In vitro fertilization 21, 123, 124, 207
Incision laparoscopic surgery 132
Indigestion 206
Infections 47, 100, 102
    natural 214
    recurrent 226
    secondary 47
Inflammatory sites 230
Infundibulopelvic ligament, division of 183, 184f
Inherited disorder 106
Inositols 208, 209
Insemination 122
In-situ carcinoma 215
Instrumental delivery algorithm 85f
Insulin
    resistance 204, 209
    sensitivity, peripheral 206
    sensitizing drugs 204, 205
Intensive care unit 29, 30
Internal iliac 192
Interstitial cystitis 228
Intracorporeal knotting 182
Intracytoplasmic sperm injection 21, 122
Intrafascial hysterectomy 187
Intrapartum hypertension, developing 17
Intraperitoneal transfusion 117
Intrauterine 45
    balloon tamponade 71, 73f
    growth retardation 46
    intravascular transfusion 117f
    transfusion 116-118
Intravascular transfusion 117
Intravesical glycosaminoglycan layer 232
Invasive testing 106

Ischemic placenta 18
Isoimmunized mother, rhesus negative 114
Isotonic crystalloids 69

K

Karyotyping 107
Kidney
    function test 31
    transplant 44, 45
Kitazato thawing kit 122
Kleihauer-Betke
    acid elution test 113
    test 113
Korotkoff sounds 23

L

Labetalol 26
Labor
    and delivery 42, 51
    room 78
Lactate dehydrogenase 31
Lactation 220
Lactobacilli 230, 232
Laparoscope 183
Laparoscopic hysterectomy 189
    complications of 189b
Laparoscopic supracervical hysterectomy 180
Laparoscopic tower 182
Laparoscopy
    caries 131
    one-step 133
Laryngeal papillomatosis 214
Laser therapy 179
Leflunomide 49
Left atrium 12
Leiomyomas, multiple 145f
Leukemia 135
Leukorrhea 177
Levator ani 238
Lifestyle factors 36
Ligaments, round 183
Limb movements 195
Liver
    calcification 104f
    disease 178
    function test 31, 82
Living tissue 139
Local estrogen therapy protocols 232t
Local vaginal estrogen treatment 174

Lubrication, lack of 170
Lung 155
   hypoplasia 103
Luteinizing hormone 61, 122
Lymph nodes 154
Lymphadenopathy 142

M

Magnesium sulfate 27, 28t, 29, 31, 32, 38, 38t, 43
   monitoring of 29t
Magnesium toxicity 93
Masked hypertension 17
Massive pleural effusion, unilateral 105f
Maternal collapse 88, 91
Maternal heartbeat 198
Maternal hypothyroidism 21
Maternal perception 196
Maternal preeclampsia 18
Maternal serology, role of 106
Maternal side effects 38
Maternal syndrome 18
Maternal-fetal medicine 51
Maturation index 172
Medicine mycophenolate mofetil, category D 50
Membranes, preterm premature rupture of 38
Menopause 166-168, 170, 179
   causes 168
   surgical 169
Menstrual abnormalities 44
Menstrual cyclicity, worsening of 206
Metabolic acidosis 189
Metabolic disorder 202
Metabolic health 209
Metabolism, inborn error of 101, 102
Metformin 205-209
   addition of 207
   compared to 208
   treatment, long-term 206
Methyldopa 26
Methylprednisolone 49
Meticulous sonographic examination 105
Microbial confirmation 229
Microhematuria, asymptomatic 230
Middle cerebral artery 5, 7, 11, 11f, 114, 115f
   Doppler 11
   peak systolic velocity measurement, technique for 114
   use of 114
Mini-laparotomy 133

Mirror syndrome 104
   treatment of 104
Miscarriage 48
Mitral regurgitation 111
Mitral stenosis 92
Mitral valve 111
Monopolar hook 186
Mouth metallic taste 206
Multidrug resistant organisms 225
Multifetal gestation 114
Multinodular goiter 63
Multivessel Doppler 5
Myasthenia gravis 27
Mycophenolate mofetil 49, 50
Myocardial ischemia 91
Myoinositol 208
Myometrial invasion 144
Myometrium 142

N

Nail changes 206
Nalidixic acid 233
National Transplantation Pregnancy Registry 46
Nausea 177, 206, 209
Neonatal death 48
Neurogenic bladder 226
Neuroprotection 43
Neutrophil count, absolute 31
Nifedipine 26
Nitric oxide 19f
Nitrofurantoin 47, 233
N-methyl d-aspartate receptors 38
No fetal movements 202
Nonavalent vaccine 215
Noncervical cancers 212
Nongenital infection 213
Non-Hodgkin lymphoma 135
Nonhormonal treatment 174, 175t, 179
   use of 179
Nonimmune hydrops fetalis 99
   etiopathogenesis of 99t
Non-pharmacological treatment 178
Nonpneumatic antishock garment 71, 73, 74f
Non-shockable rhythm 95
Nonstress test 30, 31

O

Obstetric
   Doppler 2, 4, 5, 7, 8f
   emergencies 84

practice 1
skill drill 78, 79
units 201
Omental injury 189, 192
Oocyte 122
cryopreservation 120, 126
optimal timing of 123
denudation 122
freezing 122
immature 122
retrieval 121
thawing 122
use of stored 125
Optic nerve sheath diameter 32
Optimum placental perfusion 25
Oral nutritional supplementation 208
Oropharyngeal cancer 214, 215
Oropharyngeal infection 213
Ovarian biopsy 132
Ovarian cancer 141
Ovarian cortex biopsy 132
Ovarian cyst, complex 142f
Ovarian failure, premature 168
Ovarian function recovery 133
Ovarian hyperstimulation syndrome, mild-to-moderate 124
Ovarian stimulation protocol 121
controlled 121
Ovarian tissue
freezing 133f
grafted 134
preservation protocols 130
replacing 132
transplantation 134, 134f, 137
Ovarian tissue cryopreservation 128-131
procedure 132
success rate of 137
technique 128
Ovarian torsion 140
Ovarian transposition 129
Ovarian tumor 134, 135
Overt hyperthyroidism 63
Overt hypothyroidism 61
Oxytocin 69

P

Paclitaxel 154
Pain, chronic 225
Papillomaviridae family, virus of 213
Paralytic ileus 189
Paraovarian cysts 142
Paratubal cysts 142

Parvovirus 106
Patellar reflex, loss of 29
Patients exhibit symptoms 61
Pelvic
examination 171
floor muscle 168
training 175
floor, hypertonic 170
infection 189
inflammatory disease 72
masses, uspicious 181
pain 170
radiation 129
Pelvis 151, 153
Penile cancer 215
Pericardial effusion 103
Perineal muscle 238
Perineal tears 236
complete 236
fourth degree 236
superficial 238
Peripartum cardiomyopathy 92
Pertussis 219
Pheochromocytoma 93
Pioglitazone 209
Pituitary hormones, anterior 61
Pivmecillinam 231
Placenta 112
manual removal of 114
previa 114
Placental growth factor, abnormal 17
Placental lesions 101
Placental origin 30
Placental pathology, severity of 10f
Placentomegaly 98, 104f, 113
Plasma concentrations 29
Pleural effusion 113
Pneumothorax 189
Point-of-care ultrasound 32
Polycystic ovary syndrome 204
Polyhydramnios 98, 104
Postcoital bleeding 170
Postnatal management 109
Postpartum collapse 88, 97
causes of 91t
Postpartum hemorrhage 67, 67t, 71, 72, 76, 83fc
bundle 68, 69
care bundles 67, 69
management 81f
Postpartum hypertension, developing 17
Postpartum hypertensive disorders 32
Post-resuscitation care 96

Prednisone 49, 50
Preeclampsia 17*f*, 24*t*, 45, 91
    angiogenesis of 20
    diagnosis of 31*fc*
    late-onset 18
    monitoring 80*f*
    till delivery decision 31*fc*
Pregnancy 45, 48, 58, 59, 207, 220
    complications during 89
    gestosis score 21*t*
    induced hypertension 208
    management of 44
    medical risks of 124
    primary sensitized 112
    rate 133
    risk of complications during 45
Preterm birth 35*t*, 36, 38*t*, 45
    classification of 35
    risk factors for 36*t*
Preterm infants 38
Preterm labour 35, 42
    established 36
    management of 36
    threatened 37
Primary healthcare 80
Primigravida 21, 236*f*
Progesterone receptor 158
Prolactin 61
Prophylactic antimicrobial treatment 228
Prophylaxis 220
Proteases 18
Psychological impact 127
Pulmonary embolism 92, 189
Pulmonary hypertension 93
Pulse
    repetition frequency 6
    wave Doppler, acquisition of 48
Pyrexia 89

R

Radiation 154
    therapy 151, 152
Radiofrequency current 139
Rapamycin 49
Recessive disorder 106
Rectovaginal fascia 185, 185*f*
Red cells, smear of 113
Reduced fetal movements despite normal
    testing, repeat episodes of 201
Regulation incentivizes, type of 126
Reinfection 214
Renal disease, end-stage 44

Renal failure 27
    chronic 58
Renal function, deteriorating 48
Renal transplantation, pregnancy after 44
Respiratory
    depression 90
    disorders 103
    papillomatosis 215
Rhesus isoimmunization 99
Rhesus negative mother 98
Rhesus positive
    fetus 112
    neonates 98
Rituximab 47
Rosiglitazone 209
Round ligaments, division of 184*f*
Rubella 106
Ruptured aneurysms 90

S

Salpingo-oophorectomy, bilateral 149
School-based Programs 220
School-based Vaccination Programs 221
Second trimester Dopplers 5, 15
Seizure 23
    control 29
    prevention 27
Sentinel lymph node 156*f*
    evaluation 155
Sepsis 89, 189
Septate uteri 143
Septic shock 92
    management 89
Serosa 153
Serosal surface 143
Serous tumor, neu-positive 148
Serum
    electrolytes 94
    estradiol levels 172
Sex hormone-binding globulin 206
Sex-cord tumors, development of 137
Sexual activity 44
Sexual intercourse 168, 227
Sexual partner, absorption by 177
Sexual violence, victims of 237
Sexually transmitted disease 221
Shockable rhythm 95
Shoulder dystocia 85*fc*
Sirolimus 49, 51
Sjögren's syndrome 106
Skeletal dysplasia 102
Skill laboratories 84

Social egg freezing 120, 121
   medical risks of 124
   process of 124
Spare fertility 151
Sperm exposure, short duration of 21
Spermicides diaphragm 227
Splenic aneurysm rupture 93
Splenomegaly 115
Spontaneous abortion, risk of 46
Spontaneous labor 51
Standard genetic testing 107
Standard ovarian stimulation 130
Staphylococci 168, 230
Stereoisomers 208
Stillbirth 48
Stomach pain 209
Stone disease 226
Streptococci 168, 230
Stroke 178
Structural cardiac abnormalities 107
Submucous leiomyomas 145*f*
Sudden postpartum cardiorespiratory collapse, causes of 92*t*
Sulfamethoxazole 233
Suprapubic pain 170
Surgical complications, risk of 131
Surgical steps 183
Surgical technique 133
Syphilis 106
Systemic hormonal therapy 178
Systolic velocity 12

T

Tachycardia 93
Tacrolimus 49
Tamoxifen 130
Tamponade 91
Tension pneumothorax 91, 93
Testosterone, topical 177
Tetanus 219
Thiazolidinediones 209
Third trimester Dopplers 4, 15
Thoracic mass, tumors 105
Thromboembolic diseases 89
Thromboembolism 88, 89, 91
Thymic hypoplasia 50
Thyroglobulin 55, 57
Thyroglobulin antibodies 55, 57
Thyroid 55
   cancer, differentiated 57
   disease 62*fc*
      subclinical 61
   disorders 55

   function test 55, 59, 62
   gland 64
      physiology of 55
   hormone 56, 57
      beta 63
      free 59
      levels 56
   nodules 63
   peroxidase 62
      antibodies 58
   problems 65
      detection of 64
      managing 64
   receptor antibodies 58, 63
   underactive 63
Thyroid-binding globulin 56
Thyroiditis, postpartum 59
Thyroid-stimulating
   antibodies 58
   hormone 22, 56, 62
Thyrotoxicosis 60
   prediction of 58
Thyrotropin-releasing hormone 55
Thyroxine, free 55
Tiredness 209
Tissues 153
   heterotopic-transplanted 137
   transplantation of 131
Tocolysis 39, 42*t*
   indications for 39
   pre-procedure 117
Tocolytic agents 40*t*
Tocolytic therapy, contraindications for 39
Total abdominal hysterectomy 149
Total laparoscopic hysterectomy 180, 192
   steps of 183*b*
Toxicity 90, 91
Toxoplasmosis 106
Transabdominal sonography 23
Transabdominal technique 9
Transthyretin 56
Transvaginal sonography 23
Transvaginal technique 10
Trendelenburg position 183
Trichomonas species 168
Tricuspid regurgitation 5, 111
Trigone, squamous metaplasia of 172
Tri-iodothyronine 55
Trimethoprim 233
Trocar placement 182
Troglitazone 209
Tuboovarian 183, 184*f*
   abscess 140

Tumor
 high-grade 153
 size 155
 solid 136
 stage 155
Tumor-node-metastasis 150
Twins 101

U

Umbilical arterial Doppler 10
Umbilical artery 5, 7, 12, 201
 Doppler 3*fc*, 10
  technique 10
  waveforms 10*f*
Umbilical cord 10
Umbilical Doppler 8
Unconsciousness 23
Ureteric injury 190
 management of 191*fc*
 site of 190
Urethra 167, 168
Urinalysis, microscopic 229
Urinary bladder 237
Urinary symptoms 228
Urinary tract
 anatomic abnormality 227
 obstruction 227
Urinary tract infections 175, 179, 225, 229
 complicated 226
 diagnosis of 228
 differential diagnosis of 228
 etiology of recurrent 226
 factors predisposing to 227*t*
 nonantibiotic interventions for 232
 prevention of recurrent 226
 recurrent 225
 treatment of uncomplicated symptomatic 231*t*
 uncomplicated 226
Urine 229
 acidic 228
 analysis, interpretation of 230
 collected 230
 culture 229
 dipstick 229
 output 29
Urological injuries 189, 190
Uterine
 abnormalities 36
 contraction 237
 Doppler 8
 inversion 92
 manipulator 183
 massage 71
 natural killer cells 18
 rupture 92
 souffle 198
 vessel ligation 185, 186*f*
Uterine artery 7, 9, 9*f*, 184
 Doppler 5, 9, 10, 23
 pulsatility index 23
Uterotonic 69
 drugs 72*t*
Uterovesical fascia 184, 185*f*
Uterus 151
 absence of 143
 entire 152
 large 181
 retrieval 187, 188*f*

V

Vaccination, facility-based 220
Vaccines, types of 214
Vagina 167
Vaginal acidity 168
Vaginal atrophy, symptoms of 167
Vaginal brachytherapy 151
Vaginal cancer 215
Vaginal childbirth, absence of 168
Vaginal cream 232
Vaginal deliveries 236, 236*f*
Vaginal dilators 175
Vaginal discomfort 177
Vaginal douching 181
Vaginal dryness 174
Vaginal epithelium 167
Vaginal health index 173, 173*t*
Vaginal hysterectomy, laparoscopic-assisted 180
Vaginal involvement 144
Vaginal lubricants 175
Vaginal moisturizers 175
 long-acting 174
Vaginal pain 177
Vaginal ring 176, 232
Vaginal smear, microscopic examination of 172
Vaginal tablet 232
Vaginitis 177
Vascular injury 189, 192
 management of 192*b*
Vault closure 187, 188*f*
Vault prolapse 189
Venous Doppler 8
Ventricular function failure, acute 91

Village Health Nurse 80
Voiding dysfunction 227
Vomiting 177, 206
Vulva 167
Vulval cancer 215
Vulvovaginal pruritus 177

W

Water-based personal lubricants 174
Weight gain, sudden 23
Weight loss 207
Wound infection 189